Dennis B. Worthen, PhD
Editor in Chief

Dictionary of Pharmacy

Pre-publication
REVIEWS,
COMMENTARIES,
EVALUATIONS . . .

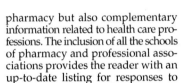

"**T**his book is a unique compilation of information for all strata of practice, from professional pharmacy students to specialized practitioners. It includes a convenient listing of all schools/colleges of pharmacy and professional associations, and a thorough, comprehensive listing of medical abbreviations. It is a convenient medical, law, statistics, and pharmaceutical dictionary 'all in one.' *Dictionary of Pharmacy* is a great reference for beginning professional pharmacy students to have for the duration of their education in pharmacy school and has value as an appropriate reference for practicing pharmacists as well."

Nicholas G. Popovich, PhD
Professor and Head,
Department of Pharmacy Administration,
University of Illinois at Chicago

Pharmaceutical Products Press®
The Haworth Reference Press®
Imprints of The Haworth Press, Inc.
New York • London • Oxford

Dictionary of Pharmacy

PHARMACEUTICAL PRODUCTS PRESS

Pharmaceutical Heritage:
Pharmaceutical Care Through History
Mickey C. Smith, PhD
Dennis B. Worthen, PhD
Senior Editors

Dictionary of Pharmacy

Dennis B. Worthen, PhD
Editor in Chief

Julian H. Fincher, PhD
L. Clifton Fuhrman, PhD
Linda L. Krypel, PharmD
Kenneth A. Lawson Jr., PhD
W. Steven Pray, PhD
Jenelle Sobotka, PharmD
Victor D. Warner, PhD

Contributing Editors

Pharmaceutical Products Press®
The Haworth Reference Press®
Imprints of The Haworth Press, Inc.
New York • London • Oxford

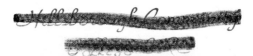

Published by

Pharmaceutical Heritage Editions, a series from Pharmaceutical Products Press®, and
The Haworth Reference Press®, imprints of The Haworth Press, Inc., 10 Alice Street,
Binghamton, NY 13904-1580.

Cover design by Lora Wiggins.

Library of Congress Cataloging-in-Publication Data

Dictionary of pharmacy / Dennis B. Worthen, editor-in-chief; Julian H. Fincher . . .
[et al.], contributing editors.
     p. ; cm. — (Pharmaceutical heritage editions)
  ISBN 0-7890-2328-8 (soft : alk. paper)
  1. Pharmacy—Dictionaries. I. Worthen, Dennis B. II. Series: Pharmaceutical
heritage.
    [DNLM: 1. Pharmacy—Dictionary—English. 2. Pharmacology—Dictionary—
English. QV 13 D55355 2004]

RS51.D482 2004
615'.1'03—dc22

                                           2004001894

To pharmacy students and practicing pharmacists
for their work to ensure positive medication outcomes
in the patients they serve

CONTENTS

About the Editor in Chief

Dennis B. Worthen, PhD, is Lloyd Scholar at the Lloyd Library and Museum in Cincinnati, Ohio. He is an adjunct professor at the University of Cincinnati College of Pharmacy, where he teaches the history of pharmacy. He retired from Procter & Gamble Health Care in 1999 after 23 years of service, most recently as Director of Pharmacy Affairs.

Dr. Worthen received a BA from the University of Michigan, and from Case Western Reserve University he earned two MS degrees and a PhD. From 1986 to 1989, he was awarded an Allied Irish Bank visiting professorship at the College of Pharmacy at Queen's University in Belfast, Northern Ireland. In 1996 he received the American Institute of the History of Pharmacy Fischelis Grant for his research on pharmacy in World War II.

Dr. Worthen is the co-author of *Pharmaceutical Education in the Queen City: 150 Years of Service 1850-2000* (Haworth) and the author of *Pharmacy in World War II* (Haworth). He is the editor of *A Road Map to a Profession's Future: The Millis Study Commission on Pharmacy,* to which he also contributed, and is editor in chief of the *Procter & Gamble Pharmacist's Handbook.* He has published more than 60 papers in professional journals.

Dr. Worthen is a contributing author to the *International Journal of Pharmaceutical Compounding* and is the author of the "Heroes of Pharmacy" series for the *Journal of the American Pharmaceutical Association.* In 1998, he was the founding co-editor of the Pharmaceutical Heritage book series of The Haworth Press, Inc., a series devoted to publishing books covering historical aspects of pharmacy, and is editor in chief of Haworth's Pharmaceutical Products Press.

Contributing Editors

Julian H. Fincher, PhD, Professor and Dean Emeritus, College of Pharmacy, University of South Carolina.

L. Clifton Fuhrman, PhD, Associate Professor and Assistant Dean, College of Pharmacy, University of South Carolina.

Linda L. Krypel, PharmD, Associate Professor, College of Pharmacy and Health Sciences, Drake University.

Kenneth A. Lawson Jr., PhD, Associate Professor, College of Pharmacy, University of Texas at Austin.

W. Steven Pray, PhD, Bernhardt Professor, School of Pharmacy, Southwestern Oklahoma State University.

Jenelle Sobotka, PharmD, Manager of Pharmacy Relations, Procter & Gamble.

Victor D. Warner, PhD, Professor, College of Pharmacy, University of Cincinnati.

Acknowledgments

A special acknowledgment is due to Julian H. Fincher, Robert L. Beamer, James M. Plaxco Jr., and C. Eugene Reeder. Their earlier *Dictionary of Pharmacy* served as an important starting point for this work.

The contributions of six students of pharmacy members of the Alpha Omicron chapter of Phi Lambda Sigma at the University of Cincinnati are gratefully acknowledged. These individuals served as reviewers for the definitions and abbreviations sections. Their insights and willingness to participate brought an important perspective to the current work. The individuals are Matthew Bremer, Neil Ernst, Amjad Iqbal, Shannon Malaney, Amit Patel, and Amy Phillips.

Thanks to the American Pharmacists Association for permission to incorporate the *Code of Ethics* and *Principles of Practice for Pharmaceutical Care.*

Thanks to the American Association of Colleges of Pharmacy for permission to use the "Pharmacist's Oath" and the "Pledge of Professionalism."

User's Guide

This dictionary provides a representative overview of terminology and concepts relevant to the study and practice of pharmacy. Terms and abbreviations are arranged alphabetically on a letter-by-letter basis.

Cross-references direct the reader from related terms to those with more specific definitions or comparative information; SEE, SEE ALSO, CONTRAST, and COMPARE precede the italicized, cross-referred terms. In addition, some definitions give alternative names, examples, and abbreviations. Abbreviations used within definitions are defined in that portion of the dictionary.

The abbreviation portion of the dictionary presents generally accepted shorthand for terms and phrases in common use within the fields of medicine and pharmacy. Symbols (e.g., &, >, +) are treated as punctuation marks and thus ignored in alphabetizing; solid abbreviations appear first, followed by those with numbers, then those with symbols, and finally those with standard punctuation (e.g., a hyphen or colon).

Much variation exists in the use of capital or lowercase letters in practice, so an attempt was made to standardize this list based on two general principles: all capitals are used for acronyms (made from the first letter of each word of the phrase), and lowercase letters are used for shortened terms. Alternative abbreviations, Latin equivalents, and term clarifications appear in parentheses following the relevant terms and phrases.

Definitions

a- prefix meaning absence of or without; example: achlorhydria

abatement to decrease; example: an abatement of symptoms of a disease

abbreviated new drug application (ANDA) established under the Drug Price Competition and Patent Term Restoration Act (1984) allowing the FDA to accept abbreviated new drug applications for generic versions of drugs first approved after 1962; safety and effectiveness data did not have to be submitted if the drug was generically equivalent to brand name drugs already proven to be safe and effective

abdominal packs SEE *laparotomy pack*

abdominohysterotomy caesarean section

abduction a drawing away, as an arm or leg from the middle line of the body

aberration 1: deviation from that which is normal **2:** an imperfection on an optical lens resulting in a disturbed image

abietic acid organic acid prepared by isomerization of rosin; used in the manufacture of soaps, plastics, and lacquers

abiogenesis spontaneous generation of biological cells without known biological explanation; synonym: autogenesis

abirritant an agent used to relieve irritation

ablution washing

ABO antigens innate blood group compounds important to blood typing and transfusions

abortifacient agent that induces abortion

abradant agent that scrapes or abrades

abrasion a scraping of the skin, mucous membranes, or teeth; wearing or rubbing away by friction

abrasive substance used to scrape or erode a surface; example: dental pumice

abscess pus accumulation in any part of the body

abscissa horizontal axis of a plot or graph

absolute humidity SEE *humidity, absolute*

absolute rate theory SEE *transition state theory*

absolutes 1: values or dimensions that are defined by international agreement (SEE *absolute unit*) **2:** pure substances that have been isolated from mixtures **3:** pure solvents; example: absolute alcohol

absolute temperature an expression of fundamental heat intensity; $°T = °C + 273.15$; synonym: degrees Kelvin

absolute unit a measurable dimension that is defined by internationally agreed-upon standards; examples: meter, kilogram, second

absolute zero a hypothetical temperature characterized by a complete absence of heat and approximately equivalent to $-273.15°C$ or $-459.67°F$

absorb 1: to take in and become part of an existent whole **2:** to suck up or take up (as a sponge absorbs water); to take in food and drugs from the intestinal tract

absorbance ability of a layer of a substance to absorb radiation

absorbent gauze SEE *gauze*

absorption 1: process of being absorbed **2:** biological process by which drugs and other substances are transported across body membranes (intestines, skin, cells) **3:** physicochemical process by which molecules (liquid or gaseous) are absorbed into another system such as water into a sponge or hydrogen into palladium **4:** physical interception of radiant energy or sound waves

absorption, active movement of substances through a living membrane against a concentration gradient; example: an energy requiring process catalyzed by enzymes

absorption, facilitated movement of substances through membranes aided by a carrier

absorption, passive movement of substances through membranes by simple diffusion

absorption band a region in an absorption spectrum of a substance in which the absorptivity reaches a maximum; an inflection point in the spectrum

absorption cell vessel used to hold substances for determination of their absorption spectra; example: cuvette used in spectrophotometry

absorption coefficient 1: absorption of one substance or phase into another **2:** a measure of the rate of decrease in the intensity of electromagnetic radiation after its passage through a particular substance **3:** absorptivity of a substance

absorption ointment base an ointment base capable of absorbing and holding relatively large amounts of water; example: lanolin

abstinence denying oneself a drug or some other gratification (food, drink, sexual intercourse)

abstract 1: short synopsis of a longer article **2:** that which has been separated **3:** profound, fundamental concept without units of measure

abstraction 1: removal or separation of one or more ingredients from a mixture **2:** a mental state characterized by a total isolation from one's environment

acacia gum dried gummy exudate of the acacia tree, used as a suspending or emulsifying agent; synonym: gum Arabic

Academy of Pharmaceutical Research and Sciences (APRS) a subdivision of the American Pharmacists Association established to promote research in pharmacy

Academy of Pharmacy Practice and Management (APPM) a subdivision of the American Pharmacists Association, composed of pharmacists who are providing or managing the provision of pharmaceutical services directly to patients

Academy of Students of Pharmacy (ASP) a subdivision of the American Pharmacists Association, composed of pharmacy students

accelerated stability testing SEE *stability testing; Arrhenius equation*

acceleration rate of increase in the velocity of movement of an object or particles, usually expressed in cm/sec^2

acceleration of gravity rate of increase in movement of a substance due to the attractive force of gravity; $980.665\ cm/sec^2$

accelerin blood-coagulation factor VI; synonym: accelerator globulin

acceptance sampling a statistically based quality control procedure of selecting representative parts of a lot of pharmaceutical preparations in order to assure that the whole is correctly prepared

access a patient's ability to obtain medical care; ease of access determined by components such as the availability of medical services and their acceptability to the patient, the location of health care facilities, transportation, hours of operation, and affordability of care, which is often a function of insurance coverage

accessories, health surgical supplies and convalescent aids; examples: wheelchairs, walkers, ostomy supplies, elastic supports

accommodation 1: to adapt **2:** ability of the eye to adjust to viewing objects at different distances; effected chiefly by changes in the convexity of the crystalline lens

accreditation process whereby an association or agency grants public recognition to an organization that meets certain established qualifications or standards, as determined through initial and periodic evaluations

accredited the fulfillment of minimum standards of an officially recognized group by a college, hospital, or other organization; example: a U.S. college or school of pharmacy must be accredited by the American Council on Pharmaceutical Education

accrete process of adding new enrollees to a health plan

accretion 1: growth characterized by addition of matter to the periphery of a body **2:** a growing together **3:** deposition of foreign matter on the surface of an object; example: accretion of tartar on teeth

accrual basis of accounting an accounting method whereby revenues are recognized in the period when goods or services are sold and expenses are recognized in the period when the related revenue is recorded

accrued revenues revenues that have been earned or recognized but not yet received

accumulated depreciation an account that shows the sums of depreciation charges on an asset from the time it was acquired

accumulation increase in the plasma or tissue concentration of a drug

accuracy 1: a measure of the correctness of data as these correspond to the true value **2:** freedom from mistake or error

acerbic 1: acidic or sour in taste **2:** acidic in temper or mood

acetoacetic ester condensation a special form of Claison condensation using ethylacetate and a base such as sodium ethoxide

acetylation substitution of an organic compound with an acyl group derived from acetic acid

acetylcholine 1: acetate ester of choline **2:** neurotransmitter secreted by the endings of the voluntary nervous system and the autonomic ganglia

achlorhydria absence of hydrochloric acid secretion in gastric fluid even after the administration of histamine

achymosis 1: a lack or deficiency of chyme acicular **2:** shaped like a needle; needlelike

acid 1: a type of compound that contributes a proton to a chemical reaction to form a conjugate base **2:** a type of compound that accepts electrons in a chemical reaction **3:** a type of compound that reacts with a base **4:** an electrophile **5:** a substance that has a sour taste

acid, weak an organic acid that does not completely dissociate in water

acid-base balance relative concentrations of acids and bases as in an organism or a physical system

acid-base indicator a dye solution that changes color with changes in pH

acid-base pair SEE *conjugate pair*

acid-fast a staining property exhibited by certain bacteria that are not decolorized by mineral acids after staining with aniline dyes; example organisms: bacilli of tuberculosis and leprosy

acidifying agent substance added to lower the pH of a system under observation

acidimetry method of quantitative analysis in which the total amount of acid in a sample is determined by titration with standard base

acidity constant 1: ionization constant of a weak acid **2:** pKa **3:** sigma constant of the Hammett equation **4:** equilibrium constant for the ionization of a weak acid in which water is included as a reactant and hydronium ion concentration is considered instead of proton concentration

acid number SEE *acid value*

acidophils microorganisms that grow well in an acid media

acidosis an abnormally increased concentration of acid in an organism; either compensated or uncompensated lowering of the pH of the blood below the normal of 7.4 due to an accumulation of acid metabolites

acid test ratio current assets less inventories divided by the current liabilities of a business; a strong measure of the firm's ability to meet its short-term obligations

acid value number of milligrams of potassium hydroxide required to neutralize the free fatty acids of one gram of substance

Ackerman tumor verrucous carcinoma of the larynx

acne chronic inflammatory condition of the sebaceous glands mainly involving the face, back, and chest

acneiform lesions resembling acne

acou- prefix meaning hearing

acoustic pertaining to hearing

acquired immunodeficiency syndrome (AIDS) a usually fatal disease caused by an infectious viral organism that results in a patient's loss of ability to produce antibodies against diseases

acridines group of tricyclic, nitrogen-containing, aromatic heterocycles

acromegaly chronic disease characterized by enlarged features, particularly the face and hands; result of hypersecretion of the pituitary growth hormone

actinomycosis often fatal, chronic, fungal disease characterized by multiple abscesses that form draining sinuses and lesions on face, neck, lungs, and abdomen

action potential impulse a singular electrical event that is recorded by a microelectrode placed within a cardiac cell either in vitro or in vivo

activated charcoal carbon black that has been treated with superheated steam to drive off adsorbed gases and to increase its adsorptive powers

active absorption SEE *absorption*

active immunity resistance to a disease or foreign material acquired in a host after an introduction of antigen (such as a vaccine or toxoid) into the body

actively at work a requirement of many insurers' policies stipulating that if a given employee is not actively at work on the day the policy goes into effect, medical coverage will not be provided until that employee returns to work

active site the cleft in the surface of an enzyme where a substrate binds

active transport SEE *absorption*

active tubular secretion process occurring in the kidneys in which acidic molecules are actively transported from the blood into the lumen of the renal tubules; SEE ALSO *secretion*

activities of daily living activities performed as part of a person's daily routine of self-care, such as bathing, dressing, toileting, transferring, continence, and eating

activity effective concentration or the effective number of discrete particles (molecules or ions) in a system under study; a correction for nonideal behavior in a system in which there are intermolecular or interionic attractive forces

activity coefficient correction factor to determine activity of a nonideal solution; SEE *Debye-Huckel theory*

actual acquisition cost the pharmacist's net payment for a drug product, after taking into account such items as purchasing allowances, discounts, and rebates

actual charge the amount a physician or other provider actually bills a patient for a particular medical service, procedure, or supply in a specific instance

actual damage SEE *damage*

actuarial table system for determining insurance rates and eligibility created by using probability and statistics

actuary person trained in the insurance field who determines policy rates and conducts statistical studies

actuator button a fitting attached to an aerosol valve stem that, when depressed or moved, opens the valve and directs the spray to the desired area

acu- prefix meaning needle

acute abrupt, sudden, intense, and excruciating; having a short course

acute care care for a single episode of short-term illness or an exacerbation of a chronic condition

acute-care drug medicine intended for short-term treatment of illness; example: antibiotic therapy for a severe infection

acute hepatitis SEE *hepatitis, acute*

acyl group functional group with the structure RC(O)- or ArC(O)- where R refers to an aliphatic group and Ar refers to an aromatic group such as phenyl; the functional group found in derivatives of the carbosylic acids

ad- prefix meaning toward

Adams-Stokes syndrome a slowed pulse that occurs with a form of heart block between the S-A and A-V nodes

adapter device by which one part of an apparatus may be attached to another part; examples: distilling adapters, bushing adapters

addict a person who is dependent upon drugs (including alcohol); one who suffers from addiction

addiction strong psychological or physiological dependence on a substance such as alcohol or drugs

Addison's disease adrenocortical insufficiency due to an abnormality in the adrenal cortex or in the anterior pituitary gland

additional drug benefit list a list of pharmaceutical products approved by a health plan and employer for dispensing in larger quantities than the standards covered under a benefit package in order to facilitate long-term patient use; also called "drug maintenance list"

addition reaction   a chemical reaction in which two molecules react to form a third molecule

additive 1: cooperative effort in which the total effect is the sum of the effects of each component acting independently (such effects may be pharmacological or physical) **2:** substance added to a preparation to improve its appearance, taste, or nutritional value

additive port   that part of an intravenous fluid container through which electrolytes, nutrients, or medicines may be added to the contents of the container

additive property   characteristic of a molecule that is the result of the sum of the properties of its individual atoms or functional groups; examples: mass and molecular weight; CONTRAST *constitutive property; colligative property,* respectively

adduction   clinical term denoting the movement of a limb or eye toward the median plane of the body

aden-   prefix meaning gland; same as adeno-

adenine phosphoribosyl-transferase   enzyme responsible for the resynthesis of AMP from adenine and phosphoribosylpyrophosphate

adeno-   prefix meaning gland; same as aden-

adenocarcinoma   malignant neoplasm originating in glandular or ducted epithelium

adenoma   a benign epithelial or glandular tumor that closely resembles the parent tissue upon which it grows

adenosine diphosphate   (ADP) nucleotide formed when ATP loses one phosphate group; synonym: adenosine-5'-diphosphate

adenosine monophosphate   (AMP) nucleotide of adenine; monophosphate ester of adenosine; synonym: adenosine-5'-phosphate

adenosine triphosphate   (ATP) nucleotide and coenzyme involved in energy transfer reactions and phosphorylations (phosphotransferase reactions); synonym: adenosine-5'-triphosphate

adenosyl cobalamin   form of vitamin B_{12} in which an adenosyl group is bonded to the central cobalt; believed to be the major natural form of vitamin B_{12}

adherence   SEE *compliance*

adhesion **1:** abnormal attachment of one tissue to another **2:** sticking or holding together

adhesive SEE *binder*

adhesive tape flexible band or strip of material that will stick or adhere to skin and bandages as well as prosthetic devices

adipo- prefix meaning fat

adipose tissue fatty tissue; tissue that contains fats and fat cells

adiposis an accumulation of excess fat in the body; obesity

adjudication processing a claim in order to determine proper payment

adjunct, pharmaceutical anything added to the drug to make a finished drug product or dosage form; example: lactose as a filler for capsules containing a low dose (very potent) drug

adjusted community rating insurance premium based on community rating adjusted for group specific demographics and the group's prior experience; also known as "prospective rating" and "factor rating"

adjusted expenses per inpatient day expenses incurred for inpatient care only; derived by dividing total expenses by adjusted inpatient days

adjusted inpatient days an aggregate figure reflecting the number of days of inpatient care, plus an estimate of the volume of outpatient services, expressed in units equivalent to an inpatient day in terms of level of effort

adjuvant substance added to a drug formulation to improve the manufacturing process, product quality, or pharmacological action; example: methylcellulose to aid in suspending drug particles in a liquid

administer to give a dose of medication to a patient; to provide treatment to a patient

administration **1:** act or process of administering; example: giving a drug to a patient **2:** act or process of performing managerial-related functions; example: managing a pharmacy

administrative costs the costs incurred by a carrier such as an insurance company or HMO for services such as claims processing, billing and enrollment, as well as overhead costs, including utilization review, insurance marketing, medical underwriting, agents commissions, premium collection, claims processing, insurer profit, quality assurance activities, medical libraries, and risk management

administrative services only insurance arrangement requiring the employer to be at risk for the cost of health care services provided, while a separate company delivers administrative services

admissions number of patients, excluding newborns, accepted for inpatient service during a reporting period

admissions/1,000 the number of hospital admissions per 1,000 health plan members; formula: (number of admissions/member months) × 1,000 members × number of months; also used to express the number of hospital admissions per 1,000 members of any other given population

admits the number of admissions to a hospital or inpatient facility during a reporting period (excludes newborns)

admixture parenteral preparation to which other substances are added for therapeutic reasons

adrenaline neurohormone secreted by the adrenal medulla; a potent endogenous stimulant; catechol amine compound; synonym: epinephrine

adrenergic 1: pertaining to the sympathetic neurons or nervous system **2:** a nerve or tract mediated at least in part by norepinephrine; synonym: sympathomimetic

adrenergic agent chemical compound that exerts its principal pharmacological effect by stimulation of peripheral sites of the sympathetic part of the autonomic nervous system; synonym: sympathomimetic agent

adrenergic blocking agent 1: drug that blocks impulses at the sympathetic receptor **2:** α type—blocks α-adrenergic receptors **3:** β_1 type—affects primarily the adrenergic receptors of the heart **4:** β_2 type—affects primarily the adrenergic receptors of the lungs and bronchi

adrenocortex hormones steroid secretions of the adrenal cortex that may have either glucocorticoid, mineralocorticoid, or male or female sex hormone activity

adrenocorticotrophic hormone peptide hormone secreted by the anterior lobe of the pituitary gland that stimulates the adrenal cortex to secrete adrenocorticosteroids

Adson syndrome compression of the brachial plexus leading to sensory disturbance of the upper extremity; also known as "Naffziger syndrome"

adsorbate substance that is adsorbed (held by attractive forces) on a surface of an adsorbent

adsorbent 1: material that adsorbs other substances onto its surface **2:** stationary phase in column chromatography

adsorption adhesion of molecules of a liquid, gas, or dissolved substance to the surface of another substance producing a higher molecular concentration at the surface; antonym: desorption

adsorption, chemical molecular adherence to a surface by strong chemical bonds; synonym: chemisorption

adsorption, physical molecular adherence to a surface through weak van der Waals–type interacting forces

adulterated made impure by the addition of a foreign or an inferior substance

adulteration adding inferior, impure, inert, or toxic ingredients to a drug or drug preparation for gain, deception, or concealment; contamination or decomposition of a product

advanced practice nurse (APN) an umbrella term that describes a registered nurse who has met advanced educational and clinical practice requirements beyond the basic nursing education required of all registered nurses

adverse drug reaction detrimental physiological reaction to a drug; a harmful side effect to the drug

adverse selection a situation in which a carrier disproportionately enrolls a population that is prone to higher than average utilization of benefits, thereby driving up costs and increasing financial risk

advertisement communications about a product/service that are nonpersonal, paid, firm-specific, and intended to encourage consumers' purchase or use

advertising discount SEE *promotional discount*

aer- prefix meaning air or gas; same as aero-

aero- prefix meaning air or gas; same as aer-

aeroallergen inhaled antigenic material which causes respiratory allergies in conditions such as allergic rhinitis; examples: pollen, animal dander

aerobic glycolysis the poorly regulated energy metabolism of tumor cells; involves a high rate of glycolysis and some level of oxidative phosphorylation

aerobic respiration the metabolic process in which oxygen is used to generate energy from food molecules

aerosol 1: a colloid dispersion of a solid or a liquid in air **2:** product that is packaged under pressure and contains therapeutically active ingredients that are released upon activation of an appropriate valve system; intended for topical application to the skin as well as local application into the nose (nasal aerosols), mouth (lingual aerosols), or lungs (inhalation aerosols)

aerosol, foam emulsion containing one or more active ingredients, surfactants, aqueous or nonaqueous liquids, and the propellants; if the propellant is in the internal (discontinuous) phase (i.e., of the oil-in-water type), a stable foam is discharged, and if the propellant is in the external (continuous) phase (i.e., of the water-in-oil type), a spray or a quick-breaking foam is discharged

aerosol, metered pressurized dosage form consisting of metered dose valves that allow for the delivery of a uniform quantity of spray upon each activation

aerosol, powder product that is packaged under pressure and contains therapeutically active ingredients, in the form of a powder, that are released upon activation of an appropriate valve system

aerosol, spray product that utilizes a compressed gas as the propellant to provide the force necessary to expel the product as a wet spray; applicable to solutions of medicinal agents in aqueous solvents

aerotolerant anaerobe organisms that depend on fermentation for their energy needs and possess detoxifying enzymes and antioxidant molecules that protect them from toxic oxygen metabolites

afebrile absence of fever

affect outward manifestation of a person's feelings or mood; often used interchangeably with emotion

affiliated provider a health care provider or facility that is subcontracted by a primary provider to obtain additional services for members

affinity amount of physical-chemical attraction between a drug and its receptor site; strength of the bond between a drug or endogenous substance and a receptor; reciprocal of the dissociation constant for the drug-drug receptor complex

affinity chromatography a technique in which proteins are isolated based on their biological properties, that is, their capacity to bind to a special molecule (the ligand)

affinity constant reciprocal of the dissociation constant of a chemical or enzymatic reaction described by the law of mass action or the Michaelis-Menton equation; synonym: association constant

aftercare services following hospitalization or rehabilitation

agar gelatinous colloid obtained from red alga; used as a thickening or gelling agent and as a culture medium for growing bacteria

Agency for Health Care Policy and Research SEE *Agency for Healthcare Research and Quality*

Agency for Healthcare Research and Quality (AHRQ) federal agency under Health and Human Services with the mission of providing evidence-based information on health care outcomes, quality, cost, use, and access to help people make more informed decisions and to improve the quality of health care services; formerly known as the Agency for Health Care Policy and Research

agent person who acts on behalf of another person known as the principal, and whose acts are binding on the principal

age/sex factor underwriting measurement that represents the age and sex risk of medical costs of one population relative to another

ageusia lack of taste

agglomeration process or action of collecting in a mass; synomym: aggregation

agglutinin antibody occurring in normal or immune serum that precipitates or clumps antigens on the surface of cell membranes

agglutinogen antigen that, when injected into an animal body, will stimulate synthesis of specific agglutinin antibodies

aggregated radioiodinated albumin albumin treated with iodine 131 under mild alkaline conditions so that no more than one gram atom of iodine is combined with one mole or 60,000 grams of albumin; used in diagnostic determinations of blood or plasma volumes, cardiac output, and the detection and location of brain tumors

aggregation clingling together of particles or globules in a pharmaceutical preparation in order to reduce the potential energy of the system; usually a contributor to instability of a dispersed system type of dosage form; synonym: agglomeration

agitation dryer device used to remove moisture from a solid formulation by stirring or frequent movement of particles continually exposing new surfaces; example: rotating cubic-vacuum dryer; synonym: moving-bed dryer; CONTRAST *static-bed dryer*

aglycone noncarbohydrate moiety of a glycoside; synonym: genin

agonist 1: drug that interacts with a receptor causing a response; CONTRAST *antagonist* **2:** a muscle that, by contracting, moves a part by bending a joint and is opposed by an antagonist muscle

agonist, partial drug that produces less than a maximal response when compared with full agonists

agranulocytosis blood condition in which there is an absence of or diminished number of granulocytes; synonym: granulocytopenia

air binding expression describing a vapor cavity interrupting a centrifugal pumping process; synonyms: vapor lock, air lock

air jet mixer device for mixing low-viscosity liquids by using high-velocity air streams to produce turbulence

air lock SEE *air binding*

air-suspension coating batch process of adding a covering layer to units of a solid dosage form or drug particles by suspending them in a gaseous stream within an enclosed chamber and spraying a rapidly drying material onto the surface of the floating particle units

akathisia motor restlessness; the inability to sit still

akinesia absence of muscle movements

alactasia inability to digest lactose due to total lack of lactase, usually congenital

alanine neutral amino acid commonly found in proteins; α-aminopropanoic acid

alanine aminotransferase synonym for serum glutamate pyruvic transaminase

alar crease creases on the sides of the nostrils; sites commonly affected with seborrheic dermatitis

albinism congenital absence of normal pigment (melanin) from skin, hair, and iris

Albright's syndrome metabolic bone disease characterized by rapid resorption of bone and fibrous replacement of marrow

albumin water-soluble protein found in blood, eggs, and other animal tissues or products; a protein that is soluble in water or dilute salt solution and is coagulated by heat; examples: egg albumin, serum albumin

albuminuria albumin in the urine

alcaptonuria accumulation and elimination in urine of homogentisic acid; result of a genetic disorder in phenylalanine-tyrosine metabolism

alcohol 1: organic compound containing a hydroxyl (-OH) group attached to a carbon atom not double-bonded to another oxygen **2:** organic compound with the general structure ROH **3:** without qualification, alcohol means ethyl alcohol

alcohol, primary one in which the hydroxyl group is attached to a carbon atom that is bonded to either hydrogen or only one other carbon atom

alcohol, secondary one in which the hydroxyl-bearing carbon is bonded to two other carton atoms

alcohol, tertiary one in which the hydroxyl-bearing carbon atom is bonded to three other carbon atoms

alcoholate complex formed between a substance and alcohol; usually a crystalline salt with alcohol molecules in its lattice structure; example: calcium chloride alcoholate

Alcoholics Anonymous (AA) an organization to assist an individual in overcoming addiction to or excessive use of alcoholic beverages

alcoholysis removal of a group (or cleavage of a ring structure) from a compound by a reaction of that compound with alcohol; COMPARE *hydrolysis*

aldehyde carbonyl compound containing a carbon atom double-bonded to an oxygen atom and covalently bonded to at least one hydrogen atom

aldol cleavage the reverse of aldol condensation

aldol condensation occurs when, under the influence of a dilute base or dilute acid, two molecules of an aldehyde or a ketone combine to form beta-hydroxyaldehyde or beta-hydroxyketone

aldose a monosaccharide with an aldehyde functional group

aldosterone mineralocorticosteroid hormone (secreted by the adrenal cortex) that regulates electrolytes in body function; hormone of the adrenal cortex that causes the kidney to retain sodium ions and excrete potassium ions

algin any of various hydrophilic colloidal substances (carboxyhydroxylated carbon chain) from marine algae, often used as stabilizers, emulsifiers, and thickeners; synonym: alginic acid

alginate salt or ester of alginic acid; SEE *algin*

algometer instrument to measure the degree of pain suffered by an individual; synonyms: algoscope, algesimeter, odynometer

algorithm prescribed set of well-defined rules or processes for the solution of a problem in a finite number of steps

algoscope SEE *algometer*

alimentary pertaining to food or the digestive tract

aliphatic organic compounds that do not contain aromatic rings (no benzene rings, etc.); examples: ethane, propane, propene, cyclohexane, acetylene

aliphatic hydrocarbon a nonaromatic hydrocarbon such as methane or cyclohexane

alkali 1: a base **2:** type of chemical compound that donates hydroxyl groups to a chemical reaction **3:** metallic element from Group I of the periodic table; example: sodium

alkalinizing agent substance that raises pH; example: sodium lactate

alkaloid 1: alkali-like or like a base; examples: morphine, strychnine, ephedrine **2:** bitter-tasting nitrogen-containing base obtained from plants **3:** any of several naturally occurring amines **4:** nitrogenous, carbon compound, derived from the vegetable kingdom and capable of neutralizing acids

alkalosis abnormally increased concentration of base in an organism; manifested by a blood pH above 7.4

alkene compound that contains a carbon-to-carbon double bond within its structure; example: ethylene; synonym: olefin

alkylating agent 1: compound capable of substituting an alkyl group on another compound **2:** group of anticancer drugs; example: nitrogen mustard

alkylation reaction in which a hydrocarbon radical or a derivative of a hydrocarbon radical is substituted for a hydrogen atom on an organic molecule

alkyl group functional group that contains only single-bonded carbon atoms plus hydrogens; a simple hydrocarbon group formed when one hydrogen from the original hydrocarbon is removed

alkyne compound with a carbon-to-carbon triple bond in its structure

allergen 1: substance capable of producing an allergy **2:** purified protein(s) of some food, bacterium, or pollen used to treat or test for allergy

allergist a physician who specializes in the diagnosis and treatment of allergies

allergy hypersensitivity to an allergen due to a previous exposure

allied health personnel specially trained and licensed (when necessary) health workers other than physicians, dentists, pharmacists, optometrists, chiropractors, podiatrists, and nurses; sometimes used synonymously with paramedical personnel, all health workers who perform tasks that must otherwise be performed by a physician, or health workers who do not usually engage in independent practice

alligation an arithmetical method often used in pharmacy for solving problems in which solutions or solid preparations of different concentrations are mixed

alligation alternate method of alligation in which the amounts of each solution or solid mixture of different concentrations needed to obtain a resultant mixture of desired concentrations are determined

alligation medial method of alligation in which the concentrations of a mixture resulting from the combination of various amounts of two or more solutions or mixtures of different known concentrations is determined

allocation base a systematic and rational method for providing an equitable distribution of costs from one department to several different departments in a pharmacy or other business

allogenic transfusion blood transfused into anyone other than the donor

allosteric reaction interactions in which drugs, hormones, or other therapeutic agents attach to a site other than the active site of an enzyme or drug receptor, either increasing or decreasing the effect

allotrope or allotropic form existence of an element in more than one molecular form; examples: oxygen and ozone, the allotropic forms of sulfur

allowable charge the maximum fee that a third party will reimburse a provider for a given service; may not be the same amount as either a reasonable or customary charge

allowable costs charges for services rendered or supplies furnished by a health provider which qualify for an insurance reimbursement

alloy a solution of two or more metals or of a metal and a nonmetal prepared by fusion; example: amalgam

all-payer system health care system in which all public and private third-party payers of medical bills are subject to the same rules and rates for payment; uniform fees that, in effect, bar health care providers from charging more to persons or firms who are more able to pay in order to make up losses from artificially low payment caps by some payers

alopecia baldness or loss of hair

alpha globin one of two types of protein subunits in hemoglobin A

alphameric SEE *alphanumeric*

alphanumeric pertaining to a character set that contains letters, digits, and usually other characters such as punctuation marks; synonym: alphameric

alpha particle 1: positively charged particle emitted from nuclei of very heavy radioactive elements **2:** a moving helium nucleus that consists of two protons and two neutrons

alpha-tocopherol a lipid-soluble molecule that acts as a radical scavenger; vitamin E

Alport's syndrome hereditary nephritis with nerve deafness and occasional platelet defect and cataracts

alternative care nontraditional care available in lieu of accepted medical practices

alternative delivery systems forms of health care delivery other than traditional fee-for-service and indemnity health care; sometimes applied to managed care organizations

alternative detailing a procedure utilized to contact providers in order to discuss treatment alternatives; most often used to direct compliance with a formulary or medical protocol

alternative medicine sytems of health care that differ from traditional, allopathic medicine

alum aluminum or another trivalent metallic sulfate

aluminum silvery colored, light ductile metal; abundant in nature in combination with silicates and metallic oxides; compounds of aluminum used as antacids, astringents, and antiperspirants

aluminum hydroxide gel white antacid suspension containing the equivalent of 4 percent w/v aluminum oxide in water; used to reduce gastric acidity

aluminum phosphate gel white antacid suspension containing 4.2 percent aluminum phosphate in water; used to treat peptic ulcers and other gastric irritations

aluminum subacetate solution SEE *Burow's solution*

alum-precipitated toxoid deactivated toxin in a water-insoluble complex with alum; used to produce active immunity with a single injection due to its prolonged antigenic response

alveolar bone bone sockets from which the teeth grow

Alzheimer's disease condition occurring most prevalently in the fifth or sixth decade of life and pathologically characterized by presenile cortical atrophy, loss of nerve cells, senile plaques in gray matter and neurofibular degeneration; synonyms: presenile dementia, presenile psychosis, Pick's disease

amalgam an alloy of mercury with other metals

amastia absence of a breast

amber glass glass rendered a dark reddish brown color by the addition of substances such as manganese and iron salts; used to protect drugs from light-catalyzed degradation

ambivalent coexistence of contradictory emotions, ideas, or desires

amblyopia dimness of vision not due to refractive error, but lack of use of the eye; synonym: lazy eye

ambulatory having the ability to walk

ambulatory care health care services that do not require hospitalization of a patient, such as those delivered at a physician's office, clinic, medical center, or outpatient facility

ambulatory care center part of an institution (hospital) that treats persons who are not admitted as inpatients; synonym: outpatient clinic

ambulatory patient noninstitutionalized patient who may or may not be an outpatient; includes patients who are not strictly ambulatory such as wheelchair patients

ambulatory setting an institutional health setting in which organized health services are provided on an outpatient basis, such as a surgery center, clinic, or other outpatient facility

ambulatory surgical facility a freestanding or hospital-based health care center that performs surgical services not requiring overnight confinement

ambulatory utilization review the review of care provided in ambulatory settings

amebiasis condition that occurs as the result of an infestation by amoeba (e.g., *Entamoeba histolytica, Giardia lamblia*); synonym: amebic dysentery

amebicide drug used to kill *Entamoeba histolytica*

amenorrhea absence of menses or failure of a woman to have a menstrual cycle

American Association of Colleges of Pharmacy (AACP) national organization for the promotion of pharmacy education; founded in 1900, as the Conference of Pharmaceutical Faculties (name changed in 1925)

American Association of Health Plans (AAHP) trade association created with the merger of Group Health Association of America and American Managed Care Research Association announced in February 1996 as the trade association serving HMOs, PPOs, and other managed care organizations

American Association of Preferred Providers Organizations reorganized as the Association of Managed Healthcare Organizations

American College of Apothecaries (ACA) organization of pharmacists who own and operate pharmacies that provide only prescription and closely related health care services; founded in 1942

American College of Clinical Pharmacy (ACCP) professional society of clinical pharmacists, founded in 1979, with the goals of encouraging appropriate drug therapy, promoting the practice of clinical pharmacy, and ensuring high standards of clinical pharmacy education

American Council on Pharmaceutical Education (ACPE) the national accrediting agency for professional programs of colleges and schools of pharmacy; founded in 1932

American Dental Association (ADA) national professional organization of dentists, founded in 1959, with goals of promoting dentistry and improving dental health

American Foundation for Pharmaceutical Education (AFPE) organization to support and improve pharmaceutical education by providing funds for graduate fellowships and special grants; founded in 1942

American Hospital Association (AHA) organization of hospitals designed to promote high-quality hospital care; conducts an annual survey of membership, listing composite statistical profiles of all registered hospitals

American Institute of the History of Pharmacy (AIHP) organization of individuals and businesses that promote the historical aspects of the profession of pharmacy; founded in 1941

American Medical Association (AMA) national professional organization of physicians; founded in 1847; establishes physicians' standards of practice and accredits medical schools; active lobbyist organization for physicians

American Medical Care and Review Association merged with Group Health Association of America to form the American Association of Health Plans in 1996

American Nurses Association (ANA) national professional organization of nurses; founded in 1896

American Pharmaceutical Association SEE *American Pharmacists Association*

American Pharmacists Association (APhA) national professional organization of pharmacists from all areas of practice; founded in 1852; formerly the American Pharmaceutical Association

American Public Health Association (APHA) organization of health professionals, health specialists, and consumers whose goal is to promote and protect individual and community health and the environment; founded in 1872

American Society of Consultant Pharmacists (ASCP) professional organization of pharmacists concerned with improving and promoting quality pharmaceutical services to nursing homes and other extended care facilities; founded in 1969

American Society of Health-System Pharmacists (ASHP) professional organization of institutional pharmacists; founded 1942; formerly the American Society of Hospital Pharmacists

American Society of Hospital Pharmacists SEE *American Society of Health-System Pharmacists*

American Society of Pharmacognosy (ASP) professional organization of pharmacognocists and others involved in study and research on the chemistry of natural products; founded in 1923

amethopterin a structural analogue of folate used to treat several types of cancer; also referred to as "methotrexate"

amide product resulting from the condensation of an acid with ammonia or a primary or a secondary amine; examples: acetamide, sulfonamides, acetaminophen

amination substitution of an amino group on a molecule

amine **1:** an organic compound containing nitrogen that reacts as a base **2:** an organic compound that is a derivative of ammonia

amine, primary an organic compound in which only one hydrogen of ammonia is substituted

amine, secondary an organic compound in which two hydrogens of ammonia are substituted

amine, tertiary an organic compound in which three hydrogens of ammonia are substituted

amino acid **1:** any of a number of fundamental units in a peptide or protein **2:** organic compound containing an amino group and an acid group; therefore, possessing amphoteric properties (both acidic and basic)

amino acid pool the amino acid molecules that are immediately available in an organism for use in metabolic processes

amino acid residue   an amino acid that has been incorporated into a polypeptide molecule

aminocephalosporanic acid   starting material used in the synthesis of semisynthetic cephalosporin antibiotics

aminoglycosides 1: group of antibiotics derived from the genus *Streptomyces* and used primarly to treat infections caused by gram-negative organisms **2:** substance containing one or more amino sugars connected by glycosidic linkages to a nonsugar component (aglycone)

amino group   basic radical containing nitrogen that is either bound to one or two hydrogens, or to one or two organic groups that are not acyl groups; SEE *amine*

aminopenicillanic acid   starting material used in the synthesis of semisynthetic penicillins

aminoquinoline compounds   containing an amino group attached to quinoline; example: primaquine

ammonia   gaseous compound composed of one nitrogen and three hydrogens; basic in nature; used as a reagent and a reflex stimulant (aromatic spirit of ammonia)

ammonia intoxication   elevated concentration of ammonia in the body that can cause lethargy, tremors, slurred speech, protein-induced vomiting, and death

ammonium   positively charged radical containing a tetra-substituted nitrogen; substitutions may be hydrogens or organic radicals or a combination of the two

amnesia   temporary or permanent loss of memory

amorphism   condition characterized by a lack of any organized structure of the molecules of a substance; CONTRAST *crystallization*

amorphous   without form or without an ordered molecular arrangement; CONTRAST *crystalline*

amortize   to diminish a debt by an orderly plan of payment; examples: to pay off a mortgage or to depreciate a durable business item

amphi- 1: prefix meaning on both sides or double **2:** (chemistry) designating positions or configurations

amphibolic pathway   a metabolic pathway that functions in both anabolism and catabolism

amphi-ionic surfactant   SEE *amphoteric surfactant*

amphipathic molecule molecule containing both polar and nonpolar domains

amphiphile molecule that has affinity for both aqueous and lipid media; synonym: surfactant

amphiprotic solvent solvent that is capable of donating or accepting a proton (or a pair of electrons)

ampho- prefix meaning both

ampholyte ionic substance capable of acting as an acid or a base; synonym: amphoteric electrolyte

amphoteric capable of acting as an acid and a base

amphoteric surfactant surface active agent that may exist with a positive charge, negative charge, or as a zwitterion depending on the pH of the system; example: peptide

ampule or ampul small hermetically sealed glass container, usually used to hold a single dose of a sterile parenteral medication

amygdalin white crystalline cyanogenetic glycoside found in bitter almond, wild cherry, and peach trees, among other plants; synonym: laetrile

amylase enzyme catalyzing the hydrolysis of starches

amylo- prefix meaning starch

amyloid deposit an insoluble aggregate of extracellular proteinaceous debris that occurs in the brains of Alzheimer's patients

amylopectin a type of plant starch; a branched polymer containing α-(1,4)- and α-(1,6)-glycosidic linkages

amylose a type of plant starch; an unbranched chain of D-glucose residues linked with α-(1,4)-glycosidic linkages

amyotrophic lateral sclerosis neurological condition involving demyelination of the neurons of the voluntary nerves leading to muscle groups and causing atrophy of the muscles involved; synonym: Lou Gehrig's disease

an- prefix meaning without; sometimes "a-" is used with same meaning

ana- prefix meaning again, upward, or backward

anabolic steroid drug stimulating tissue growth and producing a positive nitrogen balance; example: testosterone

anabolism process by which living organisms or tissues turn simple substances into more complex compounds; the biosynthesis part of metabolism; examples: protein synthesis, glycogenesis

anaerobe organism that lives in an environment lacking oxygen

anaerobic living or occurring in the absence of oxygen

analeptic agent that stimulates the central nervous system; used to restore respiration and/or wakefulness

anal fistula abnormal opening at or near the anus

analgesic agent that relieves pain without loss of consciousness

analgesics, narcotic class of drugs used to relieve pain that are capable of causing physical and psychological dependence; examples: morphine, pentazocine

analgesics, nonnarcotic class of drugs used to relieve pain and that do not cause physical dependence; examples: aspirin, acetaminophen

analog molecule similar in many ways to another molecule

anal verge area where anal canal joins perianal skin; puckered skin at the anal orifice

analysis of variance a statistical procedure used to compare the means of two or more groups

analytical balance SEE *balance*

analytical chemistry branch of chemistry that involves qualitative and quantitative determinations

analytical ultracentrifuge SEE *ultracentrifuge*

anaphylaxis acutely exaggerated allergic reaction characterized by fluid in the lungs, large blisters, and a severe decrease in blood pressure

anaplasia reversion of a cell to a more primitive form with loss of differentiation; often associated with malignancies

anaplerotic reaction a reaction that replenishes a substrate needed for a biochemical pathway

anasarca severe generalized edema; synonym: dropsy

anastomosis intercommunication of blood vessels either naturally or by means of surgery

ancillary subsidiary, auxiliary, or supplementary

ancillary charge 1: the fee associated with additional service performed prior to and/or secondary to a significant procedure **2:** hospital charges supplementary to a hospital's daily room and board charge, e.g., for drugs, medicines and dressings, lab services, X-ray examinations, and use of the operating room

ancillary services hospital services other than room, board, and professional services; may include X-ray, laboratory, or anesthesia

Andersen's disease type 4 glycogenosis (a glycogen storage disease)

andr- prefix meaning male or masculine; same as andro-

andro- prefix meaning male or masculine; same as andr-

androgen steroid hormone responsible for secondary male characteristics; example: testosterone

-ane suffix indicating paraffin; saturated hydrocarbon

anemia state in which the number of red blood cells, amount of hemoglobin, or the volume of packed red blood cells is below normal; any of several diseases involving abnormal hemoglobins; hemoglobinopathy

anergy inability to react to specific antigens

anesthesia loss of sensation or feeling with or without loss of consciousness

anesthesiologist a physician who specializes in the use of general anesthetics before, during, and immediately after major surgery

anesthetic drug or chemical agent that produces insensitivity to pain or feeling; primarily classified as local or general in their use and/or effect

anethol active constituent of anise oil

aneurysm localized thinning and dilation of an artery or a vein, causing a bulge or ballooning effect

angi- prefix meaning blood vessel; same as angio-

angiectasis abnormal dilation or enlargement of a blood vessel

angiitis inflammation of a blood vessel; synonym: vasculitis

angina disease marked by spasmodic attacks of intense suffocating pain; SEE *angina pectoris; Vincent's angina*

angina pectoris paroxysmal chest pain with a feeling of pressure and suffocation caused by decreased oxygen supply to the heart

angio- prefix meaning blood vessel; same as angi-

angioedema a condition characterized by development of edematous areas of skin, mucous membranes, or viscera; benign and thought to be an allergic reaction, possibly to food; synonyms: angioneurotic edema, Quincke's disease

angiogenesis formation of new blood vessels (e.g., in a healing wound)

angioneurotic edema SEE *Quincke's disease; angioedema*

angiotensin family of peptides with vasoconstriction activity

angiotensin I converting enzyme inhibitor (ACE) substance that inhibits the enzyme responsible for converting angiotensin I to angiotensin II

angle of repose maximum angle between the free surface of a loosely piled conical heap of powder and the horizontal plane; used to study flow properties of powders

angstrom (Å) unit of length equal to 108 cm; used in atomic and molecular spectrometry; used in expressing interatomic and intermolecular distances

anhidrotic drug that decreases sweating; SEE *antiperspirant*

anhydride the product of a condensation reaction between two carboxyl groups or two phosphate groups in which a molecule of water is eliminated

anion negatively charged atom or radical; ion or radical that migrates to the anode of an electrical cell; examples: CL and SO_4

anionic class of compounds of which the active part is negatively charged; example: anionic surfactant

anionic surfactant surface active agent that has a negative charge on the active portion of the molecule; example: sodium stearate (toilet soap)

anisotropic exhibiting different physical properties in different directions; a characteristic of all crystalline forms except cubic

ankylosis stiff or fixed joint

anneal to heat and cool slowly; usually to render less brittle

annotation the functional identification of the genes in a genome

anode positively charged electrode of an electrical cell to which anions migrate during electrolysis

anomaly significantly different from normal; example: birth defect

anomer an isomer of a cyclic sugar that differs from another in the arrangement of groups around an asymmetric carbon

anorexia absence of or loss of appetite

anorexia nervosa psychophysiologic condition, usually in young women, characterized by severe and prolonged inability or refusal to eat

anorexic pertaining to an agent or condition that reduces the appetite; synonym: anorectic

anorexigenic denotes an agent or condition that decreases the appetite

anosmia absence of the sense of smell

anoxia absence of oxygen as to a body tissue

ant- prefix meaning against; same as anti-

antacid drug capable of neutralizing excess stomach acid

antagonist **1:** agent that opposes or cancels the action of another agent or compound **2:** drug that interacts with a receptor producing no response yet blocking the effect of another substance **3:** muscle that contracts in opposition to another muscle

ante- prefix meaning before; same as antero-

antero- prefix meaning before; same as ante-

anthelmintic drug given for the eradication of parasitic worms

anthracosis accumulation of carbon in the lungs due to breathing smoke or coal dust; synonym: black lung

anti- prefix meaning against; same as ant-

antiadherent substance that prevents a tablet formulation from sticking to punches or dies during compression; SEE ALSO *lubricant*

antiadrenergic drug blocking the effects of epinephrine or norepinephrine at the myoneural junctions of the sympathetic nervous system; synonym: sympatholytic

antiandrogen drug blocking effects of male sex hormones

antiarrhythmic procedure, instrument, or medicine used to treat irregular heartbeats and restore normal rhythms

antiasthmatic SEE *bronchodilator*

antibacterial chemical or condition that is bacteriostatic and/or bacteriocidal

antibiotic chemical produced by a microorganism or prepared partially or totally by synthetic means that inhibits growth or kills other microorganisms at low concentration

antibiotic sensitivity test laboratory test to determine the susceptibility of a microorganism to a specific antibiotic

antibody **1:** substance produced in response to an antigen **2:** substance produced by an animal to neutralize specific infectious agents or the toxins produced by the infectious agent

anticholinergic drug blocking the effects of acetylcholine at the myoneural junction of the parasympathetic nervous system; example: atropine; synonym: parasympatholytic

anticoagulant **1:** drug that decreases the clotting of blood in the body; examples: warfarin, heparin **2:** substance added to whole blood to prevent clotting; example: ACD solution

anticoagulant acid citrate and dextrose solution sterile solution of citric acid, sodium citrate, and dextrose in Water for Injection; used as an anticoagulant to preserve blood for transfusion purposes; synonym: ACD solution

anticodon a sequence of three ribonucleotides on a tRNA molecule that is complementary to a codon on the mRNA molecule; codon-anticodon binding that results in the delivery of the correct amino acid to the site of protein synthesis

anticonvulsant drug to control or prevent seizures; examples: phenytoin, phenobarbital, valproic acid

antidepressant mood-elevating drug

antidiarrheal drug used to treat diarrhea

antidiuretic agent that blocks urine formation and/or secretion

antidiuretic hormone peptide hormone (secreted by the pituitary gland) that acts to decrease urine output by increasing water reabsorption in the kidneys; synonym: pitressin

antidote agent that neutralizes or counteracts the activity of a drug or a poison; examples: activated charcoal and tannic acid to adsorb and precipitate poisonous substances

antiemetic agent that inhibits vomiting

antiestrogen drug blocking the effects of female sex hormones

antifungal substance that destroys or retards the growth of fungi

antigen foreign protein or polysaccharide capable of inducing the formation of antibodies and activating T lymphocytes in the body

antihidrotic SEE *antiperspirant*

antihistamine 1: drug acting as an antagonist to histamine **2:** H_1 type—blocks histamine effects in allergy **3:** H_2 type—blocks gastric secretions including hydrochloric acid

antihyperlipidemic drug that lowers triglyceride and/or cholesterol levels in the blood; examples: clofibrate and D-thyroxin

antihypertensive drug that lowers blood pressure

anti-inflammatory drug given primarily to suppress or reverse the inflammatory process (redness, swelling, heat, pain)

antikickback statute forbids remuneration of any kind for Medicare and Medicaid referrals

antilogarithm number corresponding to a logarithm; example: the antilogarithm of 2 is 100 when the logarithmic base is 10

antimalarial drug used in treating malaria; example: quinine

antimer optical isomer

antimetabolite compound that closely resembles a natural substrate (vitamin, food) and interferes with metabolic reactions involving the natural substrate

antimony bluish white, crystalline, metallic element; chemical compounds of which produce a toxicity similar to that of arsenic; synonym: stibium

antinauseant drug used to overcome the feeling of nausea and to prevent emesis or vomiting; synonym: antiemetic

antineoplastic agent drug used to treat cancer or neoplasms

antioxidant agent that retards oxidation of another substance by being preferentially oxidized; substance that prevents the oxidation of other molecules

antipedicular agent drug used to kill lice; synonym: pediculicide

antiperspirant substance or preparation that diminishes perspiration (sweat) usually on a local skin area; synonyms: anhidrotic, antihidrotic, antisudorific

antipruritic drug that prevents or alleviates itching

antipyretic drug that reduces fever (elevated body temperature); examples: acetaminophen, aspirin

antisense RNA RNA molecule with a sequence complementary to that of an mRNA molecule

antiseptic drug that inhibits the growth of microorganisms; usually on a localized area of the body

antiserum antibody containing serum from previously immunized animal (including humans)

antisialagogue drug that prevents or decreases the flow of saliva; example: atropine

antisudorific SEE *antiperspirant*

antithyroid drug that reduces thyroid function; example: thiouracil

antitoxin substance produced by an animal body (including the human) in response to an injected toxin and capable of neutralizing that toxin; example: tetanus antitoxin

antitussive drug that suppresses or prevents cough

antivenin serum containing an antitoxin specific for an animal or insect venom; synonym: antivenom

antivenom SEE *antivenin*

antiviral drug that destroys or retards the spread of viral infection; example: acyclovir

anuria condition in which no urine is excreted

anxiety uneasy or apprehensive feeling usually from anticipated deleterious events, the origins of which are unknown or unrecognized

anxiolytic drug that relieves anxiety

any willing provider a requirement that a health insurance plan or a health maintenance organization sign a contract for the delivery of health care services with any provider in the area that would like to provide services to the plan's or HMO's enrollees

apathy indifference or lack of feeling

aperient very mild laxative

aperture opening or hole; usually a part of an instrument

aphagia inability to swallow

aphasia inability to use or understand words

apheresis a blood donation technique that allows for the donation of one or more bood components (e.g., platelets) while returning the others immediately to the donor

aphonia loss of voice or the power of speech

aphrodisiac drug that stimulates sexual desires and ability to perform sexual intercourse

aphthae round, whitish colored patches in the mouth, gastrointestinal tract, and on the lips caused by *Candida albicans;* synonym: thrush

aphthous stomatitis circular, intraoral lesions of unknown etiology; synonym: canker sore

aplastic anemia anemia caused by a lack of development of the bone marrow or its destruction by chemical agents or physical factors

apnea temporary cessation of breathing

apoenzyme protein part of an enzyme; one without its prosthetic groups or coenzymes

apoplexy sudden loss of consciousness characterized by paralysis; caused by loss of blood supply to or hemorrhage into the brain; synonyms: stroke, cerebrovascular accident (CVA)

apoprotein a protein without its prosthetic group

apoptosis programmed cell death

apothecary 1: one who procures, stores, and compounds dosage forms and dispenses drugs; synonym: pharmacist **2:** pharmacy (drugstore)

apothecary system one of several systems of weights and measures used by the apothecary or pharmacist; basic units are the grain (weight) and the minim (volume)

apothem SEE *apozema*

apozema strong infusion or decoction of vegetable drugs; also known as "apothem," "apozemata"

apozemata SEE *apozema*

apparent density SEE *density, apparent*

appeal a formal request by a covered person or provider for reconsideration of a decision, such as a utilization review recommendation, a benefit payment, or an administrative action

appendicitis inflammation of the vermiform appendix

Apple, William Shoulden (1918-1983) executive director of the American Pharmaceutical Association from 1959-1983; an early PhD having specialty expertise in pharmacy administration; pioneer of concepts of professional fees and drug product selection; Remington Honor Medal recipient in 1967

apprentice archaic term in pharmacy denoting one who works for an extended period of time under the tutelage of an experienced preceptor (pharmacist)

approved health care facility or program facility or program that is licensed under the laws of a state to provide health care and is approved by a health plan to provide the care described in a contract

a priori relating to deductive reasoning from self-evident facts

aqueous humor natural fluid in the anterior and posterior chambers of the eye

Arabic gum SEE *acacia gum*

arachidonic acid essential, unsaturated fatty acid that humans use to synthesize regulatory molecules such as prostaglandins

arachis oil fixed oil from peanuts; peanut oil

Archambault, George Frances (1909-2001) educator and one of the first pharmacy officers of the uniformed corps of the U.S. Public Health

Service; considered the "Father of Consultant Pharmacy"; Remington Honor Award recipient in 1969 and Whitney Award recipient in 1956

area **1:** extent of a surface **2:** length times width; cgs unit is cm^2; SI unit is m^2 **3:** part of the body that performs a highly specialized function; example: pectoral region

Area Health Education Center program to ensure adequate access to primary health care services in medically underserved communities through building and supporting an appropriately trained primary health care workforce

area under the curve pharmacokinetic, integral expression directly proportional to a specific quantity of material undergoing a change; example: area under the curve of blood level versus time is directly proportional to the amount of drug absorbed from a single dose over infinite time

arginine basic guanidino-bearing amino acid commonly found in protein; an essential amino acid for young children

Argyll Robertson pupil pupil does not respond to light, but reacts to accommodation; seen in syphilis, encephalopathy, and diabetes

argyria bluish or grayish purple discoloration of the skin from a deposition of silver into the skin; silver proteinate is responsible for the discoloration

arithmetic mean average of a series of numbers in a set

aromatic **1:** organic compounds containing a closed ring with alternate unsaturated bonds; examples: benzene and naphthalene **2:** possessing a distinctive odor (usually pleasant)

aromatic hydrocarbon a molecule that contains a benzene ring or has properties similar to those exhibited by benzene

aromatic water SEE *water, aromatic*

arrest cessation or stoppage; example: cardiac arrest

Arrhenius equation quantitative expression of changes in the degradation rate constant of a drug with changes in the absolute temperature; a useful relationship to predict shelf life (drug product stability at room temperature) using accelerated temperature studies

arrhythmia alteration of the normal rhythm of the heart muscles; example: tachycardia (rapid heartbeat)

arteriogram X-ray or fluoroscopic picture of an artery or arteries; taken immediately and repeatedly after injection of a radiopaque dye (X-ray contrast medium)

arteriole very small branch of an artery

arteriosclerosis vascular disorder characterized by degenerative changes in arteries, resulting in thickening and loss of elasticity of the walls; synonym: hardening of the arteries

arteritis inflammation of arteries

arthr- prefix meaning joint; same as arthro-

arthralgia pain in a joint

arthritis inflammation of a joint

arthro- prefix meaning joint; same as arthr-

arthropathy disease in a joint

Arthus phenomenon inflammation resulting from antigen-antibody (IgE) combining in tissues with resultant local reaction and damage

artifact or artefact change in natural state of a tissue; change in a chemical or biological system caused by the experiment or the experimenter

asbestosis fibrosis of the lungs due to inhalation of asbestos particles

ascariasis infection of *Ascaris lumbricoides;* roundworm or nematode infestation

ascaricide agent used to kill roundworms

ascites accumulation of serous fluid in the peritoneal cavity; synonym: abdominal dropsy

-ase suffix meaning enzyme

Asehoff nodules granuloma specific for rheumatic fever

aseptic free from pathogenic microorganisms; synonym: contamination-free

aseptic technique procedures designed to prevent contamination of preparations; example: use of a laminar flow hood for parenteral admixtures

Ashby technique nonradioisotope technique for determining red cell volume and red cell life span by injecting red cells of a different blood type into the recipient

-asis suffix meaning condition of

Asklepios primary Greek god of healing; his assisting daughters: Hygeia and Panacea

aspartame naturally occurring nonnutritive sweetener; methylester of a dipeptide of aspartic acid and phenylalanine; synonym: α-aspartylphenylalanine methylester

aspartate aminotransferase synonym for serum glutamate oxaloacetic transaminase

aspartic acid nonessential amino acid commonly found in proteins; synonyms: 2-aminosuccinic acid, 2-aminobutandioic acid

aspergillosis fungal infection caused by *Aspergillus*

aspermia lack of or scanty formation of sperm

asperse to sprinkle or to scatter

asphyxia condition resulting from deprivation of oxygen; synonym: suffocation

assay test to determine the presence or absence of a chemical or to determine the quantity of a component

assets 1: economic resources of a firm that have a future benefit or service potential **2:** fixed assets—durable economic resources lasting longer than one year **3:** liquid assets—cash or items that represent ready cash

assignee the person to whom the rights to a health insurance policy are assigned by the original policyholder

assignment of benefits patient directs insurance payment to a designated person or institution, usually a physician, pharmacist, or hospital

assisted-living facility group home for those who need assistance at a lower level than a nursing home facility

association constant SEE *affinity constant*

Association of Managed Healthcare Organizations national trade association for open model managed care organizations; previously known as American Association of Preferred Providers Organizations

asthenia loss of or lack of strength; synonym: debility

asthma a condition marked by recurrent attacks of paroxysmal dyspnea, with wheezing due to spasmodic contraction of the bronchi; may be an allergic manifestation or induced by irritant particles or vigorous exercise

astigmatism distorted image due to irregularity in the corneal curvature

astringent agent that causes local constriction or puckering of soft tissue by precipitating surface proteins

astro- prefix meaning star or star-shaped

asymmetry 1: condition in which there is a lack of symmetry; sides are unequal or unbalanced **2:** (chemistry) a condition in which a compound has optical activity; SEE *optical isomers*

asystolia lack of or faulty contraction of the heart

ataractic tranquilizer

ataxia muscular incoordination; inability to walk normally

atelectasis collapse of the lung

atherosclerosis form of arteriosclerosis in which plaques of cholesterol and other lipids are deposited within artery walls

athetosis condition characterized by involuntary movement, usually of the hands; synonyms: dyskinesia, Hammond's disease

athlete's foot fungal infection of the foot; synonyms: tinea pedis, ringworm of the foot

atomize to reduce a liquid to a fine spray or minute droplets

atomizer device to produce a fine spray

atopic gentically predisposed to certain conditions with an allergic component, such as asthma or dermatitis

atresia absence of or closure of an orifice, usually congenital atrium, chamber, or cavity leading to another structure; usually referring to the atrium of the heart

at risk assuming the financial liability for any loss that occurs when premiums paid are less than the cost of services provided; example: health care providers accepting prepayment as full coverage for a predetermined health care benefit

atrophy decrease in size or the stoppage of growth of an organ, structure, or tissue

atropine solanaceous alkaloid; the racemate of hyoscyamine; acts as a parasympatholytic or anticholinergic agent

attenuate to render less virulent or potent

attitude feeling, predisposition, or emotion directed toward a person, object, or fact

attractant substance that attracts or draws to itself; example: insect attractant

attrition 1: wearing or grinding down by friction **2:** act of weakening or exhausting by constant harassment or abuse **3:** decrease in numbers due to retirement, resignation, withdrawal, or death

atypical irregular, abnormal, or unusual

audit a systematic inspection of a firm's financial statements and reports to determine compliance to generally accepted accounting principles; involves analyses, tests, and confirmations

auditing process of examining and verifying the financial records of a business; SEE *audit*

aura any combination of signs and symptoms that precede the onset of a medical condition; example: visual disorders that precede a migraine headache

aural pertaining to the ear

auscultation to listen to body sounds

Auspitz's sign sign characterized by a small pinpoint of bleeding when a patient with psoriasis removes a psoriatic plaque; pathognomonic for psoriasis

aut- prefix meaning self; same as auto-

authorization the approval of care, such as hospitalization

autism the condition of being dominated by self-centered thoughts, not subject to external interactions

auto- prefix meaning self; same as aut-

autoanalyzer instrument used to perform chemical analyses automatically

autoclave device to sterilize instruments or finished pharmaceutical preparations using moist heat and pressure

autocrine refers to hormonelike molecules that are active within the tissue or organ in which they are produced

autogenesis SEE *abiogenesis*

autogenous vaccine vaccine made with cultured and treated bacteria from the patient's lesion

autoimmune disease a condition in which an immune reponse is directed against an animal's own tissues

autoinoculation giving oneself a disease; example: spreading warts from one body site to another

autointoxication belief popular in the late 1800s and early 1900s that retained feces would be reabsorbed by the body, causing medical problems

autologous transfusion patient donates own blood or blood component to be used later in surgery

autolysis breakdown of a substance caused by a reaction within itself; destruction of a tissue or organ by substances within that tissue or organ (occurs with no outside influences); synonym: self-digestion

automaticity ability of the heart to determine its own rate independent of autonomic influences; synonym: cardiac excitability

autonomic nervous system that part of the peripheral nervous system that is not subject to voluntary control; composed of the sympathetic and the parasympathetic nervous systems

autonomy a principle of ethics that states an individual's liberty of choice, action, and thought is not to be interfered with

autoradiograph image produced by radiation emitted from within an object; example: thyroid scan

auxins natural plant growth hormones

avascular lacking blood vessels

average collection period mean number of days required for the accounts receivable of a business to be collected

average cost per claim the average dollar amount of administrative and/or medical services rendered for the unit of measure within each expenditure category; calculated as dollar amount per number of units

average diameter mean particle size expression; calculated as the sum of the products of the number of particles of a specific diameter times the respective diameters divided by the total number of particles in the sample; abbreviation: dave

average gross margin parameter computed by subtracting average item acquisition cost from average item selling price

average length of stay the average number of days in a hospital for each admission

average manufacturer price average price paid by wholesalers for products distributed to the retail class of trade

average wholesale price published suggested wholesale price of a drug; used as a cost basis for pricing prescriptions

Avogadro's number number of molecules per mole of pure substance; 6.0222×10^{23}

avoirdupois system of weights and measures; the common system used in the United States

azeotrope a specific mixture of volatile substances that boils at a constant temperature; vapor composition equal to solution composition, so separation by distillation is not possible

azotemia elevation of nonprotein nitrogen waste products in the blood

azoxycompound substance containing both nitrogen and oxygen

B

Babinski sign/test/reflex test for pyramidal tract disturbance where stroking the lateral aspect of the sole of the foot normally produces plantar flexion of the great toe

Bachman test intradermal skin test for trichinosis infestation

bacill short, rodlike lozenge similar to a troche, except in shape

bacterial artificial chromosome (BAC) a derivative of a large *E. coli* plasmid used to clone DNA sequences as long as 300 kb

bactericide or bacteriocide drug that kills vegetative bacteria and some spores; synonym: germicide

bacteriophage **1:** bacteriolytic virus **2:** temperate bacteriophage—virus that becomes a part of the genome of a bacteria without lysis

bacteriostat drug that inhibits growth and multiplication of bacteria but does not necessarily kill them

bacteriostatic water for injection (BWFI) sterile water for injection containing an antimicrobial agent; maximum volume of 30 milliliters in each unit to prevent toxicity to the patient by larger amounts of the antimicrobial agent

bad debt expense account used to record estimated reductions in income caused by accounts receivable (credit sales) that will not be collected

baffle fixed, wide blade in a mixing container designed to cause formation of counter currents or turbulence in a mixing process (a disrupter of vortexes)

baffle pipe mixer cylindrical container with intermittently spaced baffles for continuous mixing processes

Baker's cyst enlargement of the popliteal bursa or herniation of the synovial membrane of the knee joint often associated with degenerative disease of the knee

baker's sugar SEE *confectioner's sugar*

baking soda sodium bicarbonate ($NaHCO_3$)

balance **1:** instrument to determine weight by utilizing a beam and a counter weight **2:** prescription balance—instrument with sufficient accuracy and precision to be used in compounding prescriptions **3:** class A balance—prescription balance with a sensitivity of 6 mg or less (minimum weighable quantity usually not less than 120 mg) **4:** class B balance—prescription balance with a sensitivity of 30 mg (not to be used for weighing less than 648 mg) **5:** analytical balance—instrument capable of weighing minute quantities (fraction of a mg)

balance billing **1:** a provider's billing of a covered person for charges above the amount reimbursed by the health plan **2:** the fee amount remaining after patient copayments

balance sheet periodic financial statement that summarizes the assets, liabilities, and owner's equity of a business at a specific point in time; synonym: statement of financial position

ballism involuntary violent jerking movement of extremities

ball mill machine used to reduce particle size by rotating a slurry or a powder in a container with pebbles or solid objects (usually porcelain or steel) that cause attrition as the container rotates; synonyms: pebble mill, rod mill, jar mill

ball valve SEE *valve*

balsam resin or oleoresin containing aromatic substances; example: balsam of tolu

Bamberger's disease saltatory spasm; polyserositis

bandage strip of cloth or adhesive used to protect wounds or apply pressure

bank statement written record of transactions in a bank account, showing deposits, withdrawals, special charges and account balances; usually prepared monthly

bar, chewable solid dosage form usually rectangular in shape that is meant to be chewed

Bárány's syndrome unilateral headache in the back of the head with recurrent deafness, vertigo, tinnitus, and abnormal pointing test; corrected by stimulating nystagmus

Bárány's test caloric test of semicircular canal

barbiturate any of several members of a group of chemical compounds that are derivatives of barbituric acid; used as a central nervous system depressant (sedative, hypnotic, anticonvulsant, and general anesthetic)

barium cocktail barium suspension taken orally to provide contrast on X-ray examinations of the gastrointestinal tract; synonym: barium meal; SEE *barium sulfate*

barium enema use of barium suspension as an enema to visualize the colon with X-rays; SEE *barium sulfate*

barium sulfate white insoluble solid used in suspension form as an X-ray opaque for examining the gastrointestinal tract

Barlow's disease infantile scurvy

baroreceptor nerve ending in the blood vessel wall sensitive to changes in blood pressure

Barraquer's disease progressive lipodystrophy; also known as "Simon's disease"

Barrett's esophagus premalignant cellular changes in tissue of esophageal region just above the lower esophageal sphincter caused by longstanding gastroesophageal reflux; chronic peptic ulcer of the lower esophagus; also known as "Barrett's ulcer," Barrett's syndrome"

barrier layer stratum corneum of the epidermis; consists of dead dermal cells forming the outer horny layer of the skin

barriers to access barriers to health care that can be financial (insufficient monetary resources), geographic (distance to providers), organizational (lack of available providers), and sociological (e.g., discrimination, language, cultural barriers)

basal lowest or least

basal metabolic rate (BMR) measure of energy required to support essential life-sustaining metabolic activities

base 1: compound that reacts with an acid **2:** compound that contributes a hydroxide ion to a chemical reaction **3:** compound that accepts a proton in a chemical reaction to form a conjugate acid **4:** compound that donates electrons in a chemical reaction (Lewis base) **5:** a nucleophile **6:** a molecule that can accept hydrogen ions

base, ionization constant SEE *ionization constant*

base, ointment vehicle of an ointment that serves to hold the active ingredient(s) for appropriate medical application

base, weak an organic base that has a small but measurable capacity to combine with hydrogen ions

base adsorption expression of the amount of liquids and solids required to encapsulate a suspension in a soft gelatin capsule (expressed as grams of liquid per one gram of solid)

base analogue a molecule that resembles normal DNA nucleotides and can substitute for them during DNA replication, leading to mutations

base capitation a stipulated dollar amount to cover the cost of health care per covered person, less mental health/substance abuse services, pharmacy, and administrative charges

Basedow's disease thyrotoxicosis

Basedow's syndrome myeloneuropathy, not due to vitamin B_{12} deficiency

baseline the abscissa of an *x-y* strip chart recorder

basic benefits package a core set of health benefits that everyone in the country should have either through their employer, a government program, or a risk pool

basophil type of white blood cell (granulocyte) in which the cytoplasmic granules are stained by a basic dye

batch specific quantity of a drug formulation of uniform quality and produced according to a single manufacturing order during the same cycle of manufacture; synonym: lot

batch dryer machine used to remove moisture from a specific quantity of pharmaceutical material in one drying operation; CONTRAST *continuous dryer*

batch mixing process of uniformly distributing a definite, manageable quantity of pharmaceutical materials

batch process a step or a series of steps involved in the preparation of a limited quantity of pharmaceutical material for dosage form production; example: mixing a quantity of powder for capsule filling; CONTRAST *continuous process*

batch processing pertaining to the technique of executing a set of computer programs such that each is completed before the next program is started

batch production record a complete history of quality control tests and processes of a manufactured lot of a drug product from raw material specifications through the finished product

bath lotion or solution intended to be added to water for general application

B cell a B lymphocyte; a white blood cell that produces and secretes antibodies that bind to foreign substances thereby initiating their destruction in the humoral immune response

bead solid dosage form in the shape of a small ball

bead, implant, extended release small sterile solid mass consisting of a highly purified drug intended for implantation in the body that would allow at least a reduction in dosing frequency as compared to the same drug presented as a conventional dosage form

Beal, George Denton (1887-1982) a pharmacy educator who spent the latter part of his career as the research director for the Mellon Institute of Industrial Research; served as a member of the *United States Pharmacopeia* Committee of Revision from 1920-1945; was influential in the establishment of the APhA Drug Standards Laboratory; Remington Medal recipient in 1941

Beal, James Hartley (1861-1945) pharmacist attorney and educator; developed the American Pharmaceutical Association's model state pharmacy practice act; served as president of APhA (1904-1905) and the American Association of Colleges of Pharmacy (1907-1908) and as chair of the United States Pharmacopeial Convention board of trustees from 1900-1930; recipient of the first Remington Honor Award in 1919

Beal Award established by the United States Pharmacopeial Convention in 2000 to recognize the outstanding contributions of volunteers who have advanced public health through commitment to the USP mission of providing quality standards for health care products and authoritative information on their use; named in honor of James Hartley Beal and George Benton Beal

Beck's triad low arterial pressure, high venous pressure, and absent apex beat; cardiac tamponade

bed day period of 24 hours during which a hospital bed is available for use by an inpatient

bed days/1,000 the number of inpatient days per 1,000 health plan members; formula: number of days/member months × 1,000 members × number of months

bedside manner appropriate interactions between a health team or an individual member of a health team and a patient or patient's family

Beeler's base ointment base consisting of an oil-in-water emulsion

Beer's law quantitative expression based on measurement of the extent of absorption of light of a specific wavelength by a substance in a solution; absorbance at a given wavelength proportional to concentration under controlled conditions

Beevor's sign upward displacement of umbilicus due to paralysis of lower rectus abdominis

behavioral health care assessment and treatment of mental and/or psychoactive substance abuse disorders

behavior modification attempts to change patients' habits that bear on health status, such as diet, exercise, smoking, etc., especially through organized health education programs; also called "lifestyle change" or "health promotion"

Bechterew-Mendel reflex a test that involves tapping the dorsum of the foot; normally causes extension of the second and fifth toes, whereas flexion indicates a pyramidal lesion; synonym: Mendel-Bechterew reflex

belief judgment, conviction, or expectation concerning the truth of some circumstance or the outcome of some event

belladonna solanaceous plant; source of atropine, hyoscyamine, scopolamine, and similar alkaloids

Bell's palsy functional disorder of facial nerves which may result in paralysis of facial muscles; caused by dysfunction of the seventh cranial nerve

Bence-Jones protein abnormal protein found in the urine of patients with multiple myeloma; consists of monoclonal light chains of the gamma globulin molecules

benchmarking a process of comparing one's own health care practice or entity to others (usually including the best practice) in order to improve the quality of services provided

Benedict's solution copper sulfate solution used to test for glycosuria; copper-containing solution used to test for the presence of reducing sugar (usually glucose) in urine; a screen for the possible presence of diabetes mellitus; SEE *Benedict's test*

Benedict's test method for qualitative or quantitative determination of reducing sugar in the urine; SEE *Benedict's solution*

beneficence a principle of ethics that states one should "do good" for another

beneficiary a person designated by an insuring organization as eligible to receive insurance benefits.

benefit service provided under an insurance policy or prepayment plan

benefit design a process of determining what level of coverage or type of service should be included within a health plan at specified rates of reimbursement based on factors such as market pressure, cost, clinical effectiveness and medical evidence, legislated mandate, medical necessity, and preventive value

benefit level the limit or degree of services a person is entitled to receive based on his/her contract with a health plan or insurer

benefit maximum clause in an insurance policy which specifies a dollar limit for total reimbursement during a benefit period

benefit package services an insurer, government agency, or health plan offers to a group or individual under the terms of a contract

benefit payment schedule list of amounts an insurance plan will pay for covered health care services

benign not malignant or not recurring

benne oil fixed oil from sesame; synonyms: sesame oil, teel oil

Bennett's fracture fracture of the base of the first metacarpal

bentonite colloidal hydrated aluminum silicate; used as a suspending agent and an adsorbent

benzocaine local anesthetic used to reduce pain and itching from insect stings, minor sunburn, dermatitis, and other minor medical conditions

benzodiazepines chemical class of drugs used primarily to treat anxiety, but which also have skeletal muscle–relaxing properties

benzomorphans chemical class of drugs used as narcotic analgesics; example: pentazocine

Berger's disease glomerulonephritis with mesangial IgA deposition

Berkefield filter unglazed porcelain filter formerly used to sterilize by filtration; example: candle filter

Besnier-Boeck disease sarcoidosis

best price greatest discount given to any purchaser

beta-blockers a category of drugs that inhibit the effects caused by stimulation of β_1- and β_2-adrenergic neurons; example: metaprolol

beta-carotene a plant pigment molecule that acts as an absorber of light energy and as an antioxidant

beta globin one of the two types of protein in hemoglobin A beta particle; SEE *beta ray; radioactivity*

beta-lactamase one of a group of enzymes (produced by various gram-positive and gram-negative bacteria) that catalyzes the hydrolysis of the beta-lactam ring of penicillins and cephalosporins

beta-oxidation the catabolic pathway in which most fatty acids are degraded; acetyl-CoA is formed as the bond between the α and β carbon atoms is broken

beta ray electron (negatron or positron) ejected from the nucleus of an atom during radioactive decay; the result of a change of an intranuclear neutron to a proton (negatron) or a proton to a neutron (positron); synonym: beta particle

bezoars concretion in the GI tract, composed of vegetable matter such as seeds or psyllium (phytobezoars), hair (trichobezoars), or other materials

bi- 1: prefix meaning two; example: bilateral **2:** prefix meaning an acidic salt; examples: sodium bicarbonate, sodium biphosphate

bilateral two-sided; pertaining to both sides

bile acid 1: acid derivative of a steroid **2:** natural constituent of bile that is an acidic metabolite of cholesterol

biliary excretion elimination of intact drug molecules or their metabolites in the bile secretions into the gastrointestinal track where reabsorption and/or excretion in the feces may occur

bilirubin bile pigment; reddish-brown breakdown product of heme and hemoglobin

billed claims the fees or costs for health care services provided to a covered person, submitted by a health care provider

bill review third-party review of medical bills for excessive or inappropriate charges; required of payers by some workers' compensation state statutes

bimetallic thermometer SEE *thermometer, bimetallic*

binder substance added to cause particles to adhere (usually for granulation and subsequent tablet compression); synonym: adhesive

Bingham bodies substances that exhibit plastic flow characteristics; SEE *plastic flow*

Bing's reflex extension of the great toe following a pricking of the dorsum of the toe or foot with a pin, seen in pyramidal tract lesions

bio- prefix meaning life

bioavailability rate and extent of absorption of a drug from a dosage form into the inner compartment(s) of the body

biochemistry study of the composition of organisms and the chemical reactions occurring within them

bioenergetics the study of energy transformations in living organisms

bioequivalent SEE *biological equivalent*

biogenic amine an amino acid derivative that acts as a neurotransmitter; example: GABA and the catecholamines

biological equivalent those chemical equivalents that, when administered in the same amounts, will provide the same biological or physiological availability, as measured by blood levels and urine levels

biological response a consequence of the interaction of a drug with a living system, causing changes in physiological processes; synonym: therapeutic response

biologicals usually refers to products of animal origin used to prevent, treat, or cure diseases and usually administered by injection; example: typhoid vaccine; synonym: biologics

biological value relative value of protein foods based on their abilities to supply essential amino acids

biologics SEE *biologicals*

biomolecule the molecules that make up living organisms

biopharmaceutics study of the relationship between physical, chemical, and biological properties of matter in relation to drugs, drug products, and drug availability and actions

biopsy removal of a small amount of tissue for microscopic examination

bioremediation the use of biological processes to decontaminate toxic waste sites

biotransformation chemical change of drug molecules occurring within and as a part of a life process; synonym: metabolism

birth control pill oral dosage form containing drug(s) to prevent pregnancy

bis- prefix in chemical nomenclature meaning two identical chemical groups are substituted in a molecule

bismuth white crystalline metal with a reddish tint, occurs in compounds that are used as antacids, antidiarrheals, antinauseants, and antiseptics

bismuth subcarbonate an odorless, tasteless, white powder that is insoluble in water or alcohol and used as a topical protectant and an intestinal astringent

bismuth subgallate insoluble yellowish powder used topically as an astringent

bismuth subnitrate insoluble, white powder used as an astringent absorbent and protective; contains 70 to 74 percent bismuth, which varies based on the conditions of preparation

bismuth subsalicylate insoluble white powder used as an astringent

bitter any bitter-tasting substance used to stimulate salivary and gastric secretions and improve the appetite (seldom used today)

bitter salt synonym for magnesium sulfate

black death disease caused by *Yersinia (Pasteurella) pestis;* synonym: bubonic plague

black lung SEE *anthracosis*

blank test   procedure used in colorimetry and other types of spectro-photometry in which the instrument is adjusted to compensate for the solvent and reagents

blastomycosis   fungal infection that may affect skin, lungs, or other parts of the body

bleach   compound or mixture of compounds capable of removing color from an object usually by an oxidative process

blend   mix thoroughly

blephar-   prefix meaning eyelid; same as blepharo-

blepharedema   edema or swelling of eyelid

blepharitis   inflammation of eyelid

blepharo-   prefix meaning eyelid; same as blephar-

bloating   feeling of distention in the abdominal cavity beyond its normal size; caused by serum, water, or gas accumulation

block   solid dosage form, usually in the shape of a square or rectangle

block-and-divide method   procedure for dividing a powdered formulation into equal segments by first forming a rectangularly shaped mass and then dividing it into approximately equal parts; a method that is useful for dispensing unit doses of a powder

blood   fluid tissue that circulates through the heart, arteries, veins, and capillaries, carrying oxygen and nutrients throughout the body; whole blood contains red blood cells, while blood cells, and platelets suspended in plasma

blood-brain barrier   specialized capillary membrane existing between circulating blood and the brain to prevent harmful substances from entering the brain; usually allows fat-soluble, but not water-soluble drugs to pass

blood cells, red   contain iron to transport oxygen throughout the body; manufactured in the bone marrow and removed by the spleen after approximately 120 days; synonym: erythrocytes

blood cells, white   produced in the bone marrow and responsible for protecting the body from foreign substances such as bacteria and visuses; granulocytes, macrophages, and lymphocytes are types of white blood cells; synonym: leukocytes

blood pressure   1: the force per unit area exerted by blood upon the walls of the arteries **2:** systolic blood pressure—blood pressure following the contraction of the heart forcing blood into the aorta and the pulmonary artery **3:** diastolic blood pressure—blood pressure when the heart is relaxed, representing the constriction of the arteries and arterioles; the force against which the heart must pump

blood urea amount of urea in the blood

blood urea nitrogen amount of nitrogen in the blood in the form of urea

bloom 1: gel strength of gelatin **2:** white powder that forms on cocoa butter suppositories (an undesirable property)

bluestone hydrated copper sulfate; synonym: blue vitriol

blue vitriol SEE *bluestone*

Blumberg's sign rebound tenderness indicating peritoneal inflammation

board certification voluntary process for those already licensed to practice pharmacy or medicine; indicates the individual has demonstrated an advanced level of education, experience, knowledge, and skills beyond what is required for licensure in a particular specialty practice area

board eligible a physician or pharmacist who is eligible to take the specialty board examination by virtue of having graduated from an approved medical school, completed a specific type and length of training, and practiced for a specified amount of time

Board of Pharmaceutical Specialities (BPS) created by the American Pharmaceutical Association in 1976 to formally recognize areas of specialty practice and certifying pharmacists in those areas

Board of Pharmacy state agency that examines and issues licenses to pharmacists and permits to drug outlets; also promulgates and enforces laws and regulations pertaining to pharmacy practice; synonyms: Board of Pharmaceutical Examiners or Commission on Pharmacy

bodying agent substance added to give bulk to a preparation; synonym: bulking agent

body mass index (BMI) calculation of height/weight ratio to determine whether a person is overweight and/or obese

body-mixing SEE *precoating*

body surface area body area, normally estimated using a nomogram (height–weight–surface area chart); used to calculate dose for a patient; SEE ALSO *dosage rules*

Bohr effect decrease in affinity of hemoglobin for oxygen with an increase in the pCO_2 of the blood

boil 1: acute inflammation of the subcutaneous layers of the skin, a gland, or a hair follicle; synonym: furuncle **2:** heat a liquid to bubbling

boiling chip pieces of broken porcelain or similar objects used to prevent "bumping" when distilling or refluxing liquids

bolus 1: volume of medication given rapidly by intravenous route **2:** a large solid dosage form; usually oval in shape and for administration to a large animal such as a horse or a cow

bona fide in good faith or without fraud or deceit; example: a bona fide prescription

Bond's theory quantitative expression for estimation of the energy requirement for particle size reduction, suggesting that it is inversely proportional to the square root of the diameter of the product

bone marrow depression a decrease in the quantity of bone marrow present or being produced; may be attributed to a disease state

borborygmus rumbling sounds emanating from the stomach or intestinal tract, usually due to gas

border brush SEE *microvilli*

bottle method SEE *Forbes method*

botulism often fatal food poisoning caused by ingestion of improperly canned food containing *Clostridium botulinum*

Bouchard's nodes seen in gout and osteoarthritis in the proximal interphalangeal joints

bougie 1: solid, insoluble bodies intended to be inserted into passages (e.g., urethra) for purposes of dilation; may be smeared with medicinal agent **2:** medicated suppositories of gelatin or wax for nasal or urethral use

Bowl of Hygeia vessel-serpent symbol of the profession of pharmacy originating in ancient Greece; Hygeia was one of the daughters of Asklepios, the Greek god of medicine

Bowman's capsule part of the nephron leading into the proximal convoluted tubule and enclosing the glomerulus

brachy- prefix meaning short

brady- prefix meaning slow

bradycardia slow heartbeat, usually fewer than 60 beats per minute

branched-chain amino acid one of a group of essential amino acids with branched carbon skeletons; examples: leucine, isoleucine, valine

brand-brand interchange the dispensing of one name brand prescription product in place of another on the basis of chemical equivalency

brand name registered name for a specific product by a manufacturer; synonym: trade name

brand-name drug a drug protected by a patent issued to the original innovator or marketer, which prohibits the manufacture of the drug by other companies without consent of the innovator, as long as the patent remains in effect

brandy alcoholic liquid distilled from fermented grapes or various other fruits (contains 48 to 53 percent alcohol); synonyms: *spiritus vini* and *spiritus vini vitis*

break-even point that condition in a business when revenue equals expenses

Bright's disease renal disease characterized by the presence of protein and sometimes blood in the urine; synonym: glomerulonephritis

Brill's disease relatively mild form of typhus caused by *Rickettsia prowazekii,* described first by Nathan E. Brill in eastern European immigrants; symptoms appear years following the initial infection; synonyms: sporadic typhus, recrudescent typhus

British Pharmacopoeia official drug compendium for the United Kingdom

British thermal unit amount of heat that must be absorbed by one pound of water to raise its temperature one degree Fahrenheit at 39.2°F

broad spectrum antibiotic category of drugs effective in the treatment of a large number of bacterial infections; examples: tetracycline, ampicillin

Brockedon, William (1787-1854) initial inventor of the compressed tableting process

broker the go-between for individuals or companies and health insurers; may help locate, negotiate, and finalize health insurance contracts; may also be an agent for a specific insurance company

brom- prefix meaning bad smell

bromhidrosis or bromidrosis offensive body smell or odor due to bacterial breakdown of components of perspiration

bromine red, volatile liquid element with a caustic, toxic, brown vapor

brominism or bromism poisoning from prolonged excessive use of bromides

Brompton's cocktail general term used for several mixtures of analgeics and stimulants given to patients with chronic pain and/or pain arising from terminal illness

bronchiectasis chronic dilation of a bronchus or bronchi as a result of inflammation or obstruction

bronchiolitis inflammation of the bronchioles

bronchitis acute or chronic inflammation of the bronchi

bronchodilator agent that shrinks mucosa of the bronchi, thereby increasing lumen size for better air passage in the lungs; synonym: antiasthmatic

bronchopneumonia inflammation of the bronchioli and air vesicles

bronchoscope instrument used to examine the interior of the bronchi; may also be used for surgical treatment of some bronchial diseases

Bronsted-Lowry theory concept that an acid is a substance that is capable of donating a proton and a base is a substance that is capable of accepting a proton, thereby resulting in a conjugate acid-base pair

Brookfield Viscometer (trademark) instrument to measure viscosity of a liquid, based on traction of a spindle rotating in the liquid

Brown, William (1752-1792) native Scotchman who became an American physician and wrote the *Lititz Pharmacopoeia,* a drug compendium used by the American forces during the Revolutionary War

Brownian movement random erratic movement of suspended microscopic particles due to kinetic motion of molecules of the dispersion medium; exhibited by particles about four micrometers (microns) in diameter or smaller

Brown's mixture mixture of opium and glycyrrhiza; a cough remedy

brucellosis infection caused by *Brucella* and characterized by intermittent or continuous fever, headache, chills, weakness, and loss of weight; synonym: undulant fever

brucine alkaloid of *Strychnos nux vomica* seed; related to strychnine

bruit abnormal swishing sound generally heard over an artery during auscultation

brush border outermost layer of the small intestinal epithelium, composed of many microvilli

bruxism teeth grinding

bubonic plague disease caused by *Yersinia (Pasteurella) pestis* and characterized by greatly enlarged lymph nodes (buboes), high fever, malaise, tachycardia, intense headache, and generalized muscle aches; synonym: black death

buccal concerning the cheek; example: buccal administration of a drug absorbed from the cheek pouch

buccal administration method of drug administration in which a soluble-solid dosage form is placed in the mouth, between the cheek and gum, for absorption into the blood

buccal tablet soluble tablet administered by placement in the mucosal pocket between the cheek and jaw; SEE *tablet, compressed*

bucco- prefix meaning cheek

budget an estimate of income and expenses over some specified future period of time or a financial plan for meeting a firm's goals and objectives

Buerger's disease inflammatory, obstructive disorder that affects the peripheral blood vessels of the lower extremities; synonym: thromboangiitis obliterans

buffer system containing chemical constituents that resist small changes in hydrogen ion and hydroxide ion concentrations, designed to keep the pH relatively constant; consists of a weak acid and its salt or a weak base and its salt

buffer capacity quantitative expression of the ability of a solution to resist pH changes either in the basic or in the acidic direction; expressed as concentrations of acid or base that can be added before the respective limits of capacity are reached and beyond which the pH is markedly altered

buffer equation quantitative expression of the pH of a system (dosage form) as a function of pKa and the log of the ratio of the concentrations of the buffer moieties; synonym: Henderson-Hasselbalch equation

bulimia 1: excessive hunger **2:** psychophysiological condition, usually observed in young women who are obsessed with weight control; manifested by excessive eating followed by self-induced vomiting

bulk chemical compound or mixtures of compounds produced and sold in large quantities (100 pounds to tons); CONTRAST *fine chemical*

bulk compounding preparing large amounts (liters, kilograms) of a formulation for multiple prescriptions or many patients

bulk density SEE *density, bulk*

bulking agent substance added to give bulk or body to a preparation; example: lactose added to a potent drug to be dispensed in capsule form; synonym: bodying agent

bulk laxative laxative that acts by providing bulk to the contents of the intestinal tract, thereby stimulating lower bowel evacuation

bulk transport mixing process of interspersing one or more substances by movement of large quantities of material from one position to another; example: a ribbon mixer for mixing wetted solids

bulla large fluid-filled vesicle

bundle branch block (BBB or bbb) abnormal conduction in the atrioventricular nerve transport system resulting in cardiac arrhythmias

bunion painful enlargement of the joint below the great toe induced by longstanding pressure against the joint from tight shoes

Burnett's syndrome milk-alkali syndrome (a chronic kidney disorder)

burnout feeling experienced by one who has been in a job or position too long without vacation or relief time thus becoming mentally and physically fatigued and less than enthusiastic in one's role

Burow's solution aluminum subacetate solution; used as a topical astringent

burr cell anemia form of anemia caused by carcinoma of the stomach or by a bleeding peptic ulcer; characterized by spiny projections on the cells

bursa fluid-filled sac that allows smooth motion of muscles or tendons over a bone or joint

bursitis inflammation of a bursa

butterfly valve SEE *valve*

butyrophenone class of drugs that act by blocking the release of dopamines; used as antipsychotics and antiemetics; example: haloperidol

buying group organization representing multiple independent buying sources for the purpose of obtaining price concessions from manufacturers and wholesalers through the combined purchasing power of its members and, in turn, redistributing that benefit to its members

B vitamins group of water-soluble nutrients required in the diet for growth and development of organisms and for prevention of certain neurological, dermatological, and hematological diseases; examples: thiamine, riboflavin, niacin, cyanocobalamin

by-product 1: something produced in addition to the principal product **2:** a secondary and oftentimes unintended result

cacao butter SEE *cocoa butter*

cachet obsolete oral dosage form in which the drug was placed between two thin wafers composed of starch (or flour and water), moistened, and sealed; to be dipped into water to soften before swallowing

cachexia severe state of malnutrition and emaciation

cafeteria plan an employee benefit plan under which all participants are permitted to choose among two or more benefit options according to their needs and/or ability to pay; also called "flexible benefit plan" or "flex plan"

cajeputol synonym for eucalyptol

cake layer of solid material collected by a surface filtration process in pharmaceutical manufacturing; usually the desired material in the separation process

caking separation and strong agglomeration of suspended particles from a colloidal dispersion or a suspension to the extent that the agglomerate cannot be redispersed easily; an undesirable process causing a physical incompatibility in a dosage form

calamine a pink powder composed of zinc oxide and a small amount of ferric oxide; used as an astringent and mild antiseptic

calcemic agent that elevates blood levels of calcium

calcination heating of a carbonate to drive off carbon dioxide, producing an amorphous oxide powder; examples: conversion of magnesium carbonate to magnesium oxide, conversion of calcium carbonate to calcium oxide

calcine process of calcination

calcined salt products of calcination; examples: calcium oxide from calcined calcium carbonate, magnesium oxide from calcined magnesium carbonate

calcitonin polypeptide hormone secreted by the thyroid gland in response to hypercalcemia; has a therapeutic effect of lowering serum calcium and phosphate, antagonizing the parathyroid hormone and inhibiting bone resorption; synonym: thyrocalcitonin

calcium electrolyte in body fluids; a component in the structure of bones and teeth

calcium channel blockers refers to a category of drugs that block the fast influx of calcium into cardiac and smooth muscle; agents beneficial in treating angina pectoris; example: verapamil

calcium oxide lime, quick lime, burnt lime, or calx

calculus 1: hardened material on the teeth occurring as a result of several days of poor dental hygiene **2:** a stone; examples: gallstone, kidney stone **3:** mathematical treatment of data involving processes with changing rates; example: mathematical computations of drug absorption, distribution, and elimination

calculus, differential determination of instantaneous rates in a changing process

calculus, integral summation of the finite or infinite instantaneous rates of a changing process

calibration establishment of a measurable scale of an instrument; example: setting the wavelength range (window) of a scintillation counter to measure a specific radiation type

calisaya bark cinchona, cinchona bark, or Peruvian bark; a source of quinine and quinidine

call schedule the schedule for physicians' and other health professionals' availability for after-hours care

callus hyperkeratinous lesion occurring as a result of friction and pressure, usually on the palm of the hand or the sole of the foot

calmodulin calcium-binding protein with a probable role in muscle contraction

calomel mercurous chloride (Hg_2Cl_2); formerly used as a cathartic

calorimeter instrument to measure changes in heat content in a process or a chemical reaction

calorimetry method of measuring changes in heat content in a process; examples: Parr bomb and Dewar flask experiments

calorimetry, differential scanning automated instrument to measure differences in heat changes in a process over a wide spectrum

Calvé-Perthes disease osteochondrosis of the vertebrae

Calvin cycle the major metabolic pathway by which CO_2 is incorporated into organic molecules

calx calcium oxide, quick lime, burnt lime, or calx usta; formula: CaO

cam rotating or sliding piece that imparts motion to a roller moving against its edge as in a rotary tablet press or in other processing equipment

camphor gum obtained from the camphor tree; used as a mild antiseptic and anesthetic; also made synthetically; synonyms: gum camphor, laurel camphor

camphorated opium tincture SEE *paregoric*

camphor spirit a 10 percent solution of camphor in alcohol; used as a counterirritant; synonym: spirit of camphor

cancer uncontrolled growth or tumor that spreads by invasion and metastasis; uncontrolled cellular multiplication contrary to and at the expense of normal body growth processes; synonym: malignant neoplasm

candidiasis fungal infection caused by *Candida albicans;* manifested as thrush, glossitis, or vaginitis

Cannon's syndrome increase in adrenaline secretion during emotional stress, resulting in palpitations and sweating

capacity an organized system's ability to meet the demands of both scheduled care and after-hours care

capacity factor parameter that is an indication of the amount of heat or energy a substance holds; example: enthalpy

capillarity spontaneous movement of water or other liquid into small openings or tubes due to surface forces

capillary **1:** a minute channel in porous material or a lumen of a small tube **2:** glass tube with a very small inner diameter; used in measuring surface tension and melting point **3:** very small blood vessel connected to larger arteries and veins in the body's circulatory system

capillary fragility method of measuring intrinsic bleeding-clotting mechanism by using a pressure cuff and observing appearances of petechiae

capillary viscometer test device consisting of a constant volume glass bulb with a small orifice through which liquid flows; used to measure relative viscosity

capitation a method of payment in which a health plan, such as an HMO, or a specific provider receives a fixed amount for each person eligible to receive services (dollars per member per month), which is made whether or not the covered person becomes an active patient and without regard to the number and mix of services used by that patient

capitation fund a fund based on the number of members multiplied by the budgeted or capitated amount each member pays

capitation rate stipulated dollar amount established to cover the cost of health care delivered for a person; usually a negotiated per capita rate to be paid prospectively and periodically, usually monthly, to a health care provider, who is responsible for delivering or arranging for the delivery of all health services required by the covered person under the conditions of the provider contract

Caplan's syndrome progressive massive necrosis of the lung, seen with rheumatoid arthritis

capping separation of a compressed tablet into two or more layers immediately after the compression process; a result of too many fines in the granulation, entrapped air during compression, and/or sticking to the tableting punches or dies

capsaicin topical medication used to produce a burning sensation in the skin; primary component of "hot pepper" creams used for postherpetic neuralgia

capsule gelatin shell designed to hold a unit dose of a powder, a compacted slug, or an oily liquid; a dosage form made of hard or soft gelatin, and containing a unit dose of a drug formulation

capsule, coated solid dosage form in which the drug is enclosed within either a hard or soft soluble container or "shell" made from a suitable form of gelatin; additionally, the capsule is covered in a designated coating

capsule, coated, extended release solid dosage form in which the drug is enclosed within either a hard or soft soluble container or "shell" made from a suitable form of gelatin; additionally, the capsule is covered in a designated coating and releases a drug (or drugs) in such a manner to allow at least a reduction in dosing frequency as compared to that drug (or drugs) presented as a conventional dosage form

capsule, coated pellets solid dosage form in which the drug is enclosed within either a hard or soft soluble container or "shell" made from a suitable form of gelatin; the drug itself is in the form of granules to which varying amounts of coating have been applied

capsule, delayed release solid dosage form in which the drug is enclosed within either a hard or soft soluble container made from a suitable form of gelatin, and which releases a drug (or drugs) at a time other than promptly after administration; example: enteric-coated articles

capsule, delayed release pellets solid dosage form in which the drug is enclosed within either a hard or soft soluble container or "shell" made from a suitable form of gelatin; the drug itself is in the form of granules to which enteric coating has been applied, thus delaying release of the drug until its passage into the intestines

capsule, extended release solid dosage form in which the drug is enclosed within either a hard or soft soluble container made from a suitable form of gelatin, and which releases a drug (or drugs) in such a manner to allow a reduction in dosing frequency as compared to that drug (or drugs) presented as a conventional dosage form

capsule, film coated, extended release solid dosage form in which the drug is enclosed within either a hard or soft soluble container or "shell" made from a suitable form of gelatin; additionally, the capsule is covered in a designated film coating and releases a drug (or drugs) in such a manner to allow at least a reduction in dosing frequency as compared to that drug (or drugs) presented as a conventional dosage form

capsule, gelatin coated   solid dosage form in which the drug is enclosed within either a hard or soft soluble container made from a suitable form of gelatin; through a banding process, the capsule is coated with additional layers of gelatin so as to form a complete seal

capsule, liquid filled   solid dosage form in which the drug is enclosed within a soluble, gelatin shell that is plasticized by the addition of a polyol, such as sorbitol or glycerin, and is therefore of a somewhat thicker consistency than that of a hard shell capsule; typically, the active ingredients are dissolved or suspended in a liquid vehicle

capsule body or capsule cup   larger portion of a hard capsule; the part that contains the powder or other dosage unit

capsule cap   top portion of a hard capsule that closes the capsule

capsule filler 1: machine designed to fill capsules **2:** bulking or bodying agent of capsule contents (diluent); example: cornstarch

caramel   burned sugar coloring; a concentrated solution obtained by controlled burning of sucrose or glucose; used as a pharmaceutical flavoring and coloring agent

carbamate   ester of carbamic acid (the semi-amide of carbonic acid)

carbolic acid   volatile crystal or liquid used as a caustic, disinfectant, and local anesthetic; synonym: phenol

carbon   nonmetallic element; occurring as diamond, graphite, lamp black, or charcoal

carbonate   salt or ester of carbonic acid

carbonation   process of charging a solution with carbon dioxide gas

carbon dioxide fixation   SEE *carboxylation*

carbonic acid   weak acid made by combining carbon dioxide and water

carbonic anhydrase   metabolic enzyme that catalyzes the combining of carbon dioxide and water to form carbonic acid in body processes

carboxylation   substitution of a carboxyl group (COOH) on a molecule; synonym: carbon dioxide fixation

carbuncle   a cluster of boils or furuncles involving infection of several hair follicles and surrounding tissues accompanied by inflammation, localized pain, and purulent sores

carcino-   a prefix pertaining to carcinoma

carcinogen   agent that produces cancer

carcinogenesis   the process whereby cells become genetically unstable and eventually cancerous

carcinoma malignant tumor or neoplasm arising in epithelial or associated tissue (such as glandular tissue); malignant cells may invade (or metastasize to) other tissue

carcinoma in situ tumor of the surface epithelium and/or underlying glandular tissue whose component cells are morphologically identical to those of frank carcinoma

card- prefix meaning heart; same as cardio-

cardamon seed source of volatile cardamon oil; used as a flavoring

cardiac referring to the heart

cardiac glycoside glycoside used to slow the rate and increase the contractile force of the heart; examples: digitalis glycoside, strophanthus glycoside, glycoside of squill

cardio- prefix referring to the heart; same as card-

cardiorrhexis rupture or breaking of the heart

cardiovascular pertaining to the heart and blood vessels

carditis inflammation of the heart

card program prescription plan using a drug benefit identification card that, when presented to a participating pharmacy, entitles those covered to receive the medication for a specified copay

care coordinator SEE *gatekeeper*

caries cavities

carminative substance used to relieve gaseous distention of the stomach; example: peppermint

carnauba wax very hard, brittle wax obtained from the leaves of the carnauba palm; used as a polishing agent in the manufacture of tablets and capsules

carotenoids a class of hydrocarbons (carotenes) and their oxygenated derivatives (xanthophylls); highly colored (red, orange, and yellow) group of fat-soluble plant pigments having antioxidant effects

carotid a primary artery supplying blood to the head

carriage, nasal condition in which patient's nasal passages are contaminated with *Staphylococcus aureus,* causing conditions such as recurrent furunculosis

carrier **1:** specific protein in membranes of cells or organelles used to transport substances across a particular membrane **2:** solid support for heterogeneous catalyst; example: charcoal for palladium **3:** vehicle used to transport a drug to its site of absorption or action **4:** person who is able to transmit a dormant disease to another person who becomes actively infected **5:** protein that binds to a hapten to form a complete antigen **6:** an entity that may underwrite or administer a range of health benefit programs; may refer to an insurer or a managed health plan

carrier-free preparation of a radioisotope to which no carrier has been added

cartridge enclosed device designed to perform a specific pharmaceutical process; example: cartridge filter

cartridge, insulin small, glass, multidose insulin containers created by several manufacturers to fit into specific insulin injection devices; referred to as "insulin pens"

carve out decision to purchase separately a service that is typically a part of an indemnity or HMO plan

cascara sagrada bark obtained from *Rhamnus pershiana* and used to prepare extracts for use as laxatives

case hardening formation of a more dense, dry outer surface (crust) of a material being dried, thereby reducing the rate of drying of its inner contents

case management **1:** process whereby covered persons with specific health care needs are identified and a plan designed to efficiently utilize health care resources is formulated and implemented to achieve the optimum patient outcome in the most cost-effective manner **2:** a utilization management program for patients who have prolonged, expensive, or chronic conditions; helps determine the treatment location (hospital, other institution, or home) and authorizes payment for such care

case manager experienced professional who works with patients, providers, and insurers to coordinate all services to provide a plan of medically necessary and appropriate health care

case mix the relative frequency and intensity of hospital admissions or services reflecting different needs and uses of hospital resources; can be measured based on patients' diagnoses or the severity of their illnesses, the utilization of services, and the characteristics of a hospital

cash basis of accounting revenues are recognized when cash is received and expenses are recognized when payments are made

cash discount price reduction extended to a customer in return for prompt payment of invoices

cash flow the difference in the amount of cash received and expended during a given period of time

Caspari, Charles J. (1850-1917) practitioner and educator; served as the general secretary of the American Pharmaceutical Association from 1894-1911

cassia oil oil of cinnamon; used as a flavoring agent

castile soap a whitish, solid cake composed of a mixture of sodium oleate, sodium palmitate, and other fatty acid salts; synonyms: soap, hard soap

castor oil fixed oil from the seed of the castor plant, *Ricinus communis;* used as a lubricating-irritant cathartic

catabolic pathway a series of biochemical reactions in which large complex molecules are degraded into smaller, simpler products

catabolism process by which a living organism breaks down complex compounds into more simple substances

catalepsy trancelike state in which there is loss of consciousness

catalysis enhancement or reduction of reaction rate by use of an added constituent called a catalyst

catalyst substance that facilitates or reduces the rate of a chemical reaction and is not apparently altered by the reaction; substance that alters the rate of a reaction without affecting its equilibrium constant

cataplasm viscous preparation intended to be warmed and applied to a body surface for the purpose of allaying pain and/or reducing inflammation; synonym: poultice

cataplexy sudden loss of muscular control and altered consciousness of short duration induced by strong emotions (e.g., laughter, anger); considered to be pathognomonic for narcolepsy

catastrophic health insurance insurance for severe and prolonged illness that poses a serious financial threat

catatonia state of immobility with muscular rigidity, sometimes with excessive excitability (a type of schizophrenia)

catechol refers to a compound which the structure consists of two adjacent hydroxyl groups attached to a benzene ring; *o*-hydroxyphenol

catecholamine class of orthodihydroxyphenethyl amines having a sympathomimetic action; examples: dopamine, norepinephrine, epinephrine

categorically needy under Medicaid, categorically needy cases are aged, blind, or disabled individuals or families and children who meet financial eligibility requirements for Temporary Aid to Needy Families, Supplemental Security Income, or an optional state supplement

catgut sheep's intestines processed to be used as absorbable sutures

catharsis cleansing or purging; usually of the lower bowel; the effects of taking a laxative

cathartic compound used to evacuate the lower bowel; SEE *laxative*

catheter flexible tube (made with varying lengths and lumen sizes) used to withdraw or introduce fluids from or into the body, to examine a specific part of the body, or to perform microsurgery in a specific place within the body

cathode negatively charged pole of an electrical cell to which cations migrate in electrolysis; a negatively charged electrode

cathode ray tube special type of vacuum tube for projecting electron beams; used to display information on a visible screen at the front of the tube; used in television, oscilloscope, and computer screens

cation positively charged ion that migrates to the cathode in electrolysis

cationic surfactant surface active agent that has a positive charge on the organic radical (the active part of the molecule) (R_4N^+); example: benzalkonium chloride

CAT scan SEE *tomography*

caustic burning or corrosive agent that will destroy living tissue; examples: silver nitrate, potassium hydroxide

caustic pencil toughened silver nitrate stick used to cauterize small ulcerations or slow healing sores

caustic soda sodium hydroxide

caustic stick SEE *caustic pencil*

Caventou, Joseph B. (1795-1877) French pharmacist-alkaloid chemist who, with Pelletier, discovered strychnine (1818), brucine (1819), quinine (1828), and other alkaloids

cavitation the collapsing of an "air lock" or "air pocket" in a pumping process as it is subjected to an area of high pressure, such as in the chamber of a centrifugal pump; a pump-damaging process

ceiling the highest amount of money that an insurance company will pay to cover a patient's care; not included in many HMO plans

cell fractionation a technique involving homogenization and centrifugation that allows the study of cell organelles

cellobiose a degradation product of cellulose; a disaccharide that contains two molecules of glucose linked by a β-(1,4)-glycosidic bond

cellular immunity immune system processes mediated by T cells, a type of lymphocyte

cellular pathology concept that diseases were located in the cells that hold life itself; proposed by Rudolph Virchow (1821-1902)

cellulase enzyme that splits cellulose into smaller molecular units (from polysaccharides to the fundamental sugar unit)

cellulose polysaccharide carbohydrate with $C_6H_{10}O_5$ as the fundamental unit; the part of cell walls of plants; differs from starch in that it consists of β-glycosidic bonds instead of α-glycosidic bonds between fundamental units; a polymer produced by plants that is composed of D-glycopyranose residues linked by β-(1,4)-glycosidic bonds

cement 1: dental preparation employed primarily as a temporary protective covering for exposed pulp; example: zinc oxide–eugenol mixture **2:** hard cake formed due to strong agglomeration of particles in a suspension or a colloidal dispersion; an undesirable dosage form phenomenon; a form of physical incompatibility that may cause ineffective therapy due to inadequate mixing **3:** substance that serves to produce solid union between two surfaces

cementum soft material covering the root of a tooth

census complete count of a population of interest

Centers for Medicare and Medicaid Services (CMS) the government agency within the Department of Health and Human Services that directs the Medicare and Medicaid programs (Titles XVIII and XIX of the Social Security Act) and conducts research to support those programs; formerly the Health Care Financing Administration (HCFA)

centers of excellence a network of health care facilities selected for specific services based on criteria such as experience outcomes, efficiency, and effectiveness

centipoise (0.01 poise) common unit to measure viscosity of liquid pharmaceutical systems; SEE *poise; viscosity; Newton's law of viscous flow*

central nervous system (CNS) part of the nervous system consisting of the brain and the spinal cord

central tendency effect the practice of giving all observations "average" ratings; avoiding high or low points on the scale

centrifugal blower/compressor/pump apparatus that utilizes a rotating grooved impeller to move liquid or air from an intake near the center outwardly through an outlet at the outer edge of the impeller; a low maintenance cost and a smooth flow of liquid or air are its primary advantages

centrifugal filter filtration system that separates particulate solids from liquids by a rotating motion (may be a continuous or a batch process)

centrifugal force force that tends to impel objects outward from the center of rotation

centrifuge machine that separates substances of different densities using centrifugal force at high revolutions per minute

cephalin phospholipid that is either a phosphatidylserine or a phosphatidylethanolamine; synonym: kephalin

cephalosporinases group of β-lactamase enzymes (produced by certain bacteria) that catalyze hydrolysis of the β-lactam ring of various cephalosporins

cephalosporin C natural antibiotic produced by the fungus *Cephalosporium acremonium*

cephalosporins 1: group of bacteriocidal antibiotics that block the final stage of cell wall biosynthesis in bacteria by inhibiting transpeptidase **2:** chemically, a type of compound in which a β-lactam ring is fused to a dihydro-1,3-thiazine ring

cephamycins group of bacteriocidal antibiotics that block the final stage of cell wall biosynthesis in bacteria by irreversibly acylating transpeptidase

cephem the vital nucleus for antibiotic activity of all cephalosporins

cerate preparation for external use having a high percentage of wax as a base that will soften but not liquefy at body temperature

cerate, Galen's cold cream, rose water ointment

cerebroside glycoside composed of a fatty acyl sphingolamide and a sugar (mainly galactose)

cerebrum the main and largest segment of the brain; the frontal part divided into two hemispheres

ceresin hard, white, odorless, solid wax used as a substitute for beeswax; synonyms: ozokerite, earth wax, mineral wax

certificate a document issued to a pharmacist upon successful completion of the predetermined level of performance of a certificate training program or of a pharmacy residency or fellowship

certificate of authority (COA) a certificate issued by state government, licensing the operation of a health maintenance organization

certificate of coverage (COC) a description of the benefits included in a carrier's plan, required by state laws

certificate of need (CON) certificate issued by a government body to an individual or organization proposing to construct or modify a health facility, acquire major new medical equipment, or offer a new or different health service; recognizes that a facility or service will meet the needs of those for whom it is intended

certificate training program a structured and systematic postgraduate continuing education experience for pharmacists, generally shorter than degree programs

certification voluntary process by which a nongovernmental agency or an association grants recognition to a pharmacist who has met certain predetermined qualifications specified by that organization; usually requires initial assessment and periodic reassessments of the individual's qualifications

certified dye color or dye permitted by the FDA to be used for drug and food formulations; specified in the federal Food, Drug, and Cosmetic Act

certified medical service representative a professionally trained field employee of a pharmaceutical manufacturer who provides detailed information to health professionals on the company's drug products; must meet standards established by the CMR Institute of Roanoke, Virginia

certified pharmacy technician one who has completed the Pharmacy Technician Certification Examination, which covers communication, organizational and interpersonal skills, pharmacy operations, pharmacy law, and calculations

cerumen solidified mixture of secretions of sweat and sebaceous glands in the external auditory canal; synonym: earwax

ceruminokinesis process by which cerumen migrates from its point of formation (proximal to the tympanic membrane) outward until it is removed by the patient

cetostearyl alcohol SEE *cetyl alcohol*

cetyl alcohol fatty alcohol containing 16 carbons in a straight chain; synonyms: 1-hexadecanol, palmityl alcohol, cetostearyl alcohol

cetylpalmitate ester of cetylalcohol and palmitic acid; a wax found in beeswax and spermaceti

chain pharmacy one of a group of pharmacies, usually four or more, under common ownership and operation

chalk calcium carbonate; $CaCO_3$

chalk, precipitated precipitated calcium carbonate prepared by mixing solutions of calcium chloride and sodium carbonate and then collecting, washing, and drying the resultant particles

chalk, prepared native form of calcium carbonate freed of most of its impurities by elutriation

chalone endogenous group of water-soluble secretions which are tissue-specific and which inhibit mitosis of cells in that tissue; such inhibitions are reversible

channeling use of incentives and plan design to encourage members to use network providers

channel lattice an ordered molecular structure with openings capable of entrapping smaller molecules

charcoal organic matter that has been partially burned to produce carbon; an amorphous form of carbon produced by destructive distillation of animal or vegetable matter; synonyms: lamp black, carbon black

Charcot-Marie-Tooth disease peroneal muscular atrophy (of the leg muscles near the fibula)

Charcot's triad intention tremor, nystagmus, and scanning speech seen in brain stem involvement in multiple sclerosis

charge-based payment system system of paying for a health care service (usually a hospital or other facility) on the basis of what the provider furnishing the service usually charges all patients

charlatan one who promotes unproven remedies or claims to have knowledge or skills that are not actually possessed; synonym: quack

charlatanry claiming to have knowledge or skills that are not actually possessed; synonym: quackery

Charles's Law SEE *gas law, ideal*

chart or charta prescription or other medication order notation for powder paper(s); used to dispense powders in unit dose quantities; used to protect balance pans when weighing

check valve SEE *valve, check*

chelate "claw" type of metallic complex in which a multiligand molecule forms a stable ring with a central metallic ion, rendering the ion inactive

Chemical Abstracts System of Nomenclature system of naming chemical compounds; a modification of the IUPAC system of nomenclature; specifically, the parent name is listed first followed by a comma and the names of attached substituents

chemical adsorption   SEE *adsorption*

chemical dependency   SEE *substance abuse*

chemical equivalents   multiple-source drug products which contain essentially identical amounts of the same active ingredients, in the same dosage forms, and which meet existing physical-chemical standards

chemical name   systematic name from which the exact structure can be derived; contrasted to the generic, trade, or trivial (common) names for a compound; CONTRAST *generic name; proprietary name*

chemiosmotic coupling theory   ATP synthesis is coupled to electron transport by an electrochemical proton gradient across a membrane

chemisorption   SEE *adsorption*

chemist 1: one who is knowledgeable of and works with chemical compounds **2:** British provider of pharmaceutical services; a pharmacist in the United Kingdom

chemoheterotroph   an organism that uses preformed food molecules as its sole source of energy

chemolithotroph   an organism that uses specific inorganic reactions to generate energy

chemonucleolysis   injection of an enzyme into a part of the body to destroy undesirable tissue that would otherwise require invasive surgery; example: injection of chymopapain (a proteolytic enzyme) to perform a laminectomy

chemosis   swelling of the conjunctiva

chemotherapy   therapeutic concept developed by Paul Ehrlich (1854-1915) in which a specific chemical or drug is used to treat an infectious disease or cancer; ideally, the chemical should destroy the pathogen or the cancer cells without harming the host

chewable tablet   SEE *tablet, compressed*

child-proof closure   an inappropriate way to refer to child-resistant closures

Children's Health Insurance Program   (CHIP) government program developed to provide health insurance to children not otherwise covered

child-resistant closure   designed to slow a child's access to medication and allow an adult time to intervene

chiral molecule   a molecule that has mirror-image forms

chiropodist   SEE *podiatrist*

chiropody   SEE *podiatry*

chiropractic medicine a system of health care that attributes disease to dysfunction of the nervous system, and attempts to restore normal function by treating the body structures, especially those of the vertebral column

chi-square test a statistical procedure used to test the association between two nominal variables

chitin an unbranched polymer in which *N*-acetylglucosamine residues are linked by β-(1,4)-glycosidic bonds; the principal structural component of the exoskeletons of arthropods

chlorophyll a green pigment molecule that resembles heme and absorbs light energy

cholelithiasis concretions in the gall bladder or bile duct

cholestyramine an anion exchange resin indicated for use as an antipruritic, an antihyperlipoproteinemic, and a cholesterol-lowering agent

cholinomimetic agent that mimics the action of acetylcholine in the body

chondr- prefix meaning cartilage; same as chondro-

chondro- prefix meaning cartilage; same as chondr-

Christensen-Krabble disease progressive cerebral poliodystrophy

Christmas disease hemophilia B; sex-linked recessive hereditary bleeding disorder

chromatin the DNA-containing component of the eukaryotic nucleus; the DNA is almost always complexed with histones

chromatography method for separation of dissolved substances or gases by use of differential adsorption; examples: liquid, paper, column, and gas chromatography

chromophore portion of a compound that absorbs electromagnetic radiation; chromophores absorbing visible light are responsible for color

chromosome the physical structure, composed of DNA and some proteins, that contains the genes of an organism

chronic persistent or of long duration, as in a diseased state

chronic care care for an individual with a long-term illness

chronic hepatitis SEE *hepatitis*

chronotropic affecting rate; usually in reference to heart rate

chylomicron lipoprotein synthesized in the intestinal epithelial cells and composed of triglycerides, fats, cholesterol, phospholipids, and proteins

cicatrix mark of a healed wound; synonym: scar

cilia small, independently moving, hairlike projections attached to cell surfaces; the cilia of the respiratory tract are responsible for mucokinesis

ciliated cells cells to which cilia are attached

cinchona drug obtained from the bark of a tree indigenous to the Andes Mountains of South America; source of quinine alkaloids; used as an antimalarial, antipyretic, analgesic, and antiarrhythmic; synonyms: Peruvian bark, Calesayo bark

cinchona alkaloids organic amines obtained from *Cinchona succirubra* (red cinchona) and its hybrids; examples: quinine, quinidine, cinchonine, cinchonidine

cinchonidine alkaloid from cinchona bark related stereochemically to quinine; synonym: 6'-desmethoxyquinine

cinchonine alkaloid from cinchona bark, a diastereoisomer of cinchonidine possessing the same stereochemistry as quinidine; synonym: 6'-desmethoxyquinidine

circadian rhythm twenty-four-hour cycling of events; synonym: diurnal variation

circular dichroism type of instrumentation in which the molar elipticity of an optically active substance is determined in solution at varying wavelengths

cistern lymph spaces in body tissue such as the brain

cisternography roentgenography of a cistern; a method of taking pictures of a cistern by injecting X-ray opaque dyes (contrast media) so that it may be visualized; often refers to X-ray visualization of the enlarged subarachnoid spaces of the brain

cis-trans **isomer** type of stereoisomer resulting from differing arrangements of groups on the same or opposite sides of a double-bond; examples: fumaric acid (*trans*-butenedioic acid) and maleic acid (*cis*-butenedioic acid); synonym: geometric isomer

citrate a salt or an ester of citric acid

citric acid hydroxytricarboxylic acid ($H_3C_6H_5O_7$); found in citrus fruits, especially lemon and lime juices; used as a pharmaceutical adjuvant and chelating agent

citric acid cycle biochemical pathway that begins with the formation of citric acid from oxaloacetic acid and acetyl coenzyme A and which ends with oxaloacetic acid, thus forming a cycle; synonyms: Krebs cycle, tricarboxylic acid cycle, TCA cycle

civil action   legal action resulting from a dispute between two or more parties or individuals

Civilian Health and Medical Program of the Uniformed Services (CHAMPUS) federally sponsored insurance program that pays for hospital and medical services provided to dependents of active military and deceased military personnel, the latter of whom died while on active duty, as well as retired military personnel and their dependents

Civilian Health and Medical Program of the Veterans Administration (CHAMPVA) federally sponsored insurance program that pays for hospital and medical services provided to dependents of disabled, retired veterans of the uniformed services

claim information   submitted by a provider or a covered person to establish that medical services were provided to a covered person, from which processing for payment to the provider or covered person is made

claims administration   review of health insurance claims submitted for payment, by individual claim or in the aggregate; an identification procedure, screening treatment, or charge pattern for subsequent peer review and adjudication

claims clearinghouse system   system that allows electronic claims submission through a single source

claims review   the method by which an enrollee's health care service claims are reviewed before reimbursement is made

Claison concentration   reaction in which an ester containing alpha-hydrogens is condensed under anhydrous conditions in the presence of a base such as sodium ethoxide

clarification   filtration process to remove particulate solid material (usually less than 1 percent) from a liquid of which the filtrate is the desired component

clarity   condition of being free from particulate matter, as with injections and other solution dosage forms

Clark's rule   SEE *dosage rules*

class A balance   SEE *balance*

class B balance   SEE *balance*

clathrate   cagelike molecular structure capable of physically trapping smaller molecules

clean room   a sterile, enclosed environment approved by the appropriate regulatory agency that is designated as a site for preparation of medications, usually parenteral medications; contains a laminar flow hood as one component

clearance complete removal by the kidneys of a compound (drug) from a specific volume of blood per unit of time

clear emulsion SEE *emulsion*

clearinghouse capability company capable of submitting electronic and/or paper claims to several third-party payers

client person who seeks and receives professional services; synonyms: patron, customer

clinical pertaining to actual observation and treatment of a patient (usually in a clinic or hospital)

clinical chemistry analytical biochemistry applied to the diagnosis of disease or the screening and monitoring of patients

clinical indicator a tool or marker used to monitor and evaluate care to ensure desirable outcomes and explain or prevent undesirable outcomes

clinical outcome the status of the patient's health, especially after receiving medical care services; outcome assessment dependent upon targeted goals, clinical markers, and the ability to provide objective measurements

clinical pharmacokinetics application of pharmacokinetics to the safe and effective therapeutic management of an individual patient

clinical pharmacy practice of pharmacy in which patient needs are emphasized; "patient-oriented pharmacy practice"; information and recommendations are provided to the physician/health care team, not directly to the patient

clinical privileging process of reviewing a practitioner's credentials for the purpose of granting and delineating the scope of clinical privileges

clinical trial tests conducted to test the effectiveness of new medicines, devices, surgeries, or other medical procedures to prove safety and efficacy

clinical trial, phase I studies involving a small group of people to test the safety and dosage of the drug

clinical trial, phase II studies continuing to test the drug safety and efficacy with larger groups than in phase I

clinical trial, phase III large-scale studies to test the effectiveness of the drug as well as potential side effects

clinical trial, phase IV studies that usually concentrate on possible new indications or long-term effects of the drug

clinician a staff member providing technical medical services, especially a physician, but also a pharmacist or nurse involved in patient care

closed access a type of health plan in which covered persons are required to select a primary care physician from the plan's participating providers, and to see the selected primary care physician for care and referrals to other health care providers within the plan; typically found in a staff, group, or network model HMO; also called "closed panel" or "gatekeeper model"

closed-panel HMO an HMO model that generally offers the service of a relatively limited number of health care providers (e.g., physicians employed by the HMO); staff- and group-model HMOs usually in this category

closed system process under observation that involves exchanges of heat and work (but not matter) with its surroundings; SEE *drug formulary*

closure part of container that caps and/or seals; examples: rubber closure for a multidose parenteral, a cap on a bottle

clyster an enema, typically administeed with a metal syringe; synonym: glyster

coacervate aggregation of colloidal particles held together by electrostatic charges

coagulation process by which blood clots; clumping together of fine particles into larger particles

coalescence combining discrete droplets of a liquid or semisolid into a larger drop or spherical globule that, when carried to an extreme, results in a separation of the pharmaceutical preparation into two or more phases; example: "cracking" or "breaking" of an emulsion

coarse dispersion two-phase system in which the particles of the dispersed phase are in the range of 25 to 100 micrometers (microns) in diameter; example: suspension

coarse filtration process to remove large particles from a liquid or an air system

coating covering a tablet or pill with one or more protective layer(s); examples: sugar-coated tablet, enteric-coated tablet, film-coated tablet, compressed-coated tablet

coating pan rounded, rotating vessel used in the process of covering (sugar coating) a batch of tablets

cobalamines various forms of vitamin B_{12}; example: cyanocobalamin

cobalt hard, gray, ductile metal; a trace mineral; the central metallic atom in cyanocobalamin

cobalt-60 radioisotope of cobalt that emits highly intense beta rays and X-rays; used to treat cancer and in radiation sterilization

cocaine local anesthetic for topical use; alkaloid from *Erythroxylon coca;* highly addicting and subject to abuse; a controlled substance with no recognized medical use (in Schedule I)

cocoa, breakfast solid similar to cocoa powder but contains more than 22 percent cocoa butter

cocoa butter low-melting-point fat from cacao beans; used as a suppository base and emollient; synonym: theobroma oil

cocoa powder brown powder with characteristic odor and taste, obtained by roasting cured seeds of *Theobroma cacao*

codeine alkaloid from opium; used to suppress the cough reflex and to relieve pain; synonym: 3-methylether of morphine

code number initial identification assigned to a new chemical entity before it is given a generic or official name; used for the compound throughout laboratory investigations

coding systems information organized around diagnosis, treatment, and/or reimbursement for further analysis; SEE *International Classification of Diseases System; Current Procedural Terminology System; National Drug Code System; Healthcare Common Procedure Coding System*

codon sequence of three nucleotides on mRNA that designates a specific amino acid for incorporation into protein

coefficient of viscosity synonym: viscosity; SEE *viscosity; Newton's law of viscous flow*

coenzyme a relatively small, organic, nonprotein molecule that functions as a reactant or a factor that must be present for an enzyme to function in its catalytic role; a "loosely bound" prosthetic group of an enzyme; a coenzyme (nonprotein) and its apoenzyme (protein) combine to form the holoenzyme (complete enzyme)

coenzyme A an acyl carrier molecule that consists of a 3'-phosphate derivative of ADP linked to pantohenic acid via a phosphate ester bond; pantothenic acid is linked to β-mercaptoethylamine by an amide bond

cofactor any one of several substances such as metallic ions or coenzymes required in an enzymatic reaction

cognitive impairment impairment in memory, reasoning, or orientation to person, place, or time; an impairment requiring a person to be supervised to protect himself/herself or others from harm

cognitive services pharmacy services that require professional judgment relating to the patients, including counseling and therapy monitoring

cohesive forces attractive tendencies for like molecules in a system

coincidence an occurrence in radiation measurement that compensates for the time during which the counter tube was insensitive to radiation

coinsurance type of cost-sharing requirement whereby the insured pays a fixed percentage of total charges for services

colander device for separating liquid from coarse solid particles; synonym: strainer

colation process of separating large solid particles from liquids through straining

cold cream emulsified ointment base, more commonly used as a cosmetic night cream; synonyms: rose water ointment, Galen's cerate

cold flow process whereby a plastic tends to return to its former configuration; after a flow rate is set using polyvinyl chloride IV sets, the amount of fluid delivered may vary over the next several hours as the plastic of the tubing narrows or enlarges due to cold flow

cold place denotes that the product should be refrigerated (between 20 and 80°C or 360 and 460°F), but not frozen

cold temperature any temperature not exceeding 8°C (46°F); in a refrigerator, between 2 and 8°C (36 and 46°F); in a freezer, between −20 and −10°C (−4 and 14°F)

colic severe, acute, and fluctuating abdominal pain

colic, infant condition of uncertain etiology occurring in young infants, characterized by intractable, continued crying

colitis inflammation of the bowel

collagen major body protein that is a chief component of connective tissues (e.g., fascia, dermis, cornea, tendon, and organic matrix of bone)

collateralize the designation of securities or assets given as a pledge by a borrower that will be given up if the loan is not repaid

Colles' fracture fracture of the lower end of the radius with displacement of the bone

colligative property characteristic of a liquid drug system that is dependent upon the number of discrete particles (ions or molecules) therein; example: osmotic pressure in ophthalmic solutions

collimator device that confines X-rays to the region under examination

collodion volatile, film-forming, liquid preparation intended for external use; a solution of pyroxylin in a mixture of alcohol and ether that once volatilized leaves a thin, impervious membrane

colloid 1: literally, "like a glue" **2:** state of matter characterized by large solvated molecules or aggregates of molecules usually considered to range in size from 1 nanometer to 500 nanometers **3:** a dispersion of particles in the size range noted in 2; example: gold colloid for injection

colloidal dispersion heterogeneous liquid or gaseous system having particles considered to range from 1 millimicron to 500 millimicrons in size

colloidal solution SEE *solution*

colloid mill machine consisting of a grooved rotor and a grooved stator, their distance of separation adjustable; used to reduce the particle size of a slurry such as a pharmaceutical suspension

collunarium a medicated wash or spray solution for instillation in the nostrils

collutorium mouthwash

collyrium ophthalmic liquid containing medications intended to be instilled into the eye; formulated with consideration for tonicity, pH, stability, viscosity, and sterility

colorant substance added to a formulation to give color and enhance eye appeal

colorimetry method of quantitative analysis that depends upon intensity of light transmitted through a colored solution

colostomy 1: surgically created opening (stoma) between the colon and the body surface **2:** surgical procedure that produces an opening in the colon

colp- prefix that means having to do with the vagina; same as colpo-

colpo- prefix that means having to do with the vagina; same as colp-

column chromatography type of chromatography in which the stationary (solid) phase is uniformly placed in a glass tube through which the solution whose components are to be separated is transported

coma a level of unconsciousness in which a person cannot be awakened

combined audit patient/medical care evaluation studies in which physicians, nurses, and/or other health care disciplines jointly choose and utilize the same topic and the same sample of records, as well as utilize the same data retrieval process

comminution a process to reduce particle size by physical or mechanical means; synonym: grinding

commission the portion of premiums or equivalent premium for self-funded groups paid to an insurance agent, sales representative, or broker as compensation for services provided

Commission for Certification in Geriatric Pharmacy (CCGH) created by the American Society of Consultant Pharmacy in 1997 to oversee the certification program in geriatric pharmacy practice

Common Procedural Coding System a listing of services, procedures, and supplies offered by physicians, pharmacists, and other providers

community pharmacy retail pharmacy, either chain or independent, serving the needs of the public in a defined area or neighborhood

community rating a method of determining a premium structure that is influenced not by the expected level of benefit utilization by specific groups, but by expected utilization by the population as a whole

community rating by class the practice of community rating impacted by the group's specific demographics; also known as "factored rating"

compaction SEE *compression* as it relates to solids

compartment separate division or section of the body as in a pharmacokinetic two-compartmental model in which the blood is one compartment and all other body tissues are considered as the central compartment

compatibility capable of being mixed in an acceptable physical-chemical and/or therapeutic combination

compendium information source that contains essential facts and details of a subject in concise form; example: *United States Pharmacopeia–National Formulary*

competence ability to perform one's duties accurately, make correct judgments, and interact appropriately with patients and colleagues, characterized by good problem-solving and decision-making abilities, a strong knowledge base, and an ability to apply knowledge and experience to diverse patient care situations

competency ability to perform a particular task or activity; possessing appropriate knowledge and skills

competitive antagonism most common type in which the agonist and antagonist each interact in a similar manner with the same receptor site; the substance in highest concentration will successfully win the competition; SEE *inhibition*

competitive medical plan (CMP) a status granted by the federal government to an organization meeting specified criteria, enabling that organization to obtain a Medicare risk contract

competitive products goods used for the same purpose and marketed in the same area, each affecting sales volume and price of the others

completed audit written display of patient/medical care evaluation study data for which variation records have been analyzed and corrective actions formulated for problems identified; not considered complete until follow-up of the problem has been planned and final reports forwarded to pertinent medical and professional staff and to the hospital governing body

complexation physical binding of a chemical with another substance resulting in a change in properties; examples: plasma protein binding of drugs, sequestration of metallic ions by clathrates (e.g., EDTA-lead)

compliance 1: the degree to which patients follow treatment recommendations **2:** determination through inspection of the extent to which a manufacturer is complying to prescribed regulations; synonyms: adherence, persistence

complication an unanticipated change in the patient's clinical status for which special clinical management is required to achieve desired patient outcomes

complication rate the percent of records in a patient/medical care evaluation study that indicate that a particular complication developed during treatment

component pure chemical substance that is part of a system

components, number of the smallest number of constituents in a system whose composition must be known to completely define the system

composite rate a group billing rate that is applied to all subscribers within a specified group, regardless of whether they are enrolled for single or family coverage

compound to mix or prepare several ingredients for a prescription

compounding error total expected potency error in a dosage formulation based on computation of the root-mean-square of the respective errors in each step of preparation; SEE *percentage error of compounding*

comprehensive benefits plan a variation of the major medical plan that carries coinsurance requirements, usually 10 to 20 percent of all health expenses and deductibles ranging from $100 to $1,000.

compressed-coated tablet a tablet covered by pressing the coating material around a previously tableted core; used for coating in the absence of water or other liquids

compressed tablet SEE *tablet, compressed*

compressibility a measure of the ease of compacting a discrete quantity of material into a nonresilient mass; granules for tableting must exhibit a high degree of compressibility; liquids exhibit low compressibility, whereas gases are highly compressible

compression process of rendering a discrete quantity of substance more dense or more compact; examples: solid granules to tablets, gases to liquids; synonym: compaction

compression coating SEE *coating; compressed-coated tablet*

compressor device or apparatus used to increase gaseous pressure in a closed system; example: refrigeration pump

compulsion insistent, repetitive urge to perform an act contrary to one's better judgment

Concato's disease polyserositis

concentration an expression of the number of parts of one component per total parts of all other components in a system; used in many ways, such as percent by volume, by weight and by weight-in-volume, molarity, normality, milligram percent, molality, and mole fraction

concentration range allowable (acceptable) variation in parts of one component per total parts of all other components of a system; example: drug concentration varying from 98 to 102 percent of labeled amount in each dosage unit

concomitant 1: at the same time **2:** joined together

concurrent drug evaluation an electronic assessment of claims at the point of service to detect potential problems that should be addressed prior to dispensing medicines to patients

concurrent monitors procedures for regular surveillance of patient care conducted while the care is being provided

concurrent review an assessment that determines medical necessity or appropriateness of services as they are being rendered

condensation 1: reaction in which two or more organic molecules are connected to form a larger molecule; synonym: polymerization **2:** a reduction in size by a coalescing or transition to a more orderly state of matter; examples: gas to liquid, gas to solid, liquid to solid

condiment a volatile oil used to flavor a pharmaceutical preparation

conditionally renewable policy a policy that can be renewed up to a certain age limit, such as 65

condition of participation statutory or regulatory provisions that a provider of services must satisfy in order to participate in a health care program; example: Medicare and Medicaid programs specify minimal services to be offered to patients in order for a provider to qualify

condom tubelike device used as a prophylactic against disease transmission and potential conception during sexual intercourse

conductance quantitative expression of the flow of an electrical current across a substance; the reciprocal of resistance

conductance, equivalent the conductance by a solution of sufficient volume so as to provide 1 gram-equivalent of solute in a suitable container with electrodes separated by 1 cm; used to measure the "degree of dissociation" of a substance in a given solvent

conduction 1: transfer of energy from one part of a system to another by a molecular interaction with no significant mass transfer involved **2:** transmission of an electric current through a medium (electrolyte solution, wire, etc.)

conductor substance that inherently possesses ability to transmit heat and/or electricity; atomic electrons move freely through such substances

cone solid dosage form bounded by a circular base and the surface formed by line segments joining every point of the boundary of the base to a common vertex; usually contains antibiotics and is normally placed below the gingiva after a dental extraction

cones cells of retina containing opsins related to rhodopsin; responsible for color vision

confabulation fabrication of facts about events not totally recalled from memory

confection paste consisting of medicinal agents and flavoring intended to be dissolved in the mouth

confectioner's sugar a mixture of sucrose and corn starch in a fine powder form

confidentiality condition of secrecy or privacy about a patient's medical records, medical history, or medications

confinement an uninterrupted stay for a defined period of time (as reflected in a benefit contract) in a hospital, skilled nursing facility, or other approved health care facility or program

conformation shape of an organic compound achieved by rotation of atoms around single bonds; example: the shape of proteins produced by twisting and/or folding peptide chains

conformational disease diseases caused by protein misfolding and aggregation

congealing range temperature interval through which a melted semisolid changes to a solid

congener compound of the same origin (synthetic scheme, plant source, etc.) as another

congenital existing before or at birth

congestion increased or pathological collection of blood or other aqueous fluids in an area of the body; examples: pulmonary edema, dropsy

congestive heart failure inability of the heart to maintain adequate circulation to meet the body's needs; characterized by breathlessness and abnormal sodium and water retention resulting in edema, with congestion of the lungs and/or peripheral circulation; synonym: dropsy

conjugate acid compound produced by the acceptance of a proton by a "Bronsted base"; SEE ALSO *Bronsted-Lowry theory*

conjugate base a compound produced by the ionization of a "Bronsted acid"; a base resulting when a "Bronsted acid" has lost a proton; SEE ALSO *Bronsted-Lowry theory*

conjugated protein a protein that functions only when it carries other chemical groups attached by covalent linkages or by weak interactions

conjugate pair an acid-base pair; example: ammonium ion and hydroxyl ion in ammonium hydroxide

conjugate redox pair an electron donor and its electron acceptor form

conjugation 1: chemical structure in which two or more double bonds alternate with a single bond **2:** attachment of a group to a drug, drug metabolite, or other xenobiotic

conjunctiva inner lining of the eyelid and outer lining covering the eye

conjunctival injection dilation of the conjunctival blood vessels; often occurs in conjunction with allergic rhinitis

conjunctivitis medicamentosa inflammation of the conjunctiva caused by overuse of ophthalmic medications (e.g., decongestants such as tetrahydrozoline)

Conn's syndrome primary aldosteronism (oversecretion of the hormone)

conserve a mixture of fresh medicinal agents and sugar or honey

consignment method of purchasing in which the title of the goods remains with the supplier until the goods are sold by the retailer

Consolidated Omnibus Budget Reconciliation Act (COBRA) federal law that, among other things, requires employers to offer continued health insurance coverage to certain employees and their beneficiaries whose group health insurance coverage has been terminated

conspergent synonym for dusting powder

constant parameter or element in a process or mathematical expression that does not change under controlled conditions

constant infusion a series of minidoses given at infinitely short dosage intervals; example: controlled pumping of insulin into the body

constant-rate period of drying that phase of drying through which temperature does not change; a condition in which the rate of diffusion of moisture from the interior to the surface of a substance is equal to the rate of evaporation of moisture from its surface

constipation abnormally infrequent and difficult evacuation of the bowel, characterized by dry, hardened feces

constitutive property characteristic of a drug molecule that is the result of the structural arrangement of its atoms; example: optical rotation

consultant an outside specialist not on regular institutional staff

consultant pharmacist practitioner of pharmacy who provides pharmaceutical expertise and advice to a health care facility of which the pharmacist usually is not a full-time employee

Consumer Healthcare Products Association (CHPA) trade assocation representing manufacturers of nonprescription products, devices, and dietary supplements; formerly known as the Proprietary Association and the Nonprescription Drug Manufacturers Association

consumer price index (CPI) formerly cost of living index; a price index constructed monthly from Bureau of Labor statistics of the retail prices of 400 goods and services sold in large cities across the country; weighs products in terms of importance (in terms of total expenditures) and compares prices to those of a selected base year; expresses current expenditures as a percentage of the base

contact angle SEE *wetting*

container device that holds a drug or article; may or may not be in direct contact with its contents

container, hermetic one that is impervious to air or any other gas under ordinary conditions of shipment and storage

container, light resistant colored or opaque container to protect its contents from the effects of light

container, multiple dose vial that permits needle puncture and withdrawal of successive portions of its contents without changing the strength, quality, or purity of the remaining portion

container, single dose single-unit container for articles intended for parenteral administration; example: one ampule and its contents

container, single unit one that is designed to hold a quantity of drug intended for administration as a single dose or a single finished device intended for use promptly after the container is opened

container, tight one that protects its contents from contamination by extraneous liquids, solids, or vapors, and from loss or damage of the article due to efflorescence, deliquescence, or evaporation under ordinary conditions of shipment and storage; capable of tight reclosure

container, unit dose single-unit container for articles intended for administration as a single dose by routes other than parenteral

container, well closed one that protects its contents from extraneous solids and from loss of the article under customary conditions of shipment and storage

container closure cap that seals the container and is a part of the container

contamination condition of having an impurity in a product that should not be present; synonym: adulteration

content uniformity test quality assurance evaluation of variability in the chemical composition in each dosage unit of a given batch; performed for tablets, capsules, and powders among other dosage formulations

continental method procedure for making an emulsion in which oil and emulsifying agent are placed in a dry porcelain mortar and mixed thoroughly and then water is added all at once and triturated rapidly until emulsification is accomplished; synonym: dry-gum method

continuation a situation whereby a covered person who would otherwise lose coverage under a health plan due to certain occurrences such as termination of employment or divorce is allowed to "continue" his/her coverage under specified conditions.

continuing education organized learning experiences and activities in which pharmacists engage after they have completed their entry-level academic education and training; experience designed to promote the continuous development of skills, attitudes, and knowledge needed to maintain proficiency, provide quality service or products, respond to patient needs, and keep abreast of change

continuity of care the coordination of diagnoses and treatment among practitioners and health care settings to maximize treatment benefits for the patient

continuous dryer machine or apparatus that removes moisture from large quantities of material as it is moved uninterrupted through the drying process; CONTRAST *batch dryer*

continuous mixing uninterrupted mixing; characterized by a steady inflow of substances to be combined and a steady outflow of combined materials; CONTRAST *batch mixing*

continuous process operational procedure or process, such as granulation, which is conducted without interruption for long periods of time; used in preparing bulk chemicals or materials; CONTRAST *batch process*

continuous quality improvement formal process of constantly seeking better ways to achieve stated goals

continuous variation method a means of determining stoichiometric ratios of molecules that are complexed using an additive property to measure molecular units involved in a specific type of complex

continuum of care range of clinical services provided to an individual or group; may reflect treatment rendered during a single inpatient hospitalization or care for multiple conditions over a lifetime

contr- prefix meaning against; same as contra-

contra- prefix meaning against; same as contr-

contraceptive an agent or a substance used to prevent pregnancy; examples: condoms, birth control medications, intrauterine devices

contract binding legal agreement between two or more parties to do or not do a specified act

contract pharmacy system pharmaceutical benefit delivery arrangement in which a health plan contracts with community pharmacies (chain or selected independents) to provide medications to members

contract year the period of time from the effective date to the expiration date of the contract

contraindication a situation in which one drug should not be used because of a patient's condition or use of another drug; examples: a patient with diabetes should not take an oral nasal decongestant and a patient with angle-closure glaucoma should not take a nonprescription antihistamine without consulting a physician

contribution margin an accounting term indicating an excess of net sales over variable expenses expressed as a dollar total, a ratio, or on a per unit basis; example: that portion of sales which contributes to meeting fixed costs and profit

contributory program a method of payment for group coverage in which part of the premium is paid by the employee and part is paid by the employer or union

controlled substance substance or drug under special controls of the Drug Enforcement Administration (DEA) because of its potential for abuse; SEE *scheduled drug*

contusion 1: process of subdividing a substance by pounding or bruising it, usually in a heavy metal mortar **2:** bruise injury in which the skin is not broken

convection transfer of energy from one part of a fluid system to another by molecular currents; contrasted to movement by outside forces as in the use of a mechanical stirrer

convenience goods consumer goods with a low unit value that the customer buys frequently and prefers to purchase with a minimum amount of effort

conversion the privilege given to a covered person to change his/her group medical care coverage to a form of individual coverage without evidence of insurability; conditions of change defined in the master group contract; usually made when a covered person leaves the group

convulsion an involuntary contraction or a series of contractions and relaxations of the voluntary muscles; usually paroxysmally

Cook, Ernest Fullerton (1879-1961) chairman of the *United States Pharmacopeia* Committee of Revision from 1920-1950; was active in international drug standardization; served as editor-in-chief of *Remington's Practice of Pharmacy* (Fourth to Sixth Editions); Remington Honor Medal recipient in 1931

cool temperature temperature between 8 and 15°C (46 and 59°F); unless otherwise stated, an article to be stored at a cool temperature may be stored in a refrigerator

Coombs' Test method to detect the presence of antibodies bound to the surfaces of erythrocytes using antisera; may be either direct or indirect

Cooper, Zada Mary (1875-1961) educator at the University of Iowa; one of the founders of Rho Chi and Kappa Epsilon

coordinate covalent bond chemical bond in which both shared electrons are provided by one of the atoms; synonym: dative bond

coordination number 1: number of nearest neighbors of a given atom in a crystal **2:** number of ligands attached to a central metal in a complex

coordination of benefits provision in a contract that applies when a person is covered under more than one group medical program and requires that payment of benefits be coordinated by all programs to eliminate overinsurance or duplication of benefits

copay or copayment a cost-sharing arrangement in which a covered person pays a specified charge for a specified service, such as $15 for an office visit or a prescription; includes the following structures: (1) two-tier copays with lower copays for multisource (generic) drugs and higher copays for single-source (brand-name) drugs; (2) three-tier copays with lower copays for multisource (generic) drugs, higher copays for preferred single-source (brand-name) drugs, and even higher copays for non-preferred single-source (brand-name) drugs; (3) four-tier copays with lower copays for low-cost multisource (generic) drugs, higher copays for high-cost multisource (generic) drugs, even higher copays for preferred single-source (brand-name) drugs, and the highest copays for non-preferred single-source (brand-name) drugs

copper trace element and a cometal for some enzymes

copperas synonym for ferrous sulfate

core, extended release an ocular system placed in the eye from which the drug diffuses through a membrane at a constant rate over a specified period

Cori cycle a metabolic process in which lactate, produced in tissues such as muscle, is transferred to liver where it becomes a substrate in gluconeogenesis

corn small, hyperkeratotic lesion on the foot, either between the toes or on the side of the foot, occurring as a result of pressure and friction (e.g., tightly fitting shoes)

corneal deposits matter on the transparent anterior part of the eye (the cornea)

corporation a legal body created by a state to operate a business with the purpose and rules of an approved charter

correlation measure of the nature and degree of relationship between two variables; example: relationship between solubility of a substance and the temperature of the solution

correlation coefficient statistical index of the linearity of a plot of two variables; an index of dependency of the two variables; when $r = 1$ there is perfect linearity and complete dependence and when $r = 0$ there is complete independence of the two variables

corticosteroid steroidal hormone secreted by the adrenal cortex; may be classed as a mineralocorticoid that controls electrolyte balance or a glucocorticoid that controls carbohydrate or fat metabolism

Cosmas Arabian Christian; along with his brother Damian, one of the patron Saints of medicine and pharmacy; martyred in A.D. 303 by subjects of the Roman Emperor Diocletian

cosmetic agent for preserving or improving appearance

cosmetic procedures those procedures that alter physical appearance but do not correct or materially improve a physiological function and are not deemed medically necessary

cosolvency use of a combination of liquids to increase the solubility of poorly soluble substances

cost-based reimbursement payment by third-party insurers in which the amount is based on the cost to the provider of delivering services

cost-benefit analysis in pharmacoeconomics, the evaluation of products or services where costs and consequences are simultaneously measured in terms of dollars

cost containment term used to refer to a variety of strategies designed to control costs of health care services

cost contract agreement to arrange for the provision of health services to plan members based on reasonable cost or prudent buyer concepts

cost of goods sold the dollar value of the beginning inventory plus purchases for the period minus the ending inventory

cost shifting the redistribution of payment sources occurring when a provider gives a discount to one payer and then increases the cost to another to make up the difference

Coste, Jean-Francois (1741-1819) chief physician of French forces participating in the American Revolution; compiled a drug formulary, the *Compendium Pharmaceuticum*

cost-effectiveness the degree to which a service meets a specified goal at an acceptable cost

cost-effectiveness analysis in pharmacoeconomics, the evaluation of products or services where costs and consequences are simultaneously measured; effectiveness measured in terms of obtaining a specified objective (e.g., year of life saved) and cost in monetary terms; example: a ratio expressed as the cost per year per life saved

Costen's syndrome dental malocclusion with associated neurologic headache

cost-minimization analysis in pharmacoeconomics, costs are analyzed and compared where two or more interventions have been demonstrated or assumed to be equivalent in terms of the outcome or consequence

cost-of-illness evaluation in pharmacoeconomics, an evaluation of the direct and indirect costs of a particular disease or condition

cost sharing provision of a medical insurance plan that requires the insured to pay some specified portion of the costs of medical services; SEE ALSO *coinsurance; copay or copayment; deductible*

cost to dispense the total expenses associated with dispensing a prescription; computed by allocating all expenses associated with the operation of the prescription department and dividing by the number of prescriptions dispensed

cost-utility analysis in pharmacoeconomics, the evaluation of products or services where costs and consequences are simultaneously measured; consequences measured in terms of quality of life, willingness to pay, or preference for one intervention over another, and costs measured in terms of dollars; example: ratio expressed in terms of cost per quality-adjusted life year saved

Coulter Counter (trademark) instrument used to count and estimate the "effective" volume of red and white blood cells and drug particles; used to determine particle diameter based on changes in electrical resistivity as individual particles, suspended in an electrolyte solution, pass through a standardized pore in a glass tube

counseling process by which pharmacists provide information regarding prescription products or perform triage for patients in regard to minor medical conditions

countercurrent distribution method of extraction and separation using two immiscible solvents in a series of tubes or separatory funnels; the solvent forming the lower layer moves in one direction and the upper layer moves in the opposite direction

counter detailing reeducating or influencing prescribers in a closed or controlled HMO plan to influence their prescribing habits to meet formulary compliance

counterirritant agent used externally to produce erythema and a sense of warmth to provide relief to an area

covalent bond chemical bond resulting from the sharing of a pair of electrons by two atoms, each atom donating one electron from its outer shell (bond energy around 100 kcal per mole)

coverage entire range of protection provided under an insurance contract

covered expenses medical and related costs that qualify for reimbursement under terms of an insurance contract

covered lives refers to the quantity of persons who are enrolled within a particular health plan, or for coverage by a provider network; includes enrollees and their covered dependents

covered person an individual who meets eligibility requirements and for whom premium payments are paid for specified benefits of the contractual agreement

covered services specific services and supplies for which a covered person will receive reimbursement

CPT-4 System SEE *Current Procedural Terminology System*

cracked emulsion emulsion in which the protective film has broken and the internal phase has coalesced

cradle cap condition usually confined to infants in which the scalp is covered with scales or a crust

Craigie, Andrew (1754-1819) appointed Apothecary General of the Continental Army in 1776; established a manufacturing laboratory for large-scale manufacture and distribution of medical supplies

Craigie Medal established in 1959 by the Military Surgeons of the United States in recognition of career achievements for the advancement of pharmacy in the federal government

cranio- prefix meaning skull

crash cart mobile drug container placed on a nursing floor; contains medicines and supplies needed for life-threatening medical emergencies

crayon dose form; SEE *pencil*

cream 1: viscous liquid or semisolid emulsion of either the oil-in-water or water-in-oil type; most are used topically; most often applied to soft, cosmetically accceptable types of preparations; example: vanishing cream **2:** liquid suspension of a hydrated inorganic hydroxide or oxide; example: cream of bismuth **3:** semisolid dosage form containing one or more drug substances dissolved or dispersed in a suitable base; more recently, restricted to products consisting of oil-in-water emulsions or aqueous microcrystalline dispersions of long-chain fatty acids or alcohols that are water washable and more cosmetically and aesthetically acceptable

creaming separation of the internal phase of an emulsion as a concentrated agglomerate of discrete, easily dispersible globules or droplets; depending on the relative density of the phases, creaming may go upward or downward

creatinine clearance removal from blood of the nitrogenous compound creatinine; a metabolic end product of creatine and creatine phosphate; a measure of kidney function

credential documented evidence of a pharmacists's qualifications; may include diplomas, licenses, certificates, and certifications

credentialing 1: process by which an organization or institution obtains, verifies, and assesses a pharmacist's qualifications to provide patient care services; **2:** review process to determine a provider's ability to participate in a health plan

credit the right side of an account; entering an amount on the credit side of an account represents a decrease in assets and expenses or an increase in liabilities, owner's equity revenues, and gains

Creutzfeldt-Jakob disease spastic pseudosclerosis with spinal degeneration

Creutzfeldt-Jakob disease, variant linked to eating contaminated beef products from animals infected with bovine spongiform encephalopathy (BSE), or mad cow disease

crib death SEE *sudden infant death syndrome*

criteria set a group of similar or related indicators of quality health care

critical micelle concentration concentration of an amphiphile above which micelles begin to form; SEE *micelle*

critical moisture content that time in a drying process when the rate of drying begins to decrease; that time when the first "dry spots" are formed on the surface of the substance being dried

critical pressure pressure required to liquefy a gas at its critical temperature

critical temperature that temperature above which a gas cannot be compressed to a liquid irrespective of the pressure applied

Crohn's disease regional enteritis (inflammation of the intestine)

cruciform a crosslike structure in DNA molecules likely to form when a DNA sequence contains a palindrome

crude drug term usually applied to a nonpurified drug obtained from a plant or an animal; synonym: natural drug; example: plant parts (senna leaves)

crutch 1: a support, usually fitting under the arm, to assist a disabled person to walk **2:** a substance or a behavioral pattern used to avoid or mitigate unpleasant circumstances; example: use of alcohol to avoid reality

cryo- prefix meaning cold

cryodesiccation SEE *freeze drying*

cryolite ore of a fluorine-containing mineral; formula: Na_3AlF_6

cryotherapy therapy utilizing cold to reduce the amount of inflammation after an acute injury (e.g., ankle sprain), thereby speeding a return to normal function; uses such modalities as ice packs, precooled gel packs, instant cold packs; a component of RICE (rest, ice, compression, elevation) therapy for acute joint or muscle injury

crystal naturally produced angular solid of definite form in which the ultimate units from which it is built up are systematically arranged; usually evenly spaced on a regular space lattice

crystal growth deposition of a solute from a solution onto the surface of a smaller crystal (or other minute particle) to form a larger one; an undesirable factor contributing to instability of a pharmaceutical suspension; a desired process for more complete separation and/or quantization of a drug component in a liquid system; SEE *crystallization*

crystal lattice repeating units of a specific molecular arrangement with accompanying spaces; exhibited by crystalline drug solids

crystalline refers to grainy particles of a substance, the molecules of which are arranged in definite geometrical or morphological patterns; may exhibit distinct cleavage planes; CONTRAST *amorphous*

crystallization process in which ions, atoms, or molecules deposit on themselves in a definite solid geometric pattern to form discrete crystals; SEE ALSO *crystal growth*

crystal violet synonym for gentian violet or methylrosaniline chloride

cubic mixer SEE *tumbling mixer*

culture propagation of microorganisms or of living tissue cells in special media conducive to their growth

cumin, sweet synonym for anise seed; a flavoring agent

cumulative log-dose response curve a plot or graph of a physiological activity parameter as a function of the log of the dose of a drug

cupric salts salts of copper in the +2 oxidation state; used as antiseptics and clinical reagents

cuprous salts salts of copper in the +1 oxidation state

curie (c) unit of radioactivity equal to 3.7×10^{10} nuclear transformations per second

current assets items that will be transformed into cash, sold, or used during a normal operating cycle (usually one year) of a business; examples: cash, marketable securities, accounts receivable, inventories, prepaid expenses

current liabilities obligations that are expected to be paid from current assets of the business or through creation of other current liabilities; usually satisfied within the normal operating cycle of the business (usually one year); examples: accounts payable, notes payable, salaries payable, taxes payable

Current Procedural Terminology System (CPT-4) a coding system used to identify physician services such as injections and surgeries; the health care industry's standard for reporting of physician procedures and services using a five-digit code

current ratio current assets divided by current liabilities for a business; a measure of a firm's ability to meet its short-term obligations

Cushing's syndrome pituitary basophilism (disorder of basophilic blood cells)

custodial care medical or nonmedical services that do not seek to cure; provided during periods when the medical condition of the patient is not changing or does not require continued administration by medical personnel

customary charge the charge a physician or supplier usually bills his patients for furnishing a particular service or supply

cutter mill machine that contains a rotating, slicing impeller and screen enclosed in heavy-duty housing and used to reduce the particle size of fibrous materials

cyan- 1: prefix meaning blue or bluish color **2:** C~N chemical group; same as cyano-

cyano- 1: prefix meaning blue or bluish color **2:** C~N chemical group; same as cyan-

cyanocobalamin most commonly used form of vitamin B_{12} in which a cyano group is attached to the central cobalt

cyanogenetic capable of producing cyanide as hydrogen cyanide

cyanogenetic glycoside glycoside that releases hydrogen cyanide on hydrolysis; example: laetrile (amygdalin)

cyanosis bluish color; generally refers to an excess of the reduced form of hemoglobin in the blood

cyclamate sodium or calcium salt of cyclamic acid; used as an artificial, nonnutritive sweetener that is no longer available in the United States but is in Canada; found to induce cancer in rats

cyclic adenosine monophosphate adenosine monophosphate in which the phosphate group bridges between the 3'- and 5'-OH groups

cyclone mill SEE *fluid energy mill*

cycloplegia loss of eye accommodation due to ciliary muscle paralysis

cyclotron electromagnetic machine designed to accelerate charged atomic particles to velocities corresponding to several million electron volts; example: Van der Graff accelerator for electrons

cylindrical mixer SEE *tumbling mixer*

cysteine sulfhydryl-containing amino acid, commonly found in proteins; synonyms: 3-thio-2-aminopropanoic acid and 3-mercaptoalanine

cystic fibrosis transmembrane conductance regulator the plasma membrane glycoprotein that functions as a chloride channel in epithelial cells

cystine oxidized form of cysteine in which the sulhydryl groups of two cysteines are joined together as a disulfide bond through the elimination of the hydrogen atoms

cystitis inflammation of the bladder; usually caused by *E. coli* infection

-cyte suffix meaning cell

cyto- prefix meaning cell

cytochrome 1: one of several iron-containing porphyroproteins **2:** any one of several respiratory pigments found in the cell **3:** pigment involved in oxidation-reduction reactions in cellular metabolism

cytochrome P-450 cytochrome of liver microsomes responsible for the nonspecific oxidation of drugs and endogenous steroids

cytokine a group of hormonelike polypeptides and proteins; also referred to as growth factors

cytoplasmic membrane thin biological membrane enclosing a cell

cytoskeleton a set of protein filaments (microtubules, macrofilaments, and intermediate fibers) that maintains a cell's internal structure and allows organelles to move

cytostatic agent substance that inhibits cell growth; example: zinc pyrithione in treating dandruff

cytotoxic agent that has adverse effects on cells

DaCosta's syndrome circulatory neurasthenia

Dakin's solution, modified diluted sodium hypochlorite (480 mg per 100 ml) solution, used as a disinfectant, cleaner, and deodorant

damage 1: monetary award granted by court action for injury or loss caused by the actions of another **2:** actual—award equal to the true value of loss or damage; **3:** punitive—award in excess of actual damage incurred which serves as punishment for a wrongful act; synonym: exemplary damage

Damian Arabian Christian; along with his brother Cosmas, one of the patron saints of pharmacy and medicine; martyred in A.D. 303 by subjects of the Roman Emperor Diocletian

Daniel B. Smith Practice Excellence Award established by the American Pharmacists Association in 1964 for outstanding performance and achievement in the recipient's community and practice setting

Dargavel, John W. (1894-1961) state pharmacy board executive of the Minnesota Board from 1923-1934; served as the executive secretary of the National Association of Retail Druggists 1933-1961; proponent of fair trade laws

Darling's disease histoplasmosis

date of service the date on which health care services were provided to a covered person

dative bond SEE *coordinate covalent bond*

days the unit of measure of the length of a hospital confinement

days/1,000 SEE *bed days/1,000*

day supply maximum the maximum amount of medication an insured person may receive at one time

de- prefix meaning down or away

dead spots merchandise space where a typical customer does not see displayed products

deamination the removal of an amino group from a molecule

debility SEE *asthenia*

debt-to-equity ratio total debt divided by total owner's equity for a business; a broad measure of the claims of creditors against the assets of the business

Debye forces SEE *induction effect*

Debye-Huckel theory basic quantitative estimates of activity and activity coefficients of an ionic species in dilute solution, and of ionic strength; a basis for the measure of effective ionic concentration

decantation process of separating a solid from a liquid by allowing the solid to settle and carefully pouring the liquid from the top of the sediment

decarboxylation loss of a carboxyl group from a molecule through removal of carbon dioxide, carbonate, or bicarbonate; reaction in which a carboxylic acid loses CO_2

deception act committed in order to make a person believe something that is not true

decision analysis a systematic approach to decision making under uncertain conditions; SEE *decision tree*

decision tree an analytic tool for decision analysis that displays the temporal and logical sequence of a clinical decision problem

decoction solution of the active (soluble) constituents of crude drugs prepared by boiling the drug in water and straining the resulting solution

decrepitation phenomenon of crackling or exploding when crystals containing interstitial water are heated

deductible specified fixed amount of the cost of his/her medical care that an insured person must pay each plan year before the insurer makes any payment (if plan so requires)

deduction scientific process of reasoning by which logical consequences are developed from a priori observations

deductions items, the dollar value of which may be subtracted from an individual's or a firm's income prior to computation of tax liability

defendant person against whom a legal action is brought

defensive medicine the medical practice of performing laboratory tests or other procedures to protect against potential malpractice lawsuits, even though such services may not be necessary to diagnose or treat

defervescence abatement of fever

definite integral synonym: integration between limits; SEE *integration*

deflocculation process of dispersing individual particles of a loosely held agglomerate more uniformly throughout a dispersion medium

defoliant agent that removes foliage from plants

degree Celsius SEE *temperature*

degree centigrade SEE *temperature*

degree Fahrenheit SEE *temperature*

degree Kelvin SEE *temperature*

degree of dissociation extent of ionization of a substance (drug) in aqueous solution; measured by determination of electrical conductance at various dilutions to infinite dilution; the ratio of electrical conductance of a solution to the electrical conductance at infinte dilution

degree of mixing a measure of the effectiveness of a mixing process; usually accomplished by random sampling and subsequent analysis of the composition of the mix

degrees of freedom 1: (statistical) the number of independent quantities in a set of numerical quantities **2:** (Gibbs' phase rule) the number of independent variables that must be fixed in order to define or describe a system under study **3:** (Lagrange's dynamics) each free particle in space has three degrees of freedom that are reduced by the number of stable bonds between the particles

dehydration reaction process or condition in which there is a loss of water

dehydrogenase enzyme that catalyzes the removal of hydrogen from a compound; type of oxidoreductase in which an acceptor for hydrogen, other than oxygen, is involved

dehydrogenation reaction in which there is a loss of hydrogen

dehydrohalogenation reaction in which there is a loss of hydrogen chloride, hydrogen bromide, or hydrogen iodide

deionized water water that has been purified by removing cationic and anionic impurities through the use of ion-exchange resins

deleterious harmful; hurtful

deliquescence phenomenon whereby a solid absorbs water vapor (moisture) to the extent that it is liquefied as an aqueous solution

delusion fixed false belief that cannot be corrected by reason

demand the amount of service a population seeks to obtain through the health delivery system

demand item one that brings people into the pharmacy or one that people will make a special effort to seek out

demethylation reaction in which a methyl group is removed from a molecule

demulcent an agent that soothes the part of the body to which it is applied; usually restricted to agents acting on mucous membranes; examples: glycerin and cold cream for skin, nonmedicated lozenges to soothe the throat

denature to alter a substance from its natural state; most often used in reference to alterations in protein structure and the rendering of alcohol solutions nondrinkable

densensitization a process in which target cells adjust to changes in stimulation by inactivating or decreasing the number of cell surface receptors

densitometer instrument used with electrophoretograms and thin-layer chromatograms to determine the amount of substance in the individual fractions (bands) by measurement of the amount of light passing through the separated material

density mass per unit volume; cgs unit: gram (g) per cm^3; apparent—usually observed; bulk—includes the volume of all void spaces, as in a powder; relative—comparison (or ratio) of the density of one substance to that of another

dent- prefix meaning tooth; same as denta-, denti-, dento-

denta- prefix meaning tooth; same as dent-, denti-, dento-

dental floss intraoral cleaning device consisting of a long thread (e.g., rayon) which is wrapped around both index fingers and directed up and down the interdental spaces

denti- prefix meaning tooth; same as dent-, denta, dento-

dento- prefix meaning tooth; same as dent-, denta-, denti-

dentrifice substance (such as toothpaste) used with a toothbrush to clean the surface of teeth

denture an artificial replacement for one or more teeth; also known as "false teeth" or "prosthetic tooth or teeth"

deoxy- prefix meaning lack of an oxygen at a particular site in a molecule when compared with a parent oxygen-containing structure; example: deoxyribase; same as desoxy-

dependent an individual who relies on a spouse, parent, or grandparent who is the covered person

dependent variable that part of a mathematical expression changed in accordance with a controlled change of another variable; CONTRAST *independent variable*

depilatory agent employed to rid the body of excessive or bothersome hair; example: calcium thioglycollate with calcium hydroxide

depolarization 1: excitation or stimulation of a nerve or muscle; caused by the influx of sodium ions from outside the membrane that shifts the membrane potential from a negative toward a positive charge 2: a reduction in the separation of a charge on a substance

depot 1: body compartment where a drug accumulates 2: an injected dosage unit from which a drug is released to the tissues

depreciation a reduction in the book value of an asset over time

depression mood that is sad and full of despair; often a normal feeling unless severe functional impairment occurs

depth filter filter device that allows partial penetration of particles from a slurry to be trapped as the channel diameters become smaller

DeQuervain's disease subacute thyroiditis

derivative instantaneous rate determined by differential calculus methods; the slope of the tangent at a given point on a curve

dermat- prefix meaning skin; same as dermato-, dermo-

dermatitis inflammation of the skin, characterized by weeping vesicles and/or dry scaling; induced by internal causes (endogenous dermatitis; atopic dermatitis) or exposure to external irritants or allergens (e.g., poison ivy)

dermato- prefix meaning skin; same as dermat-, dermo-

dermatologist medical practitioner who specializes in knowledge and treatment of skin diseases

dermatology study of the skin (dermis) and its diseases; a branch of medical practice

dermo- prefix meaning skin; same as dermat-, dermato-

desiccant a drying substance having a high affinity for water; usually packaged and placed in containers of medicaments to maintain a dry atmosphere for enhanced stability of the drug product; example: silica gel in a dry dosage form container for moisture protective packaging

desiccate   to dry using little or no external heat

desiccation   process of drying a solid substance at a low temperature; example: drying ephedrine by placing sulfuric acid and the ephedrine in a closed container separated from each other (the acid preferentially absorbs the water from the ephedrine)

designated mental health provider   health care worker who evaluates, diagnoses, refers, and/or provides mental health and substance abuse services, per contract with an insurer

desorption   separation of adsorbate from adsorbent; synonyms: opposite and reverse adsorption

desoxy-   prefix meaning lack of an oxygen at a particular site in a molecule when compared to a parent oxygen-containing substance; same as deoxy-

desquamation   to shed or scale off the surface epithelium

detail man   SEE *medical service representative*

detergent   surfactant used as a cleansing agent

determinate error   deviation from the true value that can be ascertained, eliminated, and/or corrected in data treatment

detoxification 1: rendering inactive or removing a toxic substance by one or more methods including enhanced excretion, binding by complexation, or destruction of toxic molecules **2:** medical management for an individual going through withdrawal from substance abuse

Deutschlander's disease   tumor of metatarsal bone

dew point   temperature at which a gas is saturated with water vapor and condensation to the liquid state begins

dextro-   prefix meaning right

dextrorotatory   optically active compound that rotates the plane of polarized light to the right

dextrose   a white crystalline powder ($C_6H_{12}O_6$) that occurs in many sweet fruits; synonyms: glucose, grape sugar, starch sugar

di-   prefix meaning two; example: a dipeptide (compound containing two amino acids joined by an amide bond)

Di Guglielmo's disease   acute or chronic erythroleukemia

diabetes   either diabetes insipidus or diabetes mellitus, having the common symptom of increase in urinary volume

diabetes, type I usually diagnosed in children and young adults; was previously known as juvenile diabetes; caused by the body not producing insulin

diabetes, type II the most common form of diabetes; caused by either the body not producing enough insulin or the cells ignoring the insulin

diabetes insipidus disease in which there is a larger than normal volume of urine due to the absence of antidiuretic hormone (normally secreted by the pituitary gland) or due to a defect in reabsorption of water by the tubules of the kidney

diabetes management patient care services to provide education and monitoring

diabetes mellitus a disease characterized by elevated glucose levels in the blood and the presence of glucose in the urine thus increasing urine volume; associated with a lack of or an inability to use insulin

diabetic patient with either diabetes mellitus or diabetes insipidus

diabetogenic producing diabetes

diabetogenic hormones hormones that tend to elevate blood sugar levels; examples: adrenocorticosteroids, growth hormone

diagnosis determination of the nature of a disease in a patient by using the patient's history, physical assessment, observation of the course of the disease, and other pertinent data

diagnosis-related groups (DRGs) a system of classification for inpatient hospital services based on principal diagnosis, secondary diagnosis, surgical procedures, age, sex, and presence of complications used as a financing mechanism

diagnostic center free-standing or hospital-based facility that specializes in diagnosing illness and injuries

diagnostics 1: science of diagnosis **2:** devices, reagents, and methods used in the determination of a disease

dialysance instantaneous rate of the net exchange of solute molecules passing through a membrane in dialysis

dialysis passage of a solute through a semipermeable membrane; example: kidney dialysis to remove waste products from the blood of patients whose kidneys have failed

Diamond-Blackfan syndrome congenital hypoplastic anemia characterized by progressive anemia with sparing of white cells and platelets

diaphoresis perspiration or sweat

diaphoretic drug that induces sweating

diaphragm barrier consisting of a stretched membrane or other material that is placed over a particular container or a body cavity

diaphragm, vaginal device, usually dome-shaped, worn during copulation over the cervical mouth for prevention of conception or infection

diaphragm valve SEE *valve*

diaplacental drug transfer process in which a drug in the amniotic fluid reaches fetal circulation by diffusion

diarrhea significant increase in frequency and fluid content of bowel movements

diarrheagenic inducing diarrhea (e.g., medications that increase peristalsis)

diascopy placing the finger on an area of skin with mild pressure to determine whether it can be blanched through mechanical vasoconstriction; if blanching occurs, nonprescription hydrocortisone may help the condition

diastereoisomers isomers containing more than one chiral center that are not mirror images of one another; diastereoisomers differ in their solubilities, boiling points, melting points, and the degree and direction of their rotations of polarized light; examples: ephedrine and pseudoephedrine, quinine and quinidine; synonym: diastereomers

diastole maximal expansion or period of maximal expansion of the heart; in particular, the left ventricle

diastolic measurement of the amount of pressure on the walls of blood vessels when the heart is at rest; bottom of the two blood pressure numbers

diatomaceous earth form of silica consisting of fragments of diatoms; used as a filtering medium; synonyms: kieselguhr, purified infusorial earth, diatomite

diatomite SEE *diatomaceous earth*

dichroism property shown by some pigments or crystals (double refractive) that exhibit one color in reflected light and another in transmitted light

die strongly constructed receptacle unit of a tableting machine that holds the granules as they are being compressed by lower and upper tablet punches

Diehl, Conrad Lewis (1840-1917) pharmacist active in practice and education; wrote the annual report "Progress in Pharmacy," published in the *APhA Proceedings* from 1873-1891 and 1894-1915, reports that reviewed the advances in both Europe and America and covered more than 11,000 pages in total

dielectric constant ratio of the electrical capacity of a given substance in a condenser to that occurring within a vacuum; a measure of the inherent polarity potential of a given substance

differential pressure flow meter instrument that measures flow rates of a liquid or air using a calibrated scale; reads flow rate based on pressure differences across a restricted flow region

differential scanning SEE *calorimetry*

differentiation rule any one of several procedures for obtaining the derivative of various types of algebraic equations

diffraction spreading of light waves behind a grating, leading to the production of interference patterns and the bending and breaking of the light ray into its component parts (respective wavelengths)

diffuse double layer SEE *zeta-potential*

diffusion movement of molecules (or minute particles) by internal kinetic motion from a region of higher concentration to a region of lower concentration (that is, across a concentration gradient) in order to reduce the potential energy in a system

diffusion coefficient quantitative expression of the amount of substance diffusing per unit time across a unit area, as in Fick's first law of diffusion

diffusion equilibrium biopharmaceutic term used to describe the state in which blood concentration of a drug is in a "steady state" with the concentrations of the drug in other body tissues

diffusion layer area on or near the surface of a drug particle from which dissolving molecules first escape to become a solution; a saturated layer of drug solution that envelops the surface of the solid drug particles and diffuses into the body of the solution

digestant a drug that promotes digestion

digestion 1: action or process of breaking down food into simpler chemical compounds **2:** a method of extraction in which the solute and solvent are heated gently for a long time period

Digitalis purpurea species of foxglove plant; source of cardiac glycosides, including digitoxin

digital rectal examination test for colorectal carcinoma in which the physician inserts a gloved finger rectally to detect abnormalities

digital thermometer thermometer with a digital display

dihydropteroate synthetase enzyme that catalyzes the condensation of the pteridine ring with *p*-aminobenzoic acid to yield dihydropteroic acid; an intermediate product in folic acid biosynthesis

dilatant flow characteristic exhibited by polyphasic, liquid systems in which viscosity increases as "shearing stress" increases; example: pharmaceutical suspensions for which "rate of shear" (velocity gradient) is plotted against "shearing stress" (force per unit area) using an appropriate viscometer

diluent any substance added to dilute or make less concentrated; may be a solid (sucrose, lactose, starch), a liquid (water, alcohol, glycerin), or a semiliquid (liquid glucose)

diluted acid (official) refers to 10 percent w/v solutions of all acids except diluted acetic acid which is 6 percent w/v

diluted alcohol aqueous alcoholic solution containing 41 to 42 percent w/v or 48.4 to 49.5 percent v/v ethanol at 15.56°C

dimension 1: measureable quantity or property of a substance **2:** (of performance) cluster of related work behaviors that can be recognized by other practitioners as having similar purpose

dimercaprol antidote for heavy metal poisoning; synonym: British antilewisite

Dioscorides first century A.D. Greek pharmacognocist who collected and studied medicinal plants in the Roman Empire; wrote *De Materia Medica libra quinque*

dipeptidase enzyme that catalyzes the hydrolysis of a dipeptide into its constituent amino acids

dipeptide organic compound in which two amino acids are joined by an amide bond between the carboxyl of one amino acid with the amino group of the other amino acid

diplo- prefix meaning twin or two

dipole-dipole interactions weak attractive forces between molecules in which the electronegative end of one molecule orients itself toward the electropositive end of another

dip tube hollow, cylindrical part of an aerosol container that conveys its contents from the inside to the valve release component of the same container

direct costs 1: medical—the amount spent on medical products and services to treat illness, including hospital care, professional services, drugs, and supplies **2:** nonmedical—out-of-pocket expenses for items outside the medical care sector, including transportation to the site of treatment and lodging; costs that are wholly attributable to a service

direct dryer machine to remove liquid by direct transfer of heat to the material to be dried; example: convection heat transfer; antonym: indirect dryer

direct expense expense incurred solely for the purpose of performing a specific activity (such as dispensing prescriptions); examples: fees, prescription vials, patient profile forms

direct-to-consumer advertising advertising of medications via broadcast or print media directly targeting consumers or potential consumers

disability any condition that results in functional limitations which interfere with an individual's ability to perform his/her customary work and/or substantial limitations in one or more major life activities

disability income insurance insurance that periodically pays a disabled subscriber to replace income lost during the period of disability

disability management strategy to prevent disability from occurring, and to promote a safe and appropriate return to work and achievement of optimal functional capabilities

disaccharidase enzyme catalyzing the hydrolysis of a disaccharide molecule into two monosaccharides

disaccharide carbohydrate composed of two monosaccharides joined to form a single molecule; example: sucrose

disallowance a denial by the payer for portions of the claimed amount

disc or disk circular platelike organ or structure

disc filter a series of filter pads separated by metal plates (with openings) placed in a cylindrical casing to accomplish pressure filtration

discharge planning the evaluation of patients' medical needs in order to arrange for appropriate care after discharge from an inpatient setting

discharges patients who leave an overnight health care facility per time period

disclosure information released by a managed care organization or health care insurer on (1) policies and practices affecting access to covered care; (2) the scientific and clinical basis for those policies; (3) any relevant criteria used in such decision making; and (4) the decision-making process itself, including how public input is solicited and considered as well as the timing of revisions

disc mill cutting machine that consists of circular rotating teeth or convolutions that reduce the particle size of fibrous materials passing between them

discounted charges hospital billing charges reduced by some percent for an HMO buying a significant and/or predictable amount of hospital care

discounted fee-for-service charges the amount of money a provider charges for its health services less a fixed discount, which is negotiated between the provider and the managed care plan; typical arrangement sought by preferred provider organizations (PPOs) with physicians, hospitals, and other providers that are selected for their networks

discounting in pharmacoeconomics, a procedure that adjusts for differences in the timing of costs and benefits

disease a disorder with specific cause(s) and recognizable signs and symptoms; any bodily abnormality leading to interruption, cessation, or disorder of proper physical or mental functions, systems, or organs, except those resulting directly from physical injury

disease classification a systematic arrangement of related diagnoses into a limited number of clinically homogenous categories, usually to support the analysis of the quality, access, utilization, and cost of health care services.

disease episode the entire time period in which a person has a specific disease

disease management an effort to improve patient outcomes and lower costs by organizing managed care initiatives around patients with a particular disease or condition

disease-specific insurance insurance that provides benefits should the insuree develop a specific illness such as cancer or heart disease; usually purchased as a supplement to conventional insurance policies that may have ceilings or limitations

disenrollment the process of terminating individuals or groups from their enrollment with an insurance carrier

disinfectant substance typically used on nonliving objects to render them aseptic (without contamination)

disinfection use of chemicals lethal to microorganisms; used to reduce the number of microorganisms on a surface or on the hands

disintegrant substance added to a tablet granulation during its preparation and after granulation to facilitate the breaking apart of the tablet into granules and the breaking apart of the granules, respectively, when it is subjected to the fluids of the gastrointestinal tract; synonym: disintegrating agent; examples: microcrystalline cellulose, dried starch

disintegrating agent SEE *disintegrant*

disintegration test procedure designed to measure the time it takes a tablet to disintegrate or to break into small particles (granules) and pass through mesh wire of a specified screen size

disintegration tester apparatus used to determine the time required for tablets to break apart and the small particles to pass through a specified mesh wire screen under standard fluid and temperature conditions; refer to the *United States Pharmacopeia–National Formulary* for detailed testing procedures

dismemberment loss of body parts usually stemming from accidental physical injury

dispensary a place where drugs and medical devices are dispensed; usually an institutional term

dispensatory a treatise on medicinal substances and formulations; example: United States Dispensatory

dispense to give a prescription to a patient

dispense as written (daw) directive issued by prescriber that the brand name product or specific manufacturer is not to be substituted with another

dispensing fee the amount paid to a pharmacy for each prescription, in addition to the negotiated formula for reimbursing ingredient cost; fee added to the cost of the medication; synonym: professional fee

dispensing tablet SEE *tablet, compressed*

dispersed phase particles or globules distributed throughout a medium or vehicle; example: oil globules constituting the internal phase of an oil-in-water emulsion

dispersion system or formulation that consists of one or more phases distributed as discrete particles (or globules) throughout a fluid medium (liquid or gas)

dispersion, colloidal SEE *solution, colloidal*

dispersion, coarse fluid medium containing particles larger than 0.1 micrometers; examples: emulsion, suspension

dispersion effect SEE *London forces*

dispersion medium vehicle in which particles or globules are distributed

dispersion step process to produce or effect a smooth, wetted, uniform, and easily dispersible quantity of a drug formulation using a colloid mill or other blender with surface active agents and viscosity enhancers

disposition 1: distribution of an absorbed drug into various body compartments or sites of action **2:** (legal) manner in which a matter of interest is settled

disproportionate share payment an amount added to government payment rates for providers, usually hospitals, that treat large numbers of patients unable to pay their bills

dissociation constant 1: equilibrium constant for the ionization of a weak acid or weak base; SEE *ionization constant* **2:** equilibrium constant for the separation of a drug from its drug-receptor complex **3:** equilibrium constant for the separation of a substrate from its enzyme-substrate complex

dissolution process by which a solute becomes homogeneous with a solvent; the process of dissolving (a drug must undergo dissolution before absorption can occur)

dissolution rate amount of solute dissolving per unit of time in a given solvent under specified conditions

dissolution test procedure used to measure the time for the active constituents of a drug product to dissolve; refer to the *United States Pharmacopeia–National Formulary* for detailed procedures

distal farther away from a point of reference; contrasted to proximal

distention distended or stretched

distillate liquid from condensing vapor

distillation purification process in which a liquid is heated to a vapor state and subsequently condensed into another container as the liquid state

distillation, reflux form of distillation in which the solvent of a reaction first vaporizes and subsequently condenses back into the original container; usually used to enhance a reaction or other process

distilled water water that has been purified by being heated to the vapor form and subsequently condensed into another container to form liquid water free of nonvolatile solutes; one means of preparing purified water; SEE *Water for Injection, USP*

distribution partitioning of a drug to the many locations or compartments in the body or another heterogeneous system

distribution, frequency a plot of the number of times a value (or a narrow range of values) appears in a set of data versus its value (or mean value)

distribution, normal a frequency distribution with data equally occurring on both sides of the mean value, forming a symmetrical, bell-shaped curve

distribution coefficient the ratio of the solubility (or concentration) of a substance in an organic immiscible solvent to the solubility (or concentration) of the same substance in water when observed in the same system under specified conditions at equilibrium

distribution method procedure used to analyze complexes by use of differential solubilities of the noncomplexed and complexed molecules

distributive justice a principle of ethics that refers to the equal distribution of the benefits and burdens of society among all of society's members

disulfide bridge a covalent bond formed between the sulfhydryl groups in two polypeptide chains

disulfide exchange an enzyme-catalyzed posttranslational process in which disulfide bonds are formed, resulting in a biologically active protein

diterpene hydrocarbon composed of twenty carbon atoms; four isoprene units connected in a "head-to-tail" fashion

diuresis excretion of urine

diuretic drug that increases the volume of urine thereby decreasing body fluids and electrolytes; used in treatment of congestive heart failure and hypertension

diurnal occurring during the day or a period of light; opposite of nocturnal

dividend earnings credited to a stockholder as a return on investment; may be cash or additional shares; usually paid on a periodic basis (normally each quarter)

Dixon plots five types of plots to determine enzyme kinetics and to distinguish between competitive, noncompetitive, and uncompetitive inhibition of enzyme reactions

DNA fingerprinting a laboratory technique used to compare DNA banding patterns from different individuals

DNA ligase enzyme capable of attaching the cleaved ends of DNA; useful physiologically in repair processes and useful pharmaceutically in recombinant DNA processes

DNA microarray a DNA "chip" used to analyze the expression of thousands of genes simultaneously

DNA profile consists of the pattern and number of repeats each in STR sequences; used to identify individuals

DNA typing DNA analysis technique used to identify individuals; involves the analysis of several highly variable sequences called markers

docking protein protein attached to the membrane of the rough endoplasmic reticulum that helps secrete other proteins out of the cell

doctor of dental surgery/science (DDS) professional degree required to become a dentist

doctor of pharmacy (PharmD) the entry-level, professional degree of pharmacy

doctor of philosophy (PhD) research-oriented degree program usually requiring a minimum of three collegiate years of study beyond the baccalaureate degree and an original research contribution to be reported in a dissertation

documentation creating, collecting, organizing, storing, citing, and disseminating documents or the information recorded in documents; a collection of documents or verifying information on a given subject

dodeca- prefix meaning twelve times; example: dodecahydrate, meaning 12 water molecules of hydration

dog button common name for seed of the *Nux vomica* plant; a source of strychnine

Domagk, Gerhard (1895-1964) discovered, in 1935, that Prontosil (trademark), a sulfonamide dye, was an effective systemic antibacterial for treating streptococcal infection (thus initiating the "sulfa drug era")

Donald E. Francke Medal established by the American Society of Health-System Pharmacists in 1973 to honor significant contributions to international hospital pharmacy

Donnan membrane equilibrium a steady-state condition observed with two solutions separated by a semipermeable membrane, one of which contains a protein (charged macro molecule) that will not pass through the membrane, and both of which contain ions permeable to the membrane; when the system is allowed to reach equilibrium, an unequal distribution of the diffusible ions exists in the two solutions and there is a measurable osmotic pressure even at equilibrium; a phenomenon observed in capillary beds and other places in the body; also known as "Gibbs-Donnan equation"

dosage form pharmaceutical preparation intended for use by or administration to a patient with a minimum of further processing; examples: tablet, capsule, elixir, suspension

dosage range maximum and minimum dose to achieve a therapeutic benefit without toxic effects

dosage regimen strictly regulated amount of drug and schedule for administration to a patient

dosage rules 1: rules for calculating dosage, especially for children **2:** Clark's rule—weight in pounds times adult dosage divided by the average adult weight (150 lb) equals child dose **3:** Young's rule—age in years divided by age plus 12 times adult dosage equals child dose **4:** body surface area (BSA) rule—BSA in m^2 (of child) divided by the average adult BSA (1.73 m^2) multipled by the adult dosage equals child dose

dose volume or quantity of a medicinal agent to be taken at one time (unit dose) or in a given time period; example: daily dose

dose, geriatric adjusted dose to be given to an elderly person

dose, lethal fatal dose

dose, loading initial dosage unit or regimen to establish a rapid therapeutic level

dose, maintenance dosage regimen required to continue therapeutic blood levels for the required time period

dose, pediatric adjusted dose given to an infant or a child; usually based on age, weight, or body surface area; SEE *dosage rules*

dose-dependent kinetics pharmacokinetics of a drug that differs depending on whether the drug is given in a high or a low dose

dose response curve 1: plot of the amount of drug in the body (expressed in a number of ways) as a function of time; used to determine the dose for optimal therapeutic response **2:** (in molecular pharmacology) a plot of the response of a tissue or cell to a drug versus the log of the dose (concentrations) of the drug; synonym: log dose response curve

dosing interval time elapsed between the administration of consecutive doses of a drug

double bond a binding of two atoms that share two pairs of electrons, one pair of which is a sigma bond and the other a pi bond that exists as an electron cloud around the sigma bond

double-pipe heat exchanger heat transfer system utilizing a tube within a tube as the component parts in which heat transfer occurs

double reciprocal plot a graph of the reciprocal of the rate of an enzyme-catalyzed reaction versus the reciprocal of the substrate concentration; example: a Lineweaver-Burk plot; SEE *Dixon plots*

douche aqueous solution directed against a part of or instilled into a cavity of the body for cleansing and/or antiseptic action

douche, vaginal liquid preparation, intended for the irrigative cleansing of the vagina, that is prepared from powders, liquid solutions, or liquid concentrates and contains one or more chemical substances dissolved in a suitable solvent or mutually miscible solvents

down-regulation the reduction of cell surface receptors in response to stimulation by specific hormone molecules

Down's syndrome condition in which an individual has 47 chromosomes; an extra chromosome (chromosome 21) that produces a mental defect, enlarged tongue, a mongoloid appearance, and dwarfism of the child; synonyms: trisomy 21, mongolism

draft SEE *draught*

dragee sugar-coated oral solid dose form

dram an apothecary unit of weight equal to 60 grains, 3 scruples, 1/8 apothecary ounce, or 3.5437 grams

draught liquid mixture intended to be drunk at one time; synonym: draft

Dressier's syndrome complications developing several days to weeks following a myocardial infarction; postmyocardial infarction syndrome

dressing cover placed over a wound (usually made of absorbent gauze); the application of various materials for protecting a wound

drops medications given in small doses, used especially for pediatrics when medicines are to be instilled in eyes, ears, or nose

dropsy SEE *anasarca*

drug substance (or its dosage form) intended for use in the diagnosis, mitigation, treatment, cure, or prevention of disease

drug abuse use of a drug for other than medically accepted therapeutic purposes; examples: deliberate overdose, ingestion to produce euphoria

drug detailing presenting information about pharmaceutical products to prescribers to educate them about activity, uses, side effects, proper dosage, administration, etc.

drug disposition collective expression to describe release, absorption, distribution, and elimination of a medicinal substance

Drug Efficacy Study Implementation (DESI) the program under which the FDA reviewed the effectiveness of drugs approved between 1938 and 1962; established in 1962 following amendment of the Food, Drug and Cosmetic Act to require closer regulation of drugs sold in the United States; part of the Drug Amendments of 1962 (Public Law 87-781) that dictated all new drugs must be shown by adequate studies to be both safe and effective before being marketed; applied retroactively to all drugs approved as safe from 1938 to 1962 (referred to as pre-62 drugs), which were allowed to remain on the market while evidence of their effectiveness was reviewed

drug elimination collective expression to describe metabolism and secretion, excretion, and/or exhalation of a drug from the body

drug formulary a listing of prescription medications which are preferred for use by a health plan and which will be dispensed through participating pharmacies to covered persons

druggist 1: former name for a pharmacist in America; SEE *apothecary* **2:** English name for a drug wholesaler

Drug Information Association (DIA) organization to facilitate drug information dissemination

drug interaction the pharmacological influence of one drug on another; may be beneficial or harmful

drug lag time between the introduction of a new medicine in advanced technological countries (e.g., England, Germany, or Canada) and the United States

drug metabolism biochemical alteration of a drug; SEE *detoxification, biotransformation;* reaction (or a series of reactions) with two phases: phase I = substitution of a polar group on a drug molecule; phase II = substitution of a group or moiety on a polar group of a drug or drug metabolite (from phase I)

drug metabolism, first-pass SEE *first-pass effect*

drug misadventuring includes overdosage, subtherapeutic dosage, improper drug selection, drug interactions, adverse reactions, patient noncompliance, and untreated conditions

Drug Price Competition and Patent Term Restoration Act passed in 1984, with these effects: (1) extended the patent terms for pharmaceutical products meeting certain criteria, and (2) authorized procedures for the approval of generic versions of prescription drugs first approved after 1962; also known as the "Waxman-Hatch Act"

drug product drug dosage form suitable for marketing and dispensing to consumers

drug product selection act of choosing the source or supply of a drug product in a specified dosage form; usually done by a pharmacist, a physician, or a pharmacy and therapeutics committee of a health care institution

drug receptor complex drug action where the drug molecule is weakly bound to a receptor site, such as a specific area on an enzyme or on nucleic acid

drug receptor specificity concept that a biochemical receptor will react only with a limited number of chemically similar or analogous compounds

drug room place supervised by a physician or a nurse where medicinal agents are stored for distribution in their original containers without a compounding procedure

drug selection when the pharmacist is legally authorized to decide whether to dispense brand-name drugs or generic equivalents

drugstore community or retail pharmacy; a pharmaceutical service outlet

drug use evaluation (DUE) an evaluation of prescribing patterns of prescribers to specifically determine the appropriateness of drug therapy; has three forms: prospective (before or at the time of prescription dispensing), concurrent (during the course of drug therapy), and retrospective (after the therapy has been completed); same as "drug utilization review"

drug utilization the prescribing, dispensing, administering, and ingestion or use of pharmaceutical products

drug utilization review a quantitative evaluation of medication use, prescribing patterns, or patient drug utilization to determine the appropriateness of drug therapy; applicable to an an individual or group of patients

dry-bulb temperature in a drying process, the temperature of air measured with a nonmoisture-laden thermometer over an evaporating surface that is at the wet-bulb temperature; one of the readings taken when using a hygrometer

Dry-Coater tablet press (trademark) tableting machine designed to receive lower-punch-granular coating materials, a precompressed drug dosage unit (slug), and upper-punch-granular coating materials, sequentially, and then to compress the coat onto the precompressed dosage unit; a dry process used to coat tablets

dryer instrument or machine capable of effecting a liquid removal process; examples: spray, vacuum, and freeze dryers; SEE *tray dryer; spray dryer; vacuum dryer; freeze dryer; freeze drying*

dry granulation method the process whereby tablets are formed by compacting large masses of the mixture and then crushing and sizing these pieces into smaller granules; a method that does not involve moistening or adding a binding agent; SEE *slugging*

dry-gum method SEE *continental method*

dry-heat sterilization use of an oven to render a heat-resistant substance (or device) devoid of all life forms (140°C for 2 hours or 260°C for 40 minutes is usually sufficient)

drying process to remove a liquid (usually water) from the contents of a batch of solid or liquid materials; involves heat and mass transfer processes such as heat absorption into the substance to be dried, diffusion of the liquid molecules to the surface, vaporization (heat of vaporization must be added), and diffusion into the gaseous phase

drying by expression process of removing liquids from a wet mass of material by squeezing or compressing the mass; used to prevent waste in extraction and other separation processes in pharmaceutical production

drying by sublimation SEE *freeze drying; freeze dryer*

dual choice a term used to describe a situation in which only two carriers are contracted by a specific group; example: an employer offering its employees one HMO and one PPO or two HMOs and no PPO

dual diagnosis coexistence of more than one disorder in an individual patient; commonly refers to a patient who is diagnosed with mental illness in conjunction with substance abuse

dual eligibles refers to individuals who are eligible for both Medicare and Medicaid

Dubin-Johnson syndrome chronic idiopathic jaundice

Duchenne's syndrome anterior spinal paralysis with neuritis

Duhring's disease dermatitis herpetiformis

Dunning, Henry Armitt Brown (1877-1962) partner in Hynson, Westcott & Dunning; served as the president of both the American Pharmacists Association and its Foundation; was instrumental in the building of the APhA headquarters on Constitution Ave in Washington, DC; Remington Honor Medal recipient in 1926

duodenum first division of the small intestine

duplicate coverage inquiry request to an insurance company or group medical plan by another insurance company or medical plan to find out whether coverage exists for the purpose of coordination of benefits

duplication of benefits overlapping or identical coverage of an insured person under two or more health plans, usually the result of contracts with different service organizations, insurance companies, or prepayment plans

Dupuytren's disease plantar fibromatosis (abnormal growth of fibrous tissue on the sole of the foot)

durable medical equipment (DME) equipment that can stand repeated use, primarily and customarily used to serve a medical purpose, generally not useful to a person in the absence of illness or injury, and is appropriate for use at home; examples: hospital beds, bed pans, wheelchairs, oxygen equipment

Durham, Carl (1892-1974) Congressman pharmacist who co-authored the Durham-Humphrey Amendment establishing two classes of medicines (prescription and nonprescription) and the Durham-Reynolds Bill to establish the Army's Pharmacy Corps

Durham-Humphrey Amendment 1951 amendment to the Federal Food, Drug, and Cosmetic Act that first distinguished between legend (prescription) and nonprescription (OTC) drugs

dynamic dialysis method for determinating protein binding by measuring the disappearance of a drug from one compartment of a dialysis cell; involves passage of a drug through a membrane into a compartment in which the complexation or binding to protein occurs

dyne the cgs unit of force (cm/sec^2)

dys- prefix meaning painful, abnormal, bad, or difficult: CONTRAST *eu-*

dysentery any of a number of conditions characterized by inflammation of the mucous membrane lining of the colon and attended by cramps, bloody diarrhea, and fever; examples: amoebic dysentery, bacillary dysentery, viral dysentery

dysesthesia **1:** impairment of the sense of touch **2:** abnormally painful sensation caused by being touched **3:** pricking sensations as if by needles

dyskinesia abnormal voluntary movements, usually resulting in only partial or incomplete movements; type of extrapyramidal sign or symptom; an adverse effect of certain antipsychotics

dyslexia a condition resulting from a lesion in the central brain in which there is a loss of the ability to read

dysmenorrhea pain during menstruation

dysphagia difficulty in swallowing

dysphonia difficulty in speaking

dysphoria unpleasant mood

dysplasia abnormality of the development of size, shape, or organization of adult cells; abnormal tissue development

dyspnea difficulty in breathing

dystonia acute tonic muscular spasms

dystrophy defective development caused by poor nutrition

E

Eales' disease recurrent retinal and vitreous hemorrhage of unknown etiology

Early and Periodic Screening, Diagnosis and Treatment screening and diagnostic services to determine physical or mental defects in recipients of Medicaid under age 21, as well as health care and other measures to correct or ameliorate any defects and chronic conditions discovered

earth nut oil oleaginous liquid consisting of glycerol esters of unsaturated and saturated fatty acids; sometimes used as adjuvant for pharmaceutical preparations; synonyms: peanut oil (one of a number of fixed oils or nonvolatile oils), earth wax; SEE *ceresin*

earwax SEE *cerumen*

Ebers Papyrus Egyptian parchment paper written about 1500 B.C., containing pharmaceutical and medical knowledge up to that time

Ebert, Albert Ethelbert (1840-1906) born in Germany; a graduate of the Philadelphia College of Pharmacy; spent most of his professional life in Chicago where he practiced, taught at the Chicago College of Pharmacy, and served as an editor

Ebert Prize established by the American Pharmacists Association in 1873 recognizing the author of the best report of original investigation of a medicinal substance published in the *Journal of Pharmaceutical Sciences* during the preceding year

Ebstein's disease congenital heart disorder with tricuspid valve displacement into the right ventricle; also known as "Ebstein's anomaly"

ecchymosis hemorrhagic area or bruiselike spot in subcutaneous tissues; frequently observed in hemorrhagic diseases

ecgonine alcohol part of the cocaine molecule

echolalia verbal repetition of words overheard by a patient, often accompanied by muscle twitching; a symptom of catatonic schizophrenia

echopraxia involuntary imitation of the movements of other people; synonyms: echomimia, echomotism

eclampsia coma and convulsions in pregnant women; a condition associated with hypertension, edema, and/or proteinuria

Eclectic Pharmacy and Medicine sect or school that purports to select the best from all other systems of medicine; sect activity-simulated research in pharmacy and medicine, especially on the use of natural products

ectopic occurring outside of its normal place; example: pregnancy occurring in the Fallopian tube

edema abnormal collection of large amounts of fluid in intercellular spaces; manifested by swelling and congestion in a part of the body

edentulous lacking teeth

edge filter self-cleaning filter usually made of metallic plates that are periodically scraped to remove the caked material

effective date the date a contract goes into effect

effective dose the dosage of medicine that may be expected to produce the desired effect

effector a molecule whose binding to a protein alters the protein's activity

effervescence bubbling escape of gas through a liquid occuring when an effervescent salt is placed in water

effervescent mixture SEE *effervescent salt*

effervescent salt mixture of sodium bicarbonate and citric and/or tartaric acid plus the drug; when placed in water the CO_2 released by the reaction bubbles through the liquid thereby carbonating it; synonym: effervescent mixture

effervescent tablet tablet made from effervescent granules that releases CO_2 when placed in water; used to mask undesirable taste; SEE *tablet, compressed*

efficacious effective; having the ability to produce the desired effect

efficacy the ability of a medicine or or treatment to produce the desired effect

efflorescence 1: process of losing water of crystallization, thereby converting a hydrated crystal to an amorphous powder **2:** rash or redness of the skin

effluent 1: flowing out **2:** liquid discharge from a process, such as in liquid chromatography

effusion leakage of fluid into a cavity or other part of the body

ego in Freudian theory, one of the divisions of the psychic apparatus responsible for mediation between the demands of primitive drives (the id), the internalized prohibitions (the superego), and reality

Ehlers-Danlos syndrome hyperelasticity of the skin, easy bruising, and joint extensibility, usually due to faulty collagen synthesis

Ehrlich's test method used to determine bilirubin in serum or plasma in which the sample is treated with a solution of a diazonium salt of sulfanilic acid

eicosanoid a hormonelike molecule that contains 20 carbons; most derived from arachidonic acid; examples: prostaglandins, thromboxanes, leukotrienes

Einstein's equation basic energy-mass relationship in which energy is expressed as mass times the square of the velocity of light; $E = MC_2$, where E equals energy, M equals mass, and C equals the velocity of light

ejaculation sudden discharge of fluid from a duct; example: release of semen containing spermatozoa during climax by the male

elastic deformation reversible strain (deformation); example: stress applied to a system having fluid characteristics that creates a strain or deformation that, when the stress is removed, returns to original shape

elastin scleroprotein found in connective tissue that serves to give the tissue its flexibility

electrical gradient of a cell refers to the negative charge on the intracellular surface and the positive charge on the outer cellular surface

electro- prefix meaning electricity

electrocardiogram (ECG, EKG) curve or plot composed of P, Q, R, S, and T waves and representing a summation of electrical events occuring within the heart as recorded by at least three electrodes placed on the skin surface of the body (P wave = atrial contraction, QRS interval = ventricular contraction, T wave = ventricular repolarization)

electrocautery process of directing a high-frequency electrical current through tissue

electroconvulsive therapy (ECT) electrically induced convulsions; used in treatment of some psychiatric conditions; synonym: electroshock therapy (EST)

electroencephalogram (EEG) graphic recording representing the electrical activity in the brain, obtained by placing electrodes on the scalp

electrolysis 1: method of hair removal using electricity **2:** destructive process of separation and electrical discharge of ions in a solution by using an electrical potential across electrodes placed some distance apart in the solution; cations migrate to and are discharged by the cathode (negatively charged electrode) and anions migrate to and are discharged by the anode (positively charged electrode)

electrolyte substance that is ionized in an aqueous solution enabling it to conduct electricity; strong—substance that is completely ionized in aqueous solution; weak—substance that is partially ionized in aqueous solution

electromagnetic radiation light flashes (photons) characterized by specific wavelengths and frequencies; examples: gamma ray, X-ray, UV ray, visible and infrared light, microwave, and radiowave; SEE *gamma ray; infrared light; microwaves; radiowaves; visible light; X-ray; ultraviolet light*

electron basic particle of matter having a rest mass of $9 \times 1,028$ grams and 1 electrostatic unit (esu) of charge ($1.6 \times 1,019$ coulombs)

electron, orbital one that revolves around the nucleus of an atom and is a part of its atomic structure; SEE ALSO *negatron; positron*

electronic claim insurance claim submitted to the carrier by electronic means rather than hardcopy

electronic medical record an automated, online medical record that is available to any number of providers, ancillary service departments, pharmacies, and others involved in patient treatment or care

electron paramagnetic resonance (epr) method of spectrometry that depends upon vibrational frequencies generated by a radio frequency signal in electrons precessing in a magnetic field; observed in those substances possessing impaired electrons, i.e., a free radical; synonym: electron spin resonance (esr)

electron spin resonance spectroscopy a technique that measures the differences in the energy levels of unpaired electrons occuring in a rapidly changing magnetic field

electron transport system a series of electron carrier molecules that bind reversibly to electrons at different energy levels

electrophile **1:** a substance that accepts electrons in a chemical reaction **2:** an oxidizing agent **3:** Lewis acid **4:** a substance that attacks centers of high electron density in a chemical reaction

electrophilic substitution a chemical reaction in which an electropositive atom, molecule, or radical (an electrophile) attacks a molecule

electrophoresis method of analysis involving the movement of a charged particle in an electric field; particularly important to protein chemistry and peptide separation

electrostatic interaction noncovalent attraction between oppositely charged atoms or groups

electrostatic unit (esu) basic unit of charge for an atomic electron and a nuclear proton; 1 esu = 1.6022×10^{19} coulombs

electrovalent bond a binding of atoms together by electron transfer to assume a more stable configuration; synonym: ionic bond

electuary soft preparation consisting of sweetened, soluble semisolids that melts in the mouth

element substance that cannot be subdivided or degraded further by ordinary chemical means; an atom that has a unique atomic number

eligibility date the defined date a covered person becomes eligible for benefits

eligible dependent a dependent of a covered employee who meets the requirements specified in the group contract to qualify for coverage and for whom premium payment is made

eligible employee/person one who meets the requirements specified in the contract to qualify for coverage

eligible expenses reasonable and customary charges or the agreed-upon health services fee for health services and supplies covered under a health plan

elimination **1:** removal of a drug from the body **2:** act of excretion or explusion from the body; examples: urination, defecation, exhalation, and perspiration **3:** chemical reaction leading to the loss of a radical or group from a molecule

elixir clear, pleasantly flavored, sweetened hydroalcoholic liquid containing dissolved medicinal agents; intended for oral use

elongation the polypeptide chain growth phase during translation on ribosomes

elution **1:** separation of material by washing **2:** removal of substances from a chromatogram by the use of a solvent

elutriation process of separating a substance into various particle sizes by suspending them in a liquid (usually water) and allowing the particles to settle; the heavier particles are drawn from the bottom of the suspension and the lighter particles from one or more points above the bottom; synonym: water sifting

emaciation condition in which one's body mass is abnormally low; an abnormal loss of flesh; an excessive leaness; a wasted condition of the body resulting from disease or malnutrition

embolism sudden blocking of a blood vessel by an occluding substance (may be a clot or foreign material) brought by the blood to the sight of blockage

embolus blood-borne clot or other obstructive material that lodges in a small vessel thus blocking blood flow; SEE *embolism*

embrocation a fluid liniment

emergency a serious medical condition resulting from injury, sickness, or mental illness that arises suddenly and requires immediate care and treatment, generally within 24 hours of onset, to avoid jeopardy to the life or health of a person

emergency medical technician (EMT) skilled technician who provides on-the-spot first aid and medical treatment (under a medical doctor's supervised protocol) to persons in a health crisis and away from an acute health care provider

emergi-care center SEE *free-standing emergency medical service center*

emesis vomiting or regurgitation

emetic substance that induces vomiting; example: ipecac syrup

emission **1:** involuntary discharge of semen **2:** release of electromagnetic radiation **3:** discharge of substances into the environment; example: automobile exhaust fumes

emodin type of genin from glycosides; occurs in aloe, senna, and cascara and has cathartic action

emollient agent that softens and soothes that part of the body to which applied, usually the skin; example: cold cream

emotion **1:** state of arousal determined by subjective feelings; usually accompanied by physiological changes **2:** state of feeling

empathy awareness of another person's feelings, emotions, and behavior

empirical based on experience or observations rather than on theory and controlled, basic experimentations

empirical formula chemical formula showing the relative amounts of various elements in a compound; example: $C_6H_{12}O_6$ for the glucose molecule

empirical therapy treatment of diseases based on observations only; contrasted to treatment based on theory and controlled experimentation; synonym: symptomatic therapy

employee assistance program (EAP) services designed to assist employees, their family members, and employers in finding solutions for workplace and personal problems, including family/marital concerns, legal or financial problems, elder care, child care, substance abuse, emotional/stress issues, and daily living concerns

employee benefits program health insurance and other benefits, beyond salaries, offered to employees by their employer

employee contribution the amount an employee must contribute toward the premium costs of the benefit contract

Employee Retirement Income Security Act of 1974 law (Public Law 93-406) that mandates reporting and disclosure requirements for group life and health plans; also exempts many self-insured employers from many state health insurance regulatory requirements

employer contribution the amount an employer contributes toward the premium costs of the benefit contract

empyema presence of pus in a body cavity

emulsification process of preparing an emulsion; examples: dry-gum method, wet-gum method

emulsifier or emulsifying agent substance (usually a surfactant and/or film former) that promotes the formation and stabilization of an emulsion

emulsion heterogeneous, liquid or semisolid dosage form containing at least two immiscible liquids or semisolids, one of which is dispersed as small globules throughout the other, usually with the aid of a surfactant

emulsion, clear heterogeneous system in which the dispersed globule is sufficiently small so that it appears clear under normal vision; a system in which each immiscible liquid has the same visible light refraction (refractive index)

emulsion, oil-in-water an emulsion in which the oil is dispersed as fine droplets within the water; heterogeneous system in which oil is the dispersed phase (internal phase) and water is the dispersion medium (external phase); SEE *emulsion*

emulsion, water-in-oil heterogeneous system in which water is the internal phase and oil is the external phase

enantiotropic refers to a polymorphic compound in which crystalline form transition is reversible

encapsulation process of enclosing a substance in a capsule; example: preparation of soft gelatin capsules filled with vitamin A and sealed

encephalopathy degenerative disease of the brain; usually metabolic, toxic, or neoplastic

encopresis overflow incontinence; involuntary staining of underclothes

encounter a face-to-face meeting between a covered person and a health care provider where services are rendered

encounters per member per year the number of encounters related to each member on a yearly basis; calculated as total number of encounters per year divided by total number of members per year

endergonic refers to a nonspontaneous process in which free energy is absorbed or a process that requires an energy input to make it occur

endocarditis inflammation of the endocardium

endocardium endothelial lining of the heart

endocrine refers to glands that secrete hormones into the blood or lymph; CONTRAST *exocrine*

endocytosis the process in which a cell takes up solutes or particles by enclosing them in vesicles pinched off from its plasma membrane

endodontist a dentist who specializes in the etiology, prevention, diagnosis, and treatment of conditions that affect the tooth, pulp, root, and periapical tissues

endogenous arising from within; biosynthesized by the body

endophytic growing inward (e.g., an endophytic wart, such as a plantar wart)

endoplasmic reticulum a series of membranous channels and sacs that provides a compartment separate from the cytoplasm for numerous chemical reactions

endorphin endogenous morphinelike compound; depending on the compound, may suppress pain or act as a neurohormonal regulator; a neurohormone of a polypeptide nature that is involved in blocking pain

endothermic refers to a process in which the system under study absorbs heat from its surroundings; a process in which heat is required

endotoxins lipopolysaccharide-protein complexes (normally associated with the cell wall of gram-negative bacteria) that are released upon death of bacteria and are accompanied by disintegration of the cell wall; toxic substances which are formed in the cells of bacteria, freed once the bacterial cell is destroyed, and produce deleterious effects within the host

-ene suffix meaning an olefin or alkene (a double-bonded hydrocarbon)

enediol the intermediate formed during the isomerization reactions of monosaccharides

enema pharmaceutical preparation (usually aqueous) intended to be instilled into the rectum; used to evacuate the lower bowel, to treat the lower bowel locally, to supply medication systemically, or for diagnostic purposes; example: barium enema is an opaque contrast medium used with X-ray of the lower colon

energy ability of a body to do work, usually expressed as force times length; cgs unit (g/cm^2 per sec^2) or erg; SI units (kg/m^2 per sec^2) or joule

enfleurage process of extracting volatile oils from flowers without the use of heat

Engelmann's disease progressive diaphyseal dysplasia

English method process for making an emulsion in which the emulsifying agent (usually acacia) is dissolved in water and oil is added in divided portions, triturating thoroughly after each addition, until all the oil has been added to form the primary emulsion; synonym: wet-gum method

enkephalin either of two pentapeptides, having as their C-terminus either methionine (met-enkephalin) or leucine (leu-enkephalin), each of which acts as an opioid neuropeptide hormone in the brain

enrollee an individual enrolled for a health plan contract and is eligible on his/her own behalf (not by virtue of being an eligible dependent) to receive the health services provided under the contract

enrolling unit an employer or other entity with which a contract for participation is made

enrollment **1:** the total number of covered persons in a health plan **2:** the process by which a health plan signs up groups and individuals for membership **3:** the number of enrollees who sign up in any one group

ent- prefix meaning inside or within; same as ento-

enter- prefix referring to the intestine; same as entero-

enteral **1:** within the intestinal tract; example: enteral feeding **2:** route of administration broadly defined as between the mouth and rectum; examples: oral, sublingual, rectal; CONTRAST *parenteral*

enteral nutrition the feeding of patients by introduction of foods or nutrients into the alimentary canal either in the normal manner or by use of gastric or duodenal tubes

enteric coating covering applied to tablets, capsules, or pills to protect them and prevent disintegration or dissolution in gastric fluids; dissolution occurs in the small intestine

enteritis inflammation of the small intestine

entero- prefix referring to the intestine; same as enter-

enterobiasis infestation with pinworms *(Enterobius vermicularis)*

enterohepatic circulation sequential secretion of an absorbed drug in the bile, followed by its reabsorption into the blood

enthalpy the sum of the internal energy of a body and the product of its volume multiplied by the pressure

ento- prefix meaning inside or within; same as ent-

entrapment **1:** physical occlusion in a filtration process or in the formation of a clathrate **2:** (legal) process of inducing a person to commit an illegal act that the person would not otherwise have committed **3:** process whereby a nerve becomes trapped in tissues, causing discomfort

entropy a thermodynamic measure of the disorder of molecules in a system; example: the increase in molecular disorder or entropy as a solid melts, and, conversely, the decrease in disorder or entropy as a liquid condenses to a solid; a measure of the tendency for a process to proceed from a more ordered state to a more chaotic state; also, the energy of a process not available for work

Environmental Protection Agency (EPA) branch of the federal government concerned with the protection and improvement of the environment

environmental science study of the effects of contamination in air, water, soil, and food, and of changes in their physical nature and biological behavior as these relate to man and other life-forms

enzymatic refers to a process that is catalyzed by an enzyme

enzyme biocatalyst or specialized protein necessary for a biochemical reaction to proceed at body temperature and atmospheric pressure

enzyme induction a process in which a molecule stimulates increased synthesis of a specific enzyme

enzyme kinetics the study of the rates of enzyme-catalyzed reactions

enzyme-linked immunosorbent assay (ELISA) a technique involving antibodies that is used to detect and measure hormones and other molecules; diagnostic test for AIDS; a means to detect antibiodies to the HTLV-3 virus that causes AIDS; a blood or blood product test for the presence of AIDS and the presence of other viral infections

eosinophilia condition in which there is a higher than normal number of eosinophils (acidophils) in the blood

ep- prefix meaning on, upon, or over; same as epi-

ephedrine an alkaloid that possesses sympathomimetic properties; the chief pharmacologically active principal of plants of the genus *Ephedra;* also produced synthetically

ephelides freckles

epi- prefix meaning on, upon, or over; same as ep-

epicutaneous refers to topical administration of a drug

epidemiology study of distribution and frequency of diseases in a specific geographical area and their causative factors

epidermal growth factor a protein that stimulates epithelial cells to undergo cell division

epidermis outermost layer of skin, located above the dermis

epiglottis flap of cartilage that seals the entryway to the larynx during swallowing and opens the entryway during breathing

epiglottitis inflammation of the epiglottis

epilepsy disorder often characterized by convulsive seizures; loss or impairment of consciousness due to transient paroxysmal disturbances in the electrical activity of the brain

epimer a molecule that differs from the configuration of another by one asymmetric carbon

epimerization the reversible interconversion of epimers

epinephrine catecholamine secreted by the adrenal medulla and by nerve fibers of the sympathetic nervous system; responsible for both increasing blood pressure, heart rate, cardiac output, and glycogenolysis and also for the physical manifestations of fear and anxiety; synonym: adrenaline

episode of care treatment rendered in a defined time frame for a specified disease

epistaxis nosebleed; hemorrhage from the nose

epithelium thin layer of cells that covers the internal and external surfaces of the body

epithem moist, soft poultice usually containing blistering or astringent agents and applied to the chest or abdomen

epoxide an ether in which the oxygen is incorporated into a three-membered ring

Epsom salts hydrated magnesium sulfate; used as a laxative (when ingested) and as a hypertonic soaking solution to reduce swelling in a part of the body (e.g., ankle, hand)

Epstein-Barr virus a herpetovirus found in lymphoma and mononucleosis

Epstein's disease diphtheroid; an infection suggesting diphtheria

Epstein's syndrome nephrotic syndrome; edema, proteinuria, hypoalbuminemia, and hyperlipidemia

equilateral having equal sides

equilibrium condition of a process in which the sums of all opposing forces are equal

equilibrium constant unchanging value (at constant temperature and pressure) equal to the product of the concentrations of the reaction products (raised to powers corresponding to their coefficients in the balanced equation) divided by the product of the concentrations of the reactants (raised to powers corresponding to their coefficients in the balanced equation)

equilibrium dialysis method used to determine the extent of protein binding of a drug; determined by placing the protein-bound drug solution in a dialysis bag, immersing the bag in a solvent (water), and measuring the drug in the solution at equilibrium

equilibrium moisture content the moisture content of an amorphous and/or gelatinous substance (one that holds water intimately associated with its molecular structure) at the point in a drying process when the solid exerts a vapor pressure equal to the vapor pressure of the atmosphere surrounding it; highly dependent on relative humidity of the drying air

equilibrium time time at which the drug concentration at the deposition site becomes equal to the drug concentration in the blood

equivalent weight 1: weight of acid or base that will produce or react with 1.008 g of hydrogen ion **2:** weight of an oxidizing or reducing agent that will produce or accept one electron in a chemical reaction

Erb-Charcot disease spastic diplegia (paralysis of corresponding parts on both sides of the body)

Erb-Goldflam disease myasthenia gravis

Erb's palsy progressive bulbar paralysis involving the muscles of the upper arm

erg cgs unit of energy expressed as physical work

ergocalciferol irradiated ergosterol or vitamin D_2

ergonovine water-soluble alkaloid of ergot *(Claviceps purpurea);* maleate salt used as an oxytocic

ergosterol steroid obtained from ergot that, upon irradiation, forms vitamin D_2; 24-methyl-7-dehydrocholesterol

ergot fungus *(Claviceps purpurea)* that grows on the rye plant and is a source of a number of alkaloids such as ergonovine and ergotamine

ergotamine alkaloid obtained from ergot *(Claviceps purpurea);* the tartrate salt of ergotamine is used as a vasoconstrictor in treating vascular headaches such as migraines

error difference between the observed value and the true value in a set of data

eructation belching of air

erythema redness of the skin

erythrocyte mature red blood cell; SEE *blood cells, red*

erythroleukemia form of leukemia involving the cells that give rise to the erythrocytes that produce large numbers of abnormal, immature red blood cells

erythropoiesis normal production and release of erythrocytes

erythropoietin hormone secreted by the kidney that serves to stimulate conversion of stem cells into normal erythrocytes

eschar necrotic, dead tissue (e.g., caused by a burn)

escharotic agent that causes destruction of tissues at the site of application and leaves a scar; SEE *caustic*

-esis suffix meaning condition of

essence SEE *essential oil*

essential amino acids amino acids that cannot be synthesized by humans and must be in their diet; including methionine, isoleucine, leucine, lysine, valine, arginine (essential for children only), tryptophan, threonine, phenylalanine (may be partially replaced by tyrosine), and histidine (children mainly)

essential fatty acid linoleic or linolenic acid that must be supplied in the diet because it cannot be synthesized by the body

essential hypertension blood pressure above normal for which no cause is known

essential oil volatile oil obtained from a plant or an animal

ester compound formed in a reaction between an acid and an alcohol that, on hydrolysis, yields the alcohol and either the free acid or its salt

esterification reaction between an acid (or an activated derivative of an acid) and an alcohol to form an ester; formation of an ester

ester value milligrams of potassium hydroxide required to saponify the esters in one gram of fat, oil, or wax; numerical difference between the saponification value of a fat, oil, or wax and its acid value

estimated acquisition cost an estimate of the price generally and currently paid by providers for a drug; commonly used in Medicaid programs to set the reimbursement amount for brand-name drugs and often calculated as a percentage off of average wholesale price

estrogen any one of three steroids (estrone, estradiol, and estratriol) secreted by the ovaries and the adrenal cortex; stimulates secondary female characteristics and participates with progestin in control of the menstrual cycle

estrogen, synthetic (nonsteroidal) simple phenolic compound that has estrogenic activity; example: diethylstilbestrol (DES)

ethanol ethyl alcohol; synonyms: grain alcohol, *spiritus vini rectificatus*

ethereal 1: relating to or resembling a chemical ether **2:** escaping easily **3:** intangible **4:** volatile

ethical drug dosage form (drug product) advertised and promoted to the medical professions; most require a prescription before dispensing

ethics 1: accepted standards for the practice of a profession **2:** morals dealing with what is good and bad; set of moral values or principles on which actions are based

etiology study of the causes of diseases/or disorders

eu- prefix meaning well, normal, or good; CONTRAST *dys-*

euchromatin a less condensed form of chromatin that has varying levels of transcriptional activity

eukaryotes organisms, the cells of which are nucleated; SEE *prokaryotes*

euphoria 1: an extreme state of perceived well-being **2:** absence of bodily pain or disorders

eutectic mixture physical combination of two or more solids that softens or liquifies, due to a depression of the melting point below that of each component taken separately

eutectic point lowest temperature (at constant pressure) at which a frozen (solid) mixture begins to melt; temperature and pressure at which solid and liquid states of a mixture of substances exist in equilibrium

euthyroid normal thyroid function

evaluation making judgments about the value or worth of a process or thing; does not include considerations of the intrinsic worth of individuals

evaporation process of conversion of a substance from the solid or liquid state to the vapor (gaseous) state; the rate of evaporation is related to the inherent vapor pressure of a substance and its temperature and pressure; may be a desired or an undesirable pharmaceutical process

evaporative humidifier device that humidifies air by circulation around a capillary filter that is immersed in a reservoir of water

evidence of coverage SEE *certificate of coverage*

evidence of insurability proof presented through written statements and/or a medical examination that an individual is eligible for a certain type of insurance coverage

Ewing's sarcoma a malignant tumor of the bone marrow seen in children

ex- prefix meaning without, outside, or completely

exacerbation worsening of a disorder or aggravation of symptoms

excipient nontherapeutic substance added to a drug dosage form in order to achieve a suitable size or consistency

excision repair a DNA repair mechanism that removes damaged nucleotides, then replaces them with normal ones

excitation contraction coupling; process by which depolarizations of the muscle fibers initiate its contraction

exclusion chromatography process of chromatography that includes the separation of components of a sample of molecules by size; SEE *gel filtration chromatography*

exclusions specific conditions or circumstances listed in the contract or employee benefit plan for which the policy or plan will not provide benefit payments

exclusive provider organization (EPO) agreement whereby a purchaser, usually an insurer, contracts with a specific vendor (e.g., a particular pharmacy) to be the sole outlet for services provided to the purchaser's clients

excoriation abrasion of the skin; examples: scraping trauma, chemical burn

excretion 1: movement of a drug or its metabolic products out of the body **2:** process for body elimination of waste products mostly by means of the skin, lungs, kidneys, and intestines

excretion ratio corrected renal clearance divided by the creatinine clearance

exergonic spontaneous process from which free energy is released

exfoliant topical medication that removes the upper cells from the epidermis; example: benzoyl peroxide (used for acne)

exocrine refers to glands that secrete fluids into a body cavity (e.g., bile from the liver to the duodenum)

exocytosis the process in which an intracellular vesicle fuses with the plasma membrane, thereby releasing the vesicle's contents into extracellular space

exogenous developed or derived from outside the body; arising from external causes

exogenous ochronosis abnormal discoloration of the skin, caused by overadministration of skin hyperpigmenting agents such as hydroquinone

exon the region in a split or interrupted gene that codes for RNA and ends up in the final product; example: mRNA

exonuclease enzyme that cleaves DNA chains at their ends

exophytic growing outward; example: an exophytic wart

exothermic refers to a process in which a system under study gives up heat to its surroundings

exotoxin highly toxic protein produced by a microorganism and secreted into the surrounding medium

expected claims projected claim level of a covered person or group for a defined contract period

expectorant substance which aids or promotes the removal of mucus from the respiratory tract; example: guaifenesin

expenditure limits a limit set on the total amount to be spent on various health services

expenditures the amount paid out by the payer (health plan, managed care organization, insurer, government agency) for the covered medical expenses of eligible participants

expense outflow of cash or other assets attributable to the costs of operating a business

experience rating rate setting based on previous claims experience and projected required revenues for a future policy year

experimental, investigational, or unproven procedures medical, surgical, psychiatric, substance abuse, or other health care services, supplies, treatments, procedures, drug therapies, or devices that are not proven to be effective in treating the condition, illness, or diagnosis for which their use is proposed

expiration date month and year after which a drug product is expected to be subpotent (or degraded) under designated storage conditions; most commercial products have expiration dates at two to five years after production; synonym: expiry

expiry SEE *expiration date*

explanation of benefits the statement sent to covered persons by their health plan listing services provided, amount billed, and payment made

expression juices pressed from herbs, roots, or fruits

exsiccate to dry using highly intense heat

exsiccation process of depriving a substance of its moisture by the application of strong heat

extein peptide segments that are spliced together to form a mature protein during protein splicing

extemporaneous prepared at the time in response to current need; example: prescription order compounded in the pharmacy

extended care facility a nursing home or nursing center licensed to operate in accordance with all applicable state and local laws to provide 24-hour nursing care; may offer skilled, intermediate, or custodial care, or any combination of these levels of care

extension of benefits a provision of many insurers' policies that allows medical coverage to continue past the termination date of the policy for employees not actively at work and for dependents hospitalized on that date

external energy that amount of energy in a system manifested as work; example: pressure times volume

externality situation in which a person or a group receives benefits or incurs costs from the actions taken by another person or group

external phase in an emulsion, the liquid throughout which another liquid is distributed; synonyms: continuous phase, dispersion medium; SEE *emulsion;* CONTRAST *internal phase*

extract 1: concentrated preparation from animal or vegetable drugs obtained by removal of the active constituents with a suitable solvent or solvent mixture, evaporation of all or nearly all the solvent, and adjustment of the residual mass or powder to prescribed standards **2:** to remove or draw out (as the active principle of a plant) by physical or chemical means

extract, pilular plastic mass obtained by extracting the active constituents from plants and animals and adjusting the mass to the consistency of a pill

extract, powdered dry powder obtained by extracting animal or vegetable drugs, removing the solvent, and adjusting the strength of the extract by the addition of suitable inert diluents

extraction process for removing soluble components (drug materials) from a multicomponent mass by use of a solvent or a mixture of solvents alternately mixed with and separated from the material mass

extraction, liquid-liquid process whereby one immiscible liquid is thoroughly dispersed with another for purpose of removing a component which is (or altered to be) more soluble in the extracting solvent; example: morphine in ether may be extracted by using water acidified with hydrochloric acid, morphine hydrochloride being more soluble in the aqueous phase

extraction, liquid-solid process whereby a liquid is used to remove soluble components from a solid (usually in the coarsely ground state); example: removal of atropine alkaloid from ground belladonna leaves using water and alcohol as solvents

extramural 1: outside the wall of an organ **2:** arising from outside an institution; example: extramural funding of a research grant

extraneous foreign material; impurities; not related to the organism; outside the confines of an experiment

extrapyramidal portion of the central nervous system consisting of nerve fibers outside the pyramidal tracts; responsible for coordinating and integrating certain types of body movements; includes the corpus striatum, subthalamic nucleus, substantia nigra, and red nucleus with their interconnections

extrapyramidal adverse effects side effects of dopamine-blocking medicines; mimic the signs of nervous diseases such as palsy

extravascular refers to areas outside a blood vessel

extremophile an organism capable of surviving and living under extreme conditions of temperature, pH, pressure, or ionic concentration

extremozyme an enzyme that functions under extreme conditions of temperature, pressure, pH, or ionic concentration

extrinsic 1: descriptive term meaning having an origin from the outside **2:** not part of or related to

extrinsic reward monetary and other compensations that satisfy physiological or security level needs

exudate 1: material high in protein (and having a specific gravity greater than 1.020) such as fluid, cells, or other material that have escaped the blood vessels and deposited in surrounding tissue; usually as a result of inflammation; CONTRAST *transudate* **2:** material squeezed or oozed from its source; example: resin from a pine tree

facilitated absorption SEE *absorption; facilitated diffusion*

facilitated diffusion movement of molecules across a membrane barrier in which a carrier protein is required; movement from a region of higher concentration to a region of lower concentration, the driving force being the concentration gradient; no other energy input required beyond that necessary for normal cellular function; SEE *absorption*

facultative anaerobes organisms that possess the mechanisms needed for detoxifying oxygen metabolites; can generate energy by using oxygen as an electron acceptor

falling object viscometer device used to measure the viscosity of liquids utilizing a spherical ball that passes through a controlled sample of the liquid; example: Hoppler viscometer

false-negative error in a testing procedure indicating the absence of a component or a condition that is actually present

false-positive error in a testing procedure indicating the presence of a component or condition that is actually absent

family dependent a person enrolled for coverage under a health plan contract who is the enrollee's spouse, or unmarried dependent child

family planning services use of medically approved means that enable individuals to determine the number and spacing of their children

fan device or apparatus to effect transfer of air, vapors, or gases from one place or position to another, usually for a cooling effect

Fanconi's syndrome   renal tubular dysfunction

Farber's disease disseminated lipogranulomatosis giving nodular plaques in the skin

fat a triglyceride; esterified lipid derivative of glycerol with three fatty acid molecules attached

fatty acid one of a homologous series of aliphatic acids with a long hydrocarbon chain consisting of 10 to 24 carbons attached to a carboxyl group; examples: oleic acid, stearic acid, palmitic acid; general formula: RCOOH

fatty acid binding protein an intracellular water-soluble protein whose sole function is to bind and transport hydrophobic fatty acids

fatty alcohol alcohol that corresponds to a fatty acid; example: cetyl alcohol; long hydrocarbon chain (C_{10} to C_{24}) containing a hydroxyl group

feathering graphical method for the separation of exponents; also called "residual method"

febrile having a fever; pertaining to a fever

Federal Employee Health Benefits Plan   the program that provides health benefits to federal employees

Federal Insurance Contributions Act law authorizing the tax withheld for Social Security

Federal Register publication of the federal government (published every working day) that includes proposed rules, regulations, amendments, and notices from all federal agencies

feed input material undergoing a pharmaceutical process or a series of processes; example: a slurry from which the solid particulate phase is to be separated from the dispersion medium as effected in the spray-drying process

feed frame part of a tablet machine that distributes the granular material to the dies just prior to compression

feed shoe part of a tablet machine that delivers the granular material to be tableted to the feed frame

fee-for-service reimbursement the traditional health care payment system under which physicians and other providers receive a payment that does not exceed their billed charge for each unit of service provided

fee schedule a listing of codes and related services with preestablished payment amounts that could be percentages of billed charges, flat rates, or maximum allowable amounts

fellowship an individualized postgraduate program that prepares the participant to become an independent researcher; unaccredited programs that usually last one to two years

felony crime that is usually punishable by imprisonment in a state or federal prison; a crime that is more serious than a misdemeanor

Felty's syndrome rheumatoid arthritis with splenomegaly and leukopenia

fermentation the anaerobic metabolism or degradation of sugars; an energy-yielding process in which organic molecules serve as both electron donors and acceptors

ferric refers to a compound of iron in its +3 oxidation state

ferrokinetics rate of turnover or change of iron in the body

ferrous refers to a compound of iron in its +2 oxidation state

ferrous sulfate sulfate salt of iron in the +2 oxidation state; used as a hematinic

ferruginous containing or related to iron

fever above normal body temperature (98.6°F or 37°C)

fever, factitious apparent fever that the patient causes by manipulation of the thermometer

fibrillation spontaneous rapid or irregular pulsations of fibrils (as in heart muscles); example: ventricular fibrillation

fibrous thready characteristic of materials such as dried plant parts that must be cut to reduce particle size

Fick's law quantitative expression of the rate of diffusion as a function of the difference in concentration of drug on each side of a biological membrane; used to describe passive diffusion

fidelity a principle of ethics which requires that health care professionals act in such a way as to demonstrate loyalty to their patients

Filatov's disease infectious mononucleosis

filler diluent or any inert substance added to a drug formulation to increase bulk or size; examples: lactose or calcium carbonate added to increase the size of a tablet or capsule

film thin layer or coating

film, extended release drug delivery system in the form of a film that releases the drug over an extended period in such a way as to maintain constant drug levels in the blood or target tissue

film, soluble thin layer or coating that is susceptible to being dissolved when in contact with a liquid

film coating process of applying a thin layer of material onto the surface of a tablet or other solid dosage form to protect the tablet, improve appearances, and/or mask bad taste

film coefficient value that approximates the entire thermal resistance to convection heat transfer from a solid to a fluid where a temperature differential exists between the two substances

film testing examining a film-coated product for blisters, wrinkles, sweating, "orange peel," "flaking bloom," or spotting and a determination of its strength, attrition (friability), and disintegration properties

filter device or part of a device that contains small pores, openings, or channels designed to allow a liquid or vapor to flow through and to trap solid particles by physical or chemical means

filter aid substance added to a liquid to be clarified to improve filter efficiency in removing undissolved particles; examples: talc, kieselguhr

filter cartridge cylindrical-shaped filter medium used to separate particles above one micron in size

filter cloth woven surface-type filter medium consisting of natural or synthetic fiber or metal

filter medium porous part of a filtration system that collects particulate matter from a batch of liquid or vapor being purified, clarified, or otherwise separated

filter needle sharp, pointed straining device that will eliminate broken glass and other particles of certain size from medications that are drawn into a syringe from a glass ampule

filter paper porous paper used for filtration and chromatography

filtrate liquid that has been subjected to a filtration process

filtration process of separating solid particles from a liquid or vapor with the simultaneous clarification of the liquid or vapor by passing the liquid or vapor through a filter medium

filtration sterilization physical removal of microorganisms and spores from a preparation by passing it through a filter medium; used to render pharmaceutical preparations void of life-forms if its contents are heat-labile

fine 1: a grade of particles, 40 percent of which will pass through a 100 mesh sieve **2:** particles in a tablet granulation that are under the size limitation of the granulation and are included in certain proportions with the other granules for the purpose of facilitating flow

fine chemical substance sold and used in smaller quantities (grams, ounces, and pounds); most drugs considered to be "fine" chemicals; CONTRAST *bulk chemical*

fineline class items with essentially the same end use that can be reasonably substituted by the consumer for one another

finished product control quality assurance tests conducted on a drug product that is otherwise ready for distribution to consumers

first-dollar coverage health policies that pay all medical expenses up to a predetermined limit, without a deductible charge

first in–first out (FIFO) a method of inventory valuation and determination of cost of goods sold; under the FIFO method, the cost of goods sold consists of the cost of the oldest goods in stock, and the ending inventory reflects the costs of the latest goods purchased

first-order kinetics, first-order reaction, or first-order process quantitative expression in which the rate of change is directly proportional to the concentration of one component of the reaction (or process) raised to the first power

first-pass effect metabolism of a drug in the liver before it reaches general body circulation; contrast to metabolism of a drug after it has reached general body circulation

fiscal intermediary agent that has contracted with providers to process claims for reimbursement under health care coverage

Fischelis, Robert Phillip (1891-1981) served as the executive of the American Pharmacists Association from 1945-1949; long career as an educator, editor, and state board executive; served with the War Production Board division of chemicals, drugs, and health supplies during World War II; Remington Honor Medal recipient in 1943 and Whitney Award recipient in 1966

Fisher's syndrome ophthalmoplegia, ataxia, and loss of tendon reflexes

fission splitting of large atomic nuclei resulting in the formation of two smaller nuclei (usually of unequal size) and accompanied by the release of large amounts of energy and excess neutrons

fissure groove, fold, or deep furrow in an organ

fistula abnormal opening or passage between two areas, organs, or to the surface of the body

fit 1: a seizure **2:** appropriate size and shape for an individual prosthetic device

fixed assets tangible property that cannot be expected to be sold or used within the normal operating cycle of the business (usually one year); examples: buildings, land, equipment; synonyms: long-lived assets, non-current assets

fixed costs expenses of operating a business that do not fluctuate with changes in sales volume; examples: rent, utilities, property taxes, depreciation; synonym: fixed expenses

fixed fee an established fee schedule for services allowed by third-party programs in lieu of cost-of-doing business markups

fixed oil nonvolatile oleaginous liquid containing a mixture of glyceryl esters of high molecular weight fatty acids (C_{10} to C_{18}); examples: corn oil, soybean oil

flammable capable of burning or catching on fire; synonym: inflammable

flash dryer machine that instantaneously removes moisture from an atomized fluid in the presence of high velocity superheated air in a manner similar to a spray-drying process

flashing sudden splattering that occurs when the patient heats menthol/methyl salicylate-based ointments in a microwave or boiling water; burns to the patient may result

flash point temperature at which a vapor ignites

flatulence excessive gas in the stomach and intestinal track

flavoprotein oxidizing enzyme resulting from a combination of FAD or FMN with proteins; yellow oxidizing enzyme that is bound to a riboflavin derivative as a prosthetic group

flavorant substance added to give a pleasant taste; synonym: flavoring agent

flexible benefit plan employees are presented annually with a number of options, allowing them to tailor benefits to their specific needs.

flip-flop model a case in which the half-life of the input function is longer than the half-life of the disposition function

flocculation phenonmenon whereby suspended particles in a liquid system are held together by weak electrostatic forces resulting in agglomerates floating in the system

flocculation, controlled mechanism of adjusting the zeta potential of suspended particles to achieve an acceptable balance of attractive and repulsive forces between particles to formulate a more stable suspension or colloidal system

floor stock drugs medicines commonly dispensed by the pharmacy to nursing wards or units to be administered to patients as prescribed

flow permanent deformation and mass movement when stress is applied to a system; example: liquid flowing under the force of gravity through an opening in its container

flowers of sulfur synonym for sublimed sulfur

flow meter instrument to measure the rate of transfer of a substance in a mass transfer process as in a pumping system; most common types: differential pressure, positive displacement

fluid term to describe a body or system that flows under infinitesimal stress or force

fluid-bed dryer or fluidized-bed dryer machine designed to remove moisture from a small quantity (kilograms) of particulate pharmaceutical materials by partially suspending them in an upward flow of heated air, all particles being in continuous motion during the process; synonym: air dryer

fluid dram (fluid drachm or fluidram) unit of liquid measure in the apothecary system; equal to 60 minims, 3.7 ml, and 1/8 of a fluid ounce

fluid energy mill device used to reduce particle size by rotating particles at high speeds in a bed of air against the sides of a chamber and against other particles; particles reduced in size by attrition and mostly spherical

fluidextract highly concentrated alcoholic solution of active principles of a botanical; concentrated liquid preparation of a vegetable drug, containing alcohol as a solvent or preservative, or both, and made such that each milliliter represents the active constitutents of one gram of crude drug; SEE *fluid glycerate*

fluid glycerate highly concentrated solution of active principles of a botanical; differs from fluidextract by its lack of alcohol as a solvent; SEE *fluidextract*

fluidity 1: a measure of the tendency of a liquid to flow **2:** the reciprocal of viscosity

fluid mosaic model the currently accepted model of cell membranes in which the membrane is a lipid bilayer with integral proteins buried in the lipid and peripheral proteins more loosely attached to the membrane surface

fluid retention a failure to eliminate fluids from the body, usually due to renal, cardiac, and/or metabolic disorders; SEE *dropsy*

fluid ounce unit of common measure equal to 8 fluid drams or 480 minims; 16 fluid ounces equals 1 pint

fluorescence a property of a substance that emits visible light in response to exposure to radiation from another source; the emitted light is of longer wavelength than the exciting radiation

fluorine salts (fluorides) that are toxic even in small amounts; used in dilute solution to prevent tooth decay

flushing 1: sudden redness of the skin **2:** irrigation of a body cavity or an organ

flutter an arrythmia in which there are rapid contractions; usually used to describe a heart rate of 200 to 320 beats per minute

foam a pharmaceutical dosage form consisting of a significantly larger gaseous phase dispersed in a liquid phase

foam, contraceptive a foam formulated with a spermicide that acts as a sperm barrier during and after sexual intercourse

foam, quick-breaking dosage form that is designed to rapidly deposit a layer of medicated liquid on a very sensitized area

Foiling's disease SEE *phenylketonuria*

Foix-Alajouanine syndrome subacute necrotizing myelopathy, often associated with thrombophlebitis or vascular malformation of the spinal cord

folate reductase enzyme that catalyzes the reduction of folic acid to tetrahydrofolic acid

Foley catheter urinary catheter with a separate lumen that allows health personnel to inflate a balloon after insertion with sterile water to prevent the patient from removing it

folliculitis inflammation of a follicle

fomentation a poultice made of herbs with liquids or lotions in cloth and applied hot

fomite inanimate object that transmits infections or infestations; example: a surface contamined with viral particles, bacteria, fungi, or pubic lice

Food and Drug Administration (FDA) federal agency with the responsibility of protecting the public against distribution and sale of unsafe foods, drugs, cosmetics, and devices; also responsible for the safety and efficacy of drugs, drug products, and medical devices

foramen naturally occurring passage or opening between two cavities of an organ or through bone

Forbes' disease type 3 glycogenesis; a glycogen storage disease

Forbes' method one of several procedures for preparing an emulsion; ingredients of the emulsion are placed in a dry bottle and shaken vigorously; synonym: bottle method

force (f) force equals mass times accleration; an expression of the rate of change in movement of a mass of substance per unit time; cgs unit: $f = $ g/cm per sec^2; basic unit: a dyne; SI unit: kg/m per sec^2

forced convection mechanically driven heat transfer process; example: the use of a fan to distribute heat throughout a system, as in a tray-drying process

force of adhesion an expression of attractive tendencies of two different substances

forgery illegal act of falsifying documents, such as prescriptions; imitation for purposes of deception

formulary 1: book of formulas; example: *National Formulary,* one of three official drug compendia in the United States and one that provides standards and specifications for drugs and drug products 2: compilation of medicines (drug products) considered appropriate to stock and use in an institution or in a given geographical region based on clinical and economic considerations; examples: hospital formularies or third-party prescription plans that designate drug products which may be prescribed or purchased

formulary, closed rigidly controlled drug compilation with minimal exceptions

formulary, negative list of all drugs that are excluded from use

formulary, open lack of limitations on drug products that may be used and purchased by a third party

formulary, positive list of all drugs that may be prescribed

four-corner penetration a type of pharmacy layout that promotes patron traffic to all four corners of the store

Fourier's Law a quantitative expression of heat transfer by conduction; the instantaneous rate of heat transfer is a function of the thermal conductivity of a substance, its cross-sectional area perpendicular to the direction of flow, and the temperature differential for a specific distance in the path

foveation formation of pits on the skin surface

franchise an agreement under which a firm (the franchis*ee*) may operate using the principles, trademarks, or merchandise of another firm (the franchis*or*)

Francke, Donald Eugene (1910-1978) director of hospital pharmacy at the University of Michigan hospitals; involved in international pharmacy; one of the founders of the American Society of Health-System Pharmacists and longtime editor of its journal; early supporter of the concept of clinical pharmacy; Remington Honor Medal recipient in 1970 and Whitney Award recipient in 1953

Francke, Gloria Niemeyer (1922-) joined APhA as first assistant director in the Division of Hospital Pharmacy; career in professional journalism and literature; fostered outreach initiatives to international pharmacists; Remington Honor Medal recipient in 1987 and Whitney Award recipient in 1955

fraud intentional deception or dishonesty

free drug refers to a drug which is not protein bound in the blood and which is available for distribution to other body compartments

freedom of choice legislation requiring managed care organizations to allow members to choose providers whether or not they are connected with the plans

free energy the energy in a system available to do useful work

free fatty acid fatty acid in a system (the body or body fluids) that is not esterified

free floor stock system drugs or drug products placed on each nursing floor for use and for which there is no specific patient charge

free on board price of an item or merchandise that includes freight and transportation charges to some specified destination

freestanding emergency medical service center a health care facility that is physically, organizationally, and financially separate from a hospital and whose primary purpose is the provision of immediate, short-term medical care for minor but urgent medical conditions; also called "emergi-center" or "urgi-center"

freestanding outpatient surgical center a health care facility, physically separate from a hospital, that provides prescheduled, outpatient surgical services; also called "surgi-center"

freeze-dried refers to a product that has been lyophilized; SEE *freeze dryer; freeze drying*

freeze dryer vacuum-chamber device that removes moisture from relatively small quantities of frozen pharmaceutical materials; designed to optimize vacuum levels in the chamber and to lower temperature of the sample(s) to maximize the moisture removal process with the least amount of energy expenditure; the freeze-dried substance is a very porous lyophilic cake which must be sealed to prevent moisture uptake; synonym: lyophilizer

freeze drying process of removing moisture from frozen materials; synonyms: lyophilization, cryodesiccation; SEE *freeze dryer*

freezing point temperature at which liquid and solid states of a substance exist at equilibrium under conditions of constant pressure and volume; temperature at which a liquid begins to change to a solid

freezing point lowering phenomenon whereby a solute dissolved in a solvent will reduce its freezing temperature; example: the lower freezing temperature of an aqueous sodium chloride solution compared to that for the pure water

French scale 1 fr = 1/3 mm; measurement for catheters (e.g., 16 French)

French chalk SEE *talc*

friability an index of the condition of being easily chipped and crumbled or pulverized; SEE *friability tester*

friability tester rotating, single-partitioned, cylindrical unit designed to impact tablets contained therein as they are rotated for a specified time and at a specified rate; tablet friability is measured by a determination of "chipping" weight loss

Friedreich's disease paramyoclonus multiplex

fritted glass filter filter medium or filtration support component made by a controlled fusing of glass beads (fritted) to form minute openings in the device; available in coarse, medium, or fine range; synonym: sintered glass filter

Fröhlich's syndrome adiposogenital dystrophy; pituitary tumor with obesity and sexual infantilism affecting mostly males

Froude number quantitative expression to describe the relationship between inertial and gravitational forces involved in a mixing process

fugacious lasting a short time

fugacity expression or function replacing pressure to correct for nonideal gaseous behavior; one measure of escaping tendency

fugue dissociation phenomenon characterized by amnesia and the performance of purposeful physical acts away from the customary environment

fumigant agent used to produce a gas or vapor, especially to destroy pests or to disinfect a confined area

functional antagonism physiological interaction between two agonists that act at separate receptors but cause opposite responses; synonym: physiological antagonism

functional genomics the scientific discipline devoted to elucidating how biomolecules work together within functioning organisms

functional group a group of atoms that undergoes characteristic reactions when attached to a carbon atom in an organic molecule or a biomolecule

fundamental dimensions basic units of measure from which all others are derived; namely, mass (M), length (L), and time (T); cgs units: gram, centimeter, and second; SI units: kilogram, meter, and second

funding level the amount of revenue necessary to finance a medical care program; under an insured program, usually premium rate; under a self-funded program, usually assessed per expected claim costs, plus stop loss premium, plus all related fees

funding method the means by which an employer pays for the employee health benefit plan; several funding methods shift risk from the employer to a carrier, or an employer may self-fund the employee health benefit plan; most common methods: prospective and/or retrospective premium payments, refunding products, self-funding, and shared-risk arrangements

fundus base or bottom of an organ

fungicide agent that kills fungi; example: undecylenic acid used to treat athlete's foot

fungistat agent that inhibits the growth of fungi

furuncle SEE *boil*

fusel oil mixture of amyl, butyl, and propyl alcohols with traces of other complex organic substances; by-product of ethanol fermentation process; undesirable toxic components that should be removed during the refining process

fusion 1: melting of a solid or semisolid **2:** collision of two small nuclei resulting in the formation of a larger nucleus and accompanied by a large amount of energy release; example: principle used in the hydrogren bomb and manifested in the energy of the sun

fusion method (for preparing ointments and suppositories) the combining of solid or semisolid substances by melting each, mixing, and cooling the mixture with constant stirring until congealed or solidified

fusion point SEE *melting point*

futile cycle a set of opposing reactions that can be arranged in a cycle, but usually do not occur simultaneously; functioning of such reactions in both directions is avoided by metabolic control mechanisms to prevent energy waste

G

GABA shunt biochemical pathway around the tricarboxylic acid cycle involved in both the synthesis and destruction of GABA (gamma-aminobutyric acid)

galact- prefix meaning milk; prefix referring to galactose; same as galacto-

galacto- prefix meaning milk; prefix referring to galactose; same as galact-

galactose an aldohexose derived from lactose and isomeric with glucose; empirical formula: $C_6H_{12}O_6$

Galen (ca. A.D. 131-201) Roman physician-pharmacist who utilized the "humoral pathology" theory in a systematized practice and is known for his compounded preparations, which are referred to as "galenicals," even in modern times

galenical a medicine prepared according to the formula of Galen; currently, used to denote standard preparations containing organic ingredients from natural products as contrasted with pure chemical substances; example: rose water ointment (Galen's cerate)

gallon unit of volume equal to 8 pints, 4 quarts, or 3.785336 liters

gallotannic acid SEE *tannic acid*

gamma globulin a globulin fraction of the blood appearing electrophoretically in the gamma position that contains a high concentration of antibodies against infectious diseases

gamma-aminobutyric acid (GABA) amino acid neurotransmitter having a depressant effect on the brain; compound formed by the decarboxylation of glutamic acid

gamma ray a photon or a radiation quanta emitted spontaneously by a radioactive nucleus when subnuclear particles shift to a lower energy level

Gamstorp's disease periodic paralysis, usually with hyperkalemia

garbling removal of foreign matter or unwanted parts of the plant from crude vegetable drugs before grinding

Gardner's syndrome variant of congenital polyposis of the colon

gargarism SEE *gargle*

gargle aqueous or hydroalcoholic solution used to treat the pharynx and nasopharynx by forcing air bubbles from the lungs through the liquid while it is held in the back of the throat

gas any elastic aeriform fluid in which the molecules are separated from one another and have free passage

gas constant universal thermodynamic constant derived from pressure, volume, and temperature relationships of one mole of an "ideal" gas

gas law, ideal quantitative expression of pressure, volume, and temperature relationships for any gas in which there is no measureable interaction between its molecules; synonyms: Boyle's, Charles's, and Gay-Lussac's laws

Gasser's syndrome acute transient aplasia of erythropoietic tissue in young children; also acute hemolytic uremic (HUR) syndrome in children

gas sterilization chemical sterilization process that utilizes ethylene oxide vapor under low heat and pressurized conditions to kill microorganisms; commonly used to sterilize heat-sensitive and moisture-sensitive materials

gastr- prefix meaning stomach; same as gastro-

gastric emptying rate average time required for the stomach to empty its contents into the intestines; normally, once every two to four hours

gastric inhibitory polypeptide (GIP) gastrointestinal hormone produced by the cells in the jejunum and lower duodenum in response to glucose and fat entering these areas; acts to decrease gastric secretion and also stimulates insulin secretion

gastrin hormone produced by cells in the pyloric antral region of the stomach in response to ingestion of food; induces secretion of pepsin and hydrochloric acid and increases gastric motility

gastritis inflammation of the stomach lining

gastro- prefix meaning stomach; same as gastr-

gastrocolic reflex wave of peristalsis following a meal; allows a patient to defecate more easily shortly after eating breakfast

gastroenterologist a physician who specializes in diseases of the stomach, intestine, and related structures

gastroesophageal reflux disease condition in which stomach contents reflux upward into the esophagus, usually caused by a faulty lower esophageal sphincter

gatekeeper a primary health care practitioner (1) who provides primary care services to an enrollee, (2) who is generally responsible for coordinating the enrollee's health care, and (3) with whom, other than in an emergency, a patient must consult to obtain a referral to a specialist provider in order to obtain the highest level of benefits under a health plan

gate valve SEE *valve*

gauge measurement used for needles in which higher numbers denote smaller lumens (e.g., a 26-gauge needle is smaller than an 18-gauge one)

gaultheria oil synonym for oil of wintergreen

gauze purified cotton woven in the form of plain cloth

gauze, absorbent gauze that is treated to render it an absorbent for aqueous fluids

gauze, petrolatum absorbent gauze saturated with petrolatum; used as a protectant and waterproof cover for wounds or for a pack into a body cavity to stop bleeding

gauze mops gauze sponges; SEE *laparotomy pack*

Geiger-Müller counter (GM counter) instrument to detect beta particles; consists of a cylinder containing a gas, a cathode, and an anode; ions passing into the cylinder cause a flow of current and each beta particle causes a pulse of current that is amplified and recorded

gel 1: semisolid system consisting of a suspension of small hydrated inorganic particles; example: aluminum hydroxide gel (also called a magma) **2:** semisolid system consisting of hydrated (or solvated) organic macromolecules uniformly distributed throughout a liquid; example: tragacanth gel (tragacanth mucilage)

gel, dentifrice combination of a dentifrice (formulation intended to clean and/or polish the teeth, and which may contain certain additional agents) and a gel used with a toothbrush for the purpose of cleaning and polishing the teeth

gel, jelly class of gels; semisolid systems that consist of suspensions made up of either small inorganic particles or large organic molecules interpenetrated by a liquid in which the structural coherent matrix contains a high portion of liquid, usually water

gelatin 1: glutinous material obtained from animal tissue by irreversible hydrolytic extraction **2:** type A—obtained from an acid-treated precursor;

exhibits an isoelectric point at a pH close to 9 **3:** type B—obtained from an alkali-treated precursor; exhibits an isoelectric point at a pH close to 4.7

gelatinous   1: having or exhibiting similar characteristics as gelatin **2:** polymeric material with large quantities of water (or other solvent) entrapped between and intimately associated with the molecules of the substance; a dispersed system in which both phases are continuous; example: methylcellulose mucilage

gel filtration chromatography type of chromatography used to separate proteins or other polymers; process is based on the ability of proteins to permeate the theoretical pores of a gel; a technique used to separate proteins according to their molecular weights and to determine their approximate molecular weights by comparing migrations with known standards

Gélineau's syndrome narcolepsy

gem- prefix indicating a substitution on adjacent carbon atoms in a molecule; example: ethylene bromide (a gem-dihalide)

gene a DNA sequence that codes for a polypeptide, rRNA, or tRNA

gene expression the mechanisms by which living organisms regulate the flow of genetic information

general anesthetic drug or chemical agent that produces an insensitivity to pain over the entire body

general enrollment period (GEP) specified amount of time when the opportunity to participate in an insurance plan is offered; outside of these dates one may not enroll as a participant unless specific conditions such as a physical examination are satisfied

generally regarded as safe (GRAS) term used by the FDA for substances (drugs and foods) generally regarded as safe for their intended use

general recombination recombination involving exchange of a pair of homologous DNA sequences; can occur at any location on a chromosome

generator   1: an apparatus for the formation of vapor or gas from a liquid or solid by heat or chemical action **2:** radioactive columns from which radionuclides are provided

generic drug a chemically equivalent copy of a brand-name drug whose patent has expired

generic equivalent SEE *pharmaceutical equivalent*

generic name specific designation term assigned to each new drug by the United States Adopted Name Council (USANC); usually a shorter and simpler name than the chemical name for a drug and more descriptive than its trade name; commonly used to refer to the drug in scientific and professional literature; synonyms: established name, official name; CONTRAST *chemical name; proprietary name*

Generic Pharmaceutical Industry Association (GPIA) represents the manufacturers and distributors of generic drugs; provides lawmakers, government agencies, regulators, prescribers, and pharmacists with information regarding the safety, effectiveness, and therapeutic equivalence of generic medicines

generic substitution act of dispensing a different brand or drug product for the one prescribed; dispensing of a drug that has the same potency and is the same chemical entity in the same dosage form, but is distributed by a different company

genetic code the set of nucleotide base triplets (codons) that code for the amino acids in protein as well as start and stop signals

genetics the scientific investigation of inheritance

genin nonsugar portion of a glycoside; synonym: aglycone

genito- prefix referring to the organs of reproduction

genome total genetic composition of a cell or organism involving both expressed and unexpressed characteristics

genomics the large-scale analyses of entire genomes

geometric diameter (dgeo) particle size expression calculated by taking the nth root of the product of diameters (d) represented in the sample

geometric dilution method of mixing solids whereby a small portion of one substance is added to an equal portion of another substance and mixed; repeated serially until the total amount has been mixed

geometric isomers SEE *cis-trans isomer*

George Urdang Medal established by the American Institute of the History of Pharmacy in 1953 to recognize original and scholarly publications on the historical aspects of pharmacy anywhere in the world

Gerhardt's disease erythromelalgia

Gerhardt's syndrome bilateral abductor paralysis of the larynx

geriatric refers to the elderly, or medical treatment of the elderly

germicide SEE *bactericide*

gero- prefix meaning elderly or old age; same as geronto-

geronto- prefix meaning elderly or old age; same as gero-

Gibbs adsorption equation quantitative expression of the excess amount of solute (moles/liter) at an interface (surface) over that in the body of the system; used to study surfactant effects in pharmaceutical systems

Gibbs free energy equation thermodynamic, quantitative expression of isothermally available energy as constrasted to isothermally unavailable energy; free energy changes symbolized by ΔF; SEE *Helmholtz free energy equation; Gibbs-Helmholtz equation*

Gibbs-Helmholtz equation thermodynamic quantitative expression combining free energy and external energy computations in order to measure the change of energy in a system undergoing a change at constant temperature and pressure

Gibbs phase rule quantitative expression for the number of degrees of freedom (F) or variables that must be controlled (or determined) in a system in order to completely define it; F equals the number of components (C) less the number of phases (P) in a system plus 2, or $F = C - P + 2$

Gierke's disease type I glycogenosis; a glycogen storage disorder

gingivitis inflammation of the gingiva (gums) caused by poor hygiene; may lead to periodontitis if not reversed

Giusti-Hayton equation equation for calculating the dosage of drugs in patients with decreased renal function

gland organ consisting of specialized tissue-cells capable of secreting substances (hormones) into the blood (endocrine), into a body cavity, or on the surface of the body (exocrine)

glassine paper thin, dense, transparent or semitransparent paper that is highly resistant to the passage of air and to a lesser degree water; used in weighing and preparing powder paper dosage units

Glauber's salt sodium sulfate decahydrate; used as a purgative to produce a watery evacuation of the bowel

glidant material that reduces interparticle friction and promotes the flow of granules during compression of tablets

glister SEE *clyster*

globe valve SEE *valve*

globin protein portion of hemoglobin

globular protein a protein that adopts a rounded or globular shape

globule made of pure sucrose, lactose, or other polysaccharides; formed into small globular masses of various sizes, and medicated by placing them in a vial and adding the liquid drug attenuation in a proportion not less than 1 percent (w/v); after shaking, the medicated globules are dried at temperatures not to exceed 40°C; synonyms: pellets, pilules

globules   SEE *orbicules*

globulin   type of protein that is round in structure, soluble in dilute salt solutions, insoluble in pure water, and coagulable by heat

glomerular filtration   process by which the glomerulus of the kidney conveys blood to the nephron and filters that blood with reabsorption of filtrate (water) into the peritubular capillaries and with blood waste products removed in the concentrated urine

glomerulonephritis   SEE *Bright's disease*

glomerulus   cluster of like structures, such as capillaries, usually describing those present in the kidney

glonoin   nitroglycerin; glyceryl trinitrate

Gloria Niemeyer Francke Leadership Mentor Award   established by the American Pharmacists Association in 1995 to recognize an individual who has promoted and encouraged pharmacists to attain leadership positions in pharmacy through example as a role model and mentor

gloss-   prefix meaning the tongue; same as glosso-

glossitis   inflammation (and usually infection) on the surface of the tongue

glosso-   prefix meaning the tongue; same as gloss-

glucagon   peptide hormone containing 29 amino acid residues; a hormone secreted into the blood by the alpha cells of the islets of Langerhans (pancreas) that serves as a major hormone in the regulation of carbohydrate metabolism; the hormone that raises blood glucose concentration

gluco-   prefix meaning glucose, but sometimes used to mean carbohydrate

glucocorticoid   type of adrenal corticosteroid that controls carbohydrate and fat metabolism

glucogenic amino acid   a molecule whose carbon skeleton is a substrate in gluconeogenesis

gluconeogenesis   production of glucose or glycogen from noncarbohydrates

glucose   an aldohexose; synonym: dextrose; SEE ALSO *liquid glucose*

glucose tolerance factor   a value specific for each patient based on the glucose tolerance test; indicative of the patient's ability to metabolize glucose

glucosuria the presence of glucose in urine; a symptom of diabetes mellitus

glucuronidation substitution of a glucuronic acid moiety on a molecule; a metabolic detoxification process

glucuronide derivative of glucuronic acid

glutamate or glutamic acid acidic amino acid derived from α-L-keto-glutaric acid and commonly found in proteins; amino acid neurotransmitter in the brain; 2-aminopentandioic acid

glycerin clear, colorless, sweet-tasting, hygroscopic, syrupy liquid; synonyms: 1,2,3-propanetriol, glycerol

glycerite dosage form consisting of a solution of a substance in glycerin; example: tannic acid glycerite

glycerogelatin dosage form consisting of a soft medicated mass that melts near body temperature and has a base consisting of gelatin, glycerin, and water; used for topical drug therapy or as a suppository base

glycerol SEE *glycerin*

glycerol phosphate shuttle a metabolic process that uses glycerol-3-phosphate to transfer electrons from NADH in the cytosol to mitochondrial FAD

glycine aminoacetic acid; an amino acid commonly found in proteins

glyco- prefix meaning sugar or carbohydrate; SEE ALSO *gluco-*

glycocalyx a carbohydrate-containing structure on the external surface of cells

glycogen primary carbohydrate used for storage of body energy; white tasteless polysaccharide; synonym: animal starch

glycogenesis process of conversion of glucose to glycogen for storage in the liver

glycogenolysis process whereby glycogen in the liver is cleaved to yield glucose

glycol aliphatic compound containing two hydroxyl groups on adjacent carbon atoms; examples: ethylene glycol, propylene glycol

glycolipid a glycosphingolipid; a molecule in which a monosaccharide, disaccharide, or oligosaccharide is attached to a ceramide through an *o*-glycosidic linkage

glycolysis metabolic breaking down of sugars into simpler compounds, such as lactate, pyruvate, carbon dioxide, and water

glycolysis, aerobic pathways in the metabolism of sugars in which oxygen is required

glycolysis, anaerobic metabolism of sugars in processes not requiring oxygen

glycoprotein a conjugated protein in which carbohydrate molecules are the prosthetic group

glycosaminoglycan a long, unbranched, heteropolysaccharide chain composed of disaccharide repeating units

glycoside organic compound (usually obtained from natural sources) which, on hydrolysis, produces a carbohydrate (sugar) and a noncarbohydrate (genin or aglycone); most glycosides are physiologically active; example: digitoxin

glycosuria presence of glucose in the urine

GM counter SEE *Geiger-Muller counter*

goal a specific outcome toward which behavior is directed

goblet cell cells in the respiratory tract that produce mucus

goiter enlargement of the thyroid gland (usually due to an iodine deficiency in the diet)

Goldflam disease myasthenia gravis (a chronic, progressive muscular weakness)

Golgi apparatus (complex) a series of curved membranous sacs involved in packaging and distributing cell products to internal and external compartments

Good Manufacturing Practices (GMP) regulations of the U.S. Food and Drug Administration setting standards for manufacturing equipment and production processes

Goodpasture syndrome acute glomerulonephritis with hemoptysis intrapulmonary hemorrhage and anemia

gout disease resulting from an abnormality in the metabolism and excretion of purines in which uric acid levels of the blood are elevated and urates and uric acid are deposited in the joints

G protein a protein that binds GTP, which activates the protein to perform a function; the hydrolysis of GTP to form GDP inactivates the G protein

grace period a set number of days past the due date of a premium payment during which medical coverage may not canceled and the premium payment may be made

graduate pharmacist graduate in pharmacy; a two-year degree in pharmacy; last entering class was in 1931

graft slip of skin or other tissue for implantation

grain unit of weight common to the apothecary and the avoirdupois systems and equal to 64.8 mg; about one-fifteenth of a gram

gram equivalent weight quantity of a substance in grams equal to its molecular weight divided by the number of charges on the ionoized molecule; in the case of oxidation-reduction, the gram molecular weight divided by the number of electrons gained or lost by the respective molecule in a specific chemical reaction

grand rounds a form of teaching usually done at a patient's bedside with the teacher presenting to a group of students or young practitioners

granulation process of preparing finely divided to moderate-sized particles of varying shapes (mostly spheroid) to produce a degree of structure for easy flow and compressibility, as in a granulation for tablet making

granulation tissue temporary, highly vascularized tissue that is mostly composed of fibroblasts and used as a temporary tissue during wound healing

granule particle resembling a small grain or having the characteristic of being grainy

granule, delayed release small medicinal particle or grain to which an enteric or other coating has been applied, thus delaying release of the drug until its passage into the intestines

granule, effervescenta small particle or grain containing a medicinal agent in a dry mixture usually composed of sodium bicarbonate, citric acid, and tartaric acid that, when in contact with water, has the capability to release gas, resulting in effervescence

granule, for solution small medicinal particle or grain made available in its more stable dry form, to be reconstituted with solvent just before dispensing; prepared to contain not only the medicinal agent, but the colorants, flavorants, and any other desired pharmaceutic ingredient

granule, for suspension small medicinal particle or grain made available in its more stable dry form, to be reconstituted with solvent just before dispensing to form a suspension; prepared to contain not only the medicinal agent, but the colorants, flavorants, and any other desired pharmaceutic ingredient

granule, for suspension, extended release small medicinal particle or grain made available in its more stable dry form, to be reconstituted with solvent just before dispensing to form a suspension; achieves slow release of the drug over an extended period of time and maintains constant drug levels in the blood or target tissue

granules   small sugar particles with liquid medicinals applied and then dried; frequently used in homeopathy to deliver very small doses

granulocyte   white blood cell that has granules in its cytoplasm; examples: neutrophil, basophil, eosinophil; synonym: myelocyte

granulocytopenia   SEE *agranulocytosis*

granuloma   mass of tissue derived from lymphoid cells and occurring with the chronic inflammation associated with infectious diseases such as tuberculosis or syphilis

grape sugar   SEE *dextrose*

graph   plot of values for an independent variable (x) against corresponding values of a dependent variable (y) in order to illustrate the relationship between them; example: blood concentration of a drug as a function of time

graph, linear   plot that is a straight line or exhibits a constant slope over an experimental range

graph, log-log   one in which the values of both variables are plotted as the logarithm of the actual numbers; a graphical means to attempt to find a linear expression of the relationship between variables

graph, semilog   a plot in which the logarithms of the actual values of one variable are plotted against the actual values of the other variable; a graphical means to find a linear expression of the relationship between two variables

Grave's disease   toxic goiter; hyperthyroidism

gravimetric analysis   quantitative determination of the amount of a substance present in a sample calculated by isolating a derivative compound and weighing it using an analytical balance

gravimetry   measurement of weight

gravity bag filter   use of a woven filter medium in the form of a bag and the force of gravity to separate the desired component; example: separation of magnesia magma

gravity filter   filtration setup that depends on gravitational forces only to accomplish the process; example: Nutzche gravity filter

green soap   potassium soap made by the saponification of various vegetable oils without removing the glycerin; synonym: soft soap

green vitriol ferrous sulfate; copperas

grinding reduction of a substance to a powder by friction and pressure; SEE *comminution*

grossing series of steps in tablet sugar-coating that produces a smooth, uniformly colored coat onto a previously applied subcoat

gross margin excess of sales over the costs of goods sold for a business; gross margin equals sales less cost of goods sold; synonym: gross profit

gross profit SEE *gross margin*

group a collection of individuals treated as a single entity; usually, an employer purchasing medical coverage on behalf of its full-time employees

group contract the application and addenda, signed by both the health plan and the enrolling unit, that constitutes the agreement regarding the benefits, exclusions, and other conditions between the health plan and the enrolling unit; also, the agreement with persons who obtain coverage for themselves and their children, whether under a group or individual program

Group Health Association of America merged with American Managed Care Research Association to form the American Association of Health Plans

group insurance any insurance policy or health services contract by which groups of employees (and often their dependents) are covered under a single policy or contract, issued by their employer or other group entity

group model HMO a health care model involving contracts with physicians organized as a partnership, professional corporation, or other association

group practice prepayment plan an organized group of medical care providers that offers selected medical and health services to members on a prepaid, fixed premium basis

group purchasing organization a shared service combining the purchasing power of individual hospitals to obtain lower prices for equipment, supplies, and services

growth factor an extracellular polypeptide that stimulates cells to grow and/or undergo cell division

growth hormone (GH) endocrinal peptide substance produced by the anterior pituitary gland that serves to enhance protein conversion into more complex compounds and thus into living matter

GTPase activating protein a protein molecule that hydrolyses GTP bound to a GTP binding protein

guaranteed renewability the assurance that an insurance company will continue to offer a policy to an individual or group that has made premium payments on a timely basis; prohibits an insurance company from dropping coverage due to specific circumstances, including high medical claims or illness

guild early trade or professional association in Italy, France, Germany, and England

Guillain-Barré syndrome acute idiopathic polyneuritis (simultaneous inflammation of a large number of the spinal nerves)

Gull's disease myxedema; hypothyroidism

gum substance exuded or extracted from certain plants that is sticky when moist or warmed but hardens when dried or cooled; COMPARE *mucilage*

gum, chewing sweetened and flavored insoluble plastic material of various shapes that, when chewed, releases a drug substance into the oral cavity

gum resin, natural mixture of gum and resin, usually obtained as exudations from plants

gum Arabic SEE *acacia gum; camphor*

guncotton soluble pyroxylin; a nitrate ester of cellulose

gutta percha milky sap of trees that is purified and dried; used as a substitute for collodion

gyn- prefix referring to the female sex; same as gyne-, gyneco-, gyno-

gyne- prefix referring to the female sex; same as gyn-, gyneco-, gyno-

gyneco- prefix referring to the female sex; same as gyn-, gyne-, gyno-

gynecologist a physician who specializes in diseases of the female genital tract

gynecology branch of medicine specializing in diseases of the female reproductive tract

gynecomastia overdevelopment of the male mammary glands

gyno- prefix referring to the female sex; same as gyn-, gyne-, gyneco-

gypsum calcium sulfate dihydrate

gyrus rounded elevations of the brain

H. A. B. Dunning Award established by the American Pharmacists Association in 1982 recognizing a pharmaceutical manufacturer for exemplary contributions to the practice of pharmacy

half-life the time elasped when one-half of an active substance remains, the other half having been degraded, processed, or removed from the system under study

half-life, biological time required for one-half of a drug to be metabolized or eliminated from the body

halide a chemical compound formed between a halogen and other atoms; examples: sodium chloride, potassium iodide, calcium bromide

hallucination sensory perception in the absence of external stimulus; synonym: delusion

hallucinogen agent that produces hallucinations when taken into the body

hallux the large toe

halo effect bias that occurs when performance in one dimension affects ratings of performance in another dimension

halogen any of several elements belonging to group VII of the periodic table; included in the halogens are fluorine, chlorine, bromine, iodine, and the artificially formed element astatine; each of the natural halogens were discovered by pharmacists

halogenation reaction in which a halogen is either added to carbon-carbon double bonds or substituted for a hydrogen on a hydrocarbon

Hamman-Rich syndrome idiopathic diffuse interstitial pulmonary fibrosis

hammer mill apparatus that contains rotating flat metal impellers and a screen enclosed in a heavy duty housing; used to reduce particle size of friable materials by impaction and attrition

Hammett equation used for predictions for reactions such as the strength of acids and the influence of substituents

Hammond's disease congenital athetosis

Hansen's disease leprosy (a chronic granulomatous infection of the skin)

hapten or haptene partial antigen; substance that must attach to a protein to form an antigen

hardness tester instrument designed to measure the pressure (kilograms per cm^2) required to break a tablet and determine its hardness

hard paraffin purified mixture of solid hydrocarbons obtained from petroleum; synonym: paraffin wax

hard soap SEE *castile soap*

hard water natural water containing high concentrations of di- and trivalent metals such as calcium, magnesium, and iron

Harley's disease paroxysmal hemoglobinuria

Harrison Narcotic Act of 1914 established controls on the prescribing and dispensing of opiates and their derivatives

Hartmann's solution synonym for lactated Ringer's solution

hartshorn spirit strong ammonia solution

Harvey A. K. Whitney Award established in 1950 by the Michigan Society of Hospital Pharmacists and transferred to the American Society of Hospital Pharmacists in 1963; honors outstanding contributions to hospital (health system) pharmacy and is health system pharmacy's highest honor

Hashimoto's disease lymphadenoid goiter; thyroiditis

HCPC System SEE *Healthcare Common Procedure Coding System*

headache crystals synonym for menthol

health belief model used to understand the likelihood of an individual to take action or change behavior by focusing on perceived susceptibility and severity of a disease

health benefits package the services and products (coverage) a health plan offers a group or individual

Healthcare Common Procedure Coding System a Medicare coding system for identifying a wide variety of services, including indictable drugs used in physicians' offices

Health Care Financing Administration (HCFA) the federal agency responsible for administering Medicare and overseeing states' administration of Medicaid; name changed to the Centers for Medicare and Medicaid Services (CMS) in 2001

health care prepayment plan a cost contract that prepays a health plan a flat amount per month to provide Medicare-eligible Part B medical services to enrolled members.

health coverage insurance that provides payment of benefits for covered sickness or injury and may include short- and long-term disability, dental, medical, vision, and sometimes accidental death coverage

Healthcare Distribution Management Association   organization of drug and drug-related wholesalers that exists for the purpose of improving the distribution of products from manufacturers to pharmacies; founded in 1876 (formerly National Wholesale Druggists Association)

health education   instruction provided to patients to promote and prompt better utilization of health care

health insurance   financial protection agains the medical care costs arising from sickness, disease, or accidental bodily injury; usually covers all or part of the medical costs of treatment; may be obtained on either an individual or a group basis

Health Insurance Portability and Accountability Act   passed in 1996; addressed (1) guarantees for health insurance access, portability, and renewal; (2) preventing health care fraud and abuse; (3) medical savings accounts and coverage for the self-employed; (4) enforcing group health plan provisions; and (5) revenue offset provisions; with provisions in Section 2 to protect the privacy and security of health-related information

health IRAs   (individual retirement accounts) proposed tax-deferred plans to encourage saving for future medical expenses

health maintainance organization   (HMO) organized medical care delivery system often characterized by periodic fixed prepayments rather than fee for service charges; often places at least some of the providers at risk for medical expenses and uses primary care physicians as gatekeepers

Health Plan Employer Data and Information Set   (HEDIS) (trademark) a core set of performance measures used to assist employers and other health purchasers in understanding the value of health care purchases and evaluating health plan performance

health service agreement   (HSA) the detailed procedure and benefit description given to each enrolled employer

health status   level of physical, social, and psychological well-being of an individual or group

Healthy People 2010   a national strategy for improving the health of the U.S. population; provides a framework to reduce preventable death and injury

heart 1: hollow muscular organ divided into chambers; main purpose is to pump blood to body cells against the peripheral resistance of the body **2:** the essence of one's being or the central issue in a matter under discussion

heart attack   onset of symptoms and effects caused by blockage of a coronary artery or a branch of the artery; pain may be located behind the breastbone or referred to the shoulder, neck, or an arm (more specifically the left arm); synonym: myocardial infarction

heartburn a sensation of burning in the esophagus caused by reflux of acid secretions from the stomach; synonym: gastroesophageal reflux; frequent—heartburn occurring two or more days per week (not episodic or food-related)

heart muscle cardiac muscle fibers forming a continuous network or syncytium, composed of three layers: epicardium (outer), myocardium (middle), and endocardium (inside)

heat form of energy which is transferable from one substance to another and which is measured by an intensity factor (temperature) and a capacity factor (calories per gram per degree of temperature change); heat transfer a necessary consideration in all pharmaceutical processes

heating bath container for holding a liquid heat transfer agent such as water, oil, or glycol; the heat source and the liquid bath that transfers heat to another substance in a reasonably controlled system; examples: water bath, oil bath

heating pad device used to deliver local heat to the patient; heat generated by passing electricity through wires embedded in insulation

heat-shock protein a protein synthesized in response to stress (e.g., high temperature)

heat therapy therapy utilizing continuous low-level heat for an extended period of time

Hebert, Louis (ca. 1580-1627) French pharmacist who provided for health needs of two early French colonies, one at Port Royal and the other at Quebec City, Canada; first known pharmacist in North America

Heisenberg uncertainty principle rule stating that it is not possible to determine both position and energy of a moving object; significant only for atomic particles such as orbital electrons

helicase ATP-requiring enzymes that catalyze the unwinding of duplex DNA

Helmholtz free energy equation thermodynamic quantitative expression of isothermally available internal energy; synonym: work function; contrasted to isothermally unavailable internal energy; SEE ALSO *Gibbs free energy equation*

helminthiasis disease caused by an infestation of the host with worms

hem- prefix meaning blood; same as hema-, hemat-, hemato-, hemo-

hema- prefix meaning blood; same as hem-, hemat-, hemato-, hemo-

hemat- prefix meaning blood; same as hem-, hema-, hemat-, hemo-

hematemesis vomiting of blood

hemato- prefix meaning blood; same as hem-, hema-, hemat-, hemo-

hematocrit percentage of erythrocytes in a specified volume of whole blood

hematuria the presence of blood in the urine

heme an iron compound that, when combined with globin, is responsible for oxygen-carrying properties of the blood

hemiacetal one of the family of organic molecules with the general formula RR'C(OR')(OH), formed by the reaction of one molecule of alcohol with an aldehyde

hemicellulase enzyme that splits gums (polysaccharides) into smaller units

hemiketal one of a family of organic molecules with the general formula RR'C(OR')(OH), formed by the reaction of one molecule of alcohol with a ketone

hemiplegia paralysis of one side of the body

hemiterpene isoprene; half of terpene; a hydrocarbon composed of five carbon atoms and two double bonds; 2-methylbutadiene

hemo- prefix meaning blood; same as hem-, hema-, hemat-, hemato-

hemoblastoma tumor that contains cells similar to those found in bone marrow

hemochromatosis an iron-storage disorder that results in an excessive accumulation of iron in the body resulting in a bronze skin pigmentation, hepatic cirrhosis, and diabetes mellitus

hemoglobin oxygen-carrying pigment of red blood cells

hemoglobin A_1 normal adult hemoglobin that comprises 95 percent of the hemoglobin in the normal human being; composed of $\alpha_2 \beta_2$ (two alpha globins combined with two beta globins)

hemoglobin A_{1c} glycosylated hemoglobin used to estimate blood glucose levels in diabetics

hemoglobin A_2 normal adult hemoglobin that comprises 5 percent of the hemoglobin in the normal human being; composed of $\alpha_2 \delta_2$ (two alpha globins combined with two delta globins)

hemoglobin F fetal hemoglobin; the predominant hemoglobin of the fetus that normally disappears before birth; in certain anemias, may persist after birth; composed of $\alpha_2\gamma_2$ (two alpha globins combined with two gamma globins)

hemoglobinopathies diseases involving a change in the globin structure of hemoglobin; either the alpha or the beta globin may be involved; examples: sickle cell anemia, Mediterranean anemias

hemoglobin S type of hemoglobin found in sickle cell anemia in which valine replaces the glutamic acid residue normally found in the "6" position of the β-globin chains of hemoglobin A_1

hemolysis destruction of red blood cells

hemolytic refers to a disease in which there is a destruction of red blood cells

hemolytic anemia anemia caused by the early destruction of red blood cells and the inability of the bone marrow to compensate for the red blood cell shortened life span

hemophilia genetic disorder resulting in the deficiency of clotting factor VIII and characterized by spontaneous or excessive bleeding

hemoprotein a conjugated protein in which heme, an iorn-containing organic group, is the prosthetic group

hemoptysis expulsion of blood-stained sputum; may be a sequelae of gastroesophageal reflux

hemorrhage bleeding, usually considered to be uncontrolled

hemorrhoids enlarged veins in the hemorrhoidal plexus

Henderson-Hasselbalch equation quantitative expression of the relationships between pH, pK_a, pK_b, and the log of the ratio of the concentration of ionized to unionized species in a system; for weak bases and their salts the pH equals the pK_b plus the log of the ratio of the concentration of unionized base to the concentration of ionized (salt); for weak acids and their salts pH equals the pK_a plus the log of the ratio of the the concentration of ionized salt to the concentration of the unionized acid; useful for pH-buffer computations; synonym: buffer equation; SEE ALSO *buffer*

Henry, O. (1862-1910) pseudonym for William S. Porter; began his career as a pharmacist and later became a renowned short story author

HEPA filter highly efficient, particulate air (HEPA) filter that has at least 99.97 percent efficiency in removing particles of 0.3 mm and larger

heparin mucopolysaccharide that prevents blood clotting

hepat- prefix meaning liver; same as hepato-

hepatitis inflammation of the liver

hepatitis, acute form of hepatitis producing overt symptoms of the condition that are readily observed; causes acute yellow atrophy of liver, a form of hepatic necrosis

hepatitis, chronic form of hepatitis that has a more prolonged course

hepatitis, infectious form of hepatitis caused by a virus; may be contracted when using drinking glasses or touching other objects that have been contaminated by persons infected with the disease; causative organism: hepatitis type A virus

hepatitis, serum a form of liver inflammation caused by injection of nonsterile substances into the blood or the use of nonsterile needles for injection; causative organism: hepatitis type B virus

hepato- prefix meaning liver; same as hepat-

hepatomegaly enlargement of the liver

herb leafy plant without a woody stem

herbal general title for any book on herbs; relating to herbs

herbalist one who specializes in selling herbs

herbarium 1: collection of dried herbs **2:** place that houses a collection of herbs

herbicide chemical used to kill or control weeds

hermetically sealed subjected to a heat-sealing process; examples: sealed glass or plastic containers, gelatin capsules

hermetic container SEE *container, hermetic*

Herzberg's theory theory of motivation which holds that all motivating factors can be divided into two groups (satisfiers and dissatisfiers); satisfiers are those aspects of the job which positively motivate an employee and dissatisfiers are those aspects which produce dissatisfaction if they are not fulfilled

heterogeneous nuclear RNA a primary transcript of DNA; precursor of an mRNA

heterotroph an organism that attains energy by degrading preformed food molecules obtained by consuming other organisms

hidrosis term to describe excessive wetness or perspiration

high-density lipoprotein a type of lipoprotein with a high protein content that is believed to scavenge excess cholesterol from cell membranes and transport it to the liver

high-energy compound compound that upon hydrolysis releases at least seven kilocalories of energy per mole of the compound; SEE *high-energy phosphates*

high-energy phosphates phosphate compounds that upon hydrolysis release at least seven kilocalories of energy per mole of compound; examples: phosphate and mixed-phosphate anhydrides; SEE *high-energy compound*

high-energy solids or liquids substances whose molecules are held together by valent, covalent, coordinate covalent, hydrogen, and/or dipolar attractive bonds or forces; (pharmaceutically) ionic or dipolar nonionic, inorganic or organic, hydrophilic substances

high iso-elixir synonym for high isoalcoholic elixir

Higuchi, Takeru (1918-1987) a chemist by training, a pharmacy educator, and scientist; founder of the APhA Academy of Pharmaceutical Sciences; Remington Honor Medal recipient in 1983

Hill-Burton Act federal program that provides grants to states to construct new hospitals; initiated in 1946 and has since become a part of national health planning legislation (Public Law 93-641)

Hippocrates (ca. 460-370 B.C.) Greek physician known for his healing knowledge involving the "humors of the body"; writings attributed to him are in the *Hippocratic Corpus;* attributed to him as well is a medical oath, the Hippocratic Oath; the "Father of Medicine"

Hirschsprung's disease dilation of the colon causing obstruction at the rectum with resultant constipation and growth retardation

hirsutism an abnormal increase in body hair; the growth of hair in an abnormal place on the body, as in females who grow a beard, for example

histamine an endogenous amine resulting from the decarboxylation of histidine; hormone released in response to an antigen-antibody reaction

histidine a basic amino acid commonly found in proteins; precursor to histamine; 3-(3-imidazoyl)2-aminopropanoic acid; one of ten essential amino acids

histoplasmosis disease caused by the fungus *Histoplasma capsulatum;* may infect lungs, skin, mucous membranes, bones, skin, and eyes

Hodgkin's disease anemia lymphatica; also a term for lymphoma

hog gum SEE *tragacanth gum*

holoenzyme the complete enzyme; a combination of the apoenzyme and the coenzyme

holoprotein an apoprotein combined with its prosthetic group

home health care level of health services for the ill patient in the place of residence in lieu of more expensive care in a hospital; examples: total parenteral nutrition instead of kidney dialysis

homeopathy sect of medical practice proposed by the German physician Samuel C. Hahnemann (1755-1843), indicating that medications which produce symptoms in the body that mimic those of the disease are good for treating the disease, when used in minute doses and very finely divided

homeostasis tendency toward physiological stability; a condition of a dynamic equilibrium of the environment of the body

homogenize to reduce a substance to small particles of relatively uniform size and distribute them evenly, usually in a liquid; example: to break up the fat globules of milk into very fine particles by forcing it through minute openings

homologous polypeptide a protein molecule whose amino acid sequences and functions are similar to those of another protein

honeys obsolete dosage form that used honey as a base or vehicle for medications

Hoppe-Goldflam syndrome myasthenia gravis

hopper the container on a tablet machine that holds the material to be tableted

horizontal strip placement technique in which the products are placed in ascending size order from left to right; the leading brand is placed at eye level; a merchandising expression

hormone chemical secreted by a ductless gland that has a physiological effect on other parts of the body; a product of the endocrine system of the body that produces physiological effects on the body; many used as drugs to correct an abnormal or a deficiency condition; examples: adrenal cortex hormones, insulin, sex hormones

hormone response element a specific DNA sequence that binds hormone-receptor complexes; the binding of a hormone-receptor complex either enhances or diminishes the transcription of a specific gene

hospice program of supportive care for terminally ill persons and their families; care designed to make the patient comfortable and prepare the patient and family for the impending death

hospital institution for the medical and surgical treatment of the sick and injured

hospital affiliation a contractual relationship between a health plan and one or more hospitals whereby the hospital provides the inpatient benefits offered by the health plan

hospital alliance a group of voluntary hospitals that have joined together to reduce costs by sharing common services and developing group purchasing programs

Hubert H. Humphrey Award established by the American Pharmacists Association in 1978 to recognize major contributions in government or legislative service at the local, state, or national level

Huchard's disease essential hypertension

Hugo H. Schaefer Award established by the American Pharmacists Association in 1964 to recognize outstanding voluntary contributions to society, the profession of pharmacy, and the APhA

human risk management proactive service designed to reduce the demand for treatment by identifying, assessing, and managing individuals' medical or behavioral health risks before treatment becomes imperative

humectant substance that promotes the retention of moisture; used in pharmaceuticals to prevent drying

humidifier, impeller device for providing humidity to the home by immersing a rotating impeller in a reservoir of water which breaks water into small droplets

humidifier, ultrasonic device for providing humidity to the home through the use of an ultrasonic transducer that breaks water into a fine mist

humidity relative amount of water vapor present in a gas such as air; humidity control a vital consideration in pharmaceutical production and drug stability control

humidity, absolute weight of water vapor per unit weight of dry air

humidity, relative 100 times the ratio of the quantity of water vapor present in a gas to the saturation humidity amount at a given temperature; a condition of 50 percent relative humidity means a gas (such as earth's atmosphere) has one-half the water vapor it will hold at that temperature; quantitatively, relative humidity is the ratio of the partial pressure of water vapor in air to the vapor pressure of liquid water at the same temperature

humidity, saturation a condition in which air or another gas holds the maximum amount of water vapor; a condition in which the vapor pressure of water in a gas is equal to the vapor pressure of liquid water in the system

humoral immune response immunity that results from the presence of antibodies in blood and tissue fluid; also referred to as antibody-mediated immunity

humoral pathology medical practice theory attributed to Hippocrates indicating that the body consisted of four fluids (humors) that must be in balance to have good health; Galen systematized this theory as factual and made it the basis of medical practice for over a millennium

humors body liquids that were a part of the Hippocratic concept that the body consisted of four such liquids (blood, phlegm, yellow and black bile) called "humors"

Humphrey, Hubert Horatio (1911-1978) worked in his father's drugstore and became a pharmacist himself; was attracted early to politics and became the mayor of Minneapolis and later a U.S. Senator; was Vice President of the United States during Lyndon Johnson's presidency and unsuccessfully ran for president in 1968; co-author of the Durham-Humphrey Amendment

hybridization 1: phenomenon in which lower energy orbital electrons are slightly elevated to higher levels and correspondingly higher energy electrons assume a slightly lower level thereby forming a new energy level for all electrons involved in the shifts; an explanation of the tetravalency of carbon **2:** in genetics, the offspring of parents that are of different varieties or species **3:** a new DNA resulting from the insertion of a foreign segment (from another species) of DNA into the genome of an organism by recombinant DNA methods

hybridized orbital an electron orbital resulting from the mixing of individual atomic orbitals; important for the formation of molecular orbitals; examples: sp^3 hybridization—important to the chemistry of carbon and nitrogen; $d^2 sp^3$ hybridization—important in covalent metal complexes; sp^2 hybridization—important in ethylene; sp hybridization—important in acetylene

hybrid model HMO an HMO that combines attributes of more than one of the four principal HMO models and hence is not classifiable in any one of the four categories

hydr- prefix meaning water or hydrogen; same as hydro-

hydration a type of addition reaction in which water is added to a carbon-carbon double bond

hydro- prefix meaning water or hydrogen; same as hydr-

hydroalcoholic liquid composed of water and alcohol; may be combined in any proportion

hydrocarbon a molecule that contains only carbon and hydrogen

hydrocortisone nonprescription corticosteroid that is useful for minor medical conditions such as dermatitis, genital itching, hemorrhoids, insect stings, etc.

hydrodynamic theory theory presenting a possible mechanism through which teeth become hypersensitive

hydrogen gaseous element having an atomic weight of 1.008 and an atomic number equal to one; used in hydrogenation reactions; very flammable and highly explosive gas

hydrogenation reaction in which a reactant is reduced by the catalytic addition of molecular hydrogen to easily reducible groups such as across the carbon-carbon double bonds, the carbon-oxygen double bonds of ketones, and the carbon-nitrogen double bonds of imines

hydrogenolysis removal of a group from a compound by a reaction with hydrogen in the presence of a catalyst; a type of catalytic hydrogenation; example: debenzylation

hydrolase enzyme that catalyzes the removal of a group by use of water; examples: protease, esterase, carbohydrase

hydrolysate product of hydrolysis; example: protein hydrolysate

hydrolysis a chemical reaction that involves the reaction of a molecule with water; the process by which molecules are broken into their constituents by adding water

hydrometer a graduated floating cylinder used to indicate the specific gravity of liquids by sinking in a liquid to a depth corresponding to the specific gravity of the liquid

hydrophilic having an affinity for water

hydrophil-lipophil balance (HLB) relative expression of the degree of affinity a surfactant molecule has for oil and water; sometimes expressed as a weighted percentage of hydrophilic atoms in the molecule

hydrophobic lacking an affinity for water

hydrophobic bonding type of bonding in an enzyme-substrate or in a drug-drug receptor complex formation in which the water structure of the enzyme protein (the receptor) becomes less structured and shifts to other positions on the protein (or receptor) molecule; this entropy shift is the driving force for a perturbation (shape change) in the molecule

hydrotrophy increase in water solubility of various substances due to the presence of large amounts of additives

hydroxycobalamin   form of vitamin B_{12} in which a hydroxy group is bound to the central cobalt

hydroxylase   form of oxygenase that catalyzes the substitution of a hydroxyl group on a molecule

Hygeia   Greek goddess of health, daughter of Asklepios; symbolized by the bowl and serpent; modern symbol of pharmacy

hygrometer   device used to measure relative humidity by utilization of materials that change in dimensions or intensity with different humidity conditions; electric—uses changes in electrical resistance as humidity changes; mechanical—uses a substance that expands or shrinks with humidity change

hygroscopic   able to take up moisture readily and retain it; example: glycerin's ability to absorb moisture from the atmosphere

hyoscine   alkaloid obtained from *Atropa belladonna;* synonym: scopolamine

hyoscyamine   alkaloid obtained from plants in the family Solanaceae that acts pharmacologically as a parasympatholytic or an anticholinergic; a levo-rotatory isomer of atropine

hyper-   prefix meaning above, beyond, or excessive

hyperalimentation   usually refers to parenteral hyperalimentation (IVH) in which a concentrated solution of nutrients is introduced into a large vein such as the vena cava by means of a subclavian catheter; central IVH differs from central TPN by the presence of a fat emulsion in the formulation used for TPN

hyperammonemia   a potentially fatal elevation of the concentration of ammonium ions in the blood

hyperbilirubinemia   elevated bilirubin in the blood

hypercalcemia   elevated concentration of calcium or calcium-containing compounds in the blood; the normal level of calcium is 5 mEq/L serum or 10 mg/100 mL

hyperglycemia   blood glucose levels that are higher than normal

hyperkalemia   a condition in which the potassium level in the blood is abnormally high

hypermelanosis   excessive pigmentation of the skin

hyperosmolar   possessing an osmotic pressure greater than that of normal blood plasma

hyperosmolar hyperglycemic nonketosis severe dehydration in non-insulin dependent diabetics; caused by persistent high blood glucose levels

hyperoxaluria an excess of oxalate in the urine

hyperplasia excessive size of a tissue due to an increase in the number of cells

hyperpnea abnormal increase in the depth and rate of respiration

hyperpyremia elevation of body temperature over normal

hypersensitivity pneumonitis inflammatory condition of the airways; an infrequent consequence of using a poorly cleaned home humidifier

hypertension blood pressure that is elevated above the values considered normal (70-80 diastolic and 115-125 systolic)

hypertonic solution pertaining to an increased tonicity (internal pressure) or tension above that observed in normal body fluids; solution containing a greater number of dissolved particles per unit volume than in body fluids; CONTRAST *hypotonic solution*

hypertrichosis excessive growth of hair; example: a female using 5 percent minoxidil may experience hypertrichosis on the face or other areas

hypertrophy enlargement of a tissue due to an increase in the size of the cells

hyperuricemia higher than normal levels of uric acid and urates in the blood

hypno- prefix meaning sleep

hypnosis mental phenomenon manifested by a person's ability to respond to suggestions, provided that these do not seriously conflict with a person's beliefs

hypnotic a drug that produces sleep by depressing the CNS

hypo- prefix meaning below or less than normal

hypoalbuminemia lower than normal blood levels of albumin

hypochlorite salt of hypochlorous acid

hypochlorous acid compound of chlorine formed by the reaction of chlorine with water; a compound in which the chlorine has an oxidation number of +1

hypochromic effect the decrease in the absorption of UV light (260 nm) that occurs when purine and pyrimidine bases are incorporated into base pairs in polynucleotide sequences

hypodermic tablets SEE *tablet, compressed*

hypogeusia reduced taste sensation

hypoglycemia a condition in which the glucose level in the blood is abnormally low

hypoglycemic agent agent that acts to lower blood glucose level; used in adult-onset diabetes

hypokalemia abnormally low serum potassium

hypomania excited psychopathologic state between euphoria and mania

hyposalivation saliva production below the norm, resulting in xerostomia (dry mouth)

hypotension abnormally low blood pressure

hypotensive agent drug that lowers blood pressure

hypothermia state of a lower than normal body temperature; results in a decrease in metabolism of the body that decreases the need for oxygen; usually defined as body temperature below 95°F (35°C); a dangerous, potentially fatal condition in the elderly and the severely debilitated

hypotonic solution one that has a lower osmotic pressure than another solution (usually body fluid); CONTRAST *hypertonic solution*

hypovolemia abnormal decrease in the volume of blood in the body

hypoxanthine 6-oxypurine or 6-oxopurine; an intermediate in the metabolic degradation of purines to uric acid

hypoxanthine/guanine phosphoribosyl transferase enzyme responsible for the resynthesis of guanylic acid from guanine and phosphoribosyl pyrophosphate or inosinic acid from hypoxanthine and phosphoribosyl pyrophosphate; its absence a cause of some forms of gout and Lesch-Nyhan syndrome

hypoxia deficiency of oxygen

hysteresis loop the enclosed area in a thixotropic flow curve; the greater the area, the greater the degree of thixotropic breakdown; a consideration in suspension stability

-iasis suffix meaning condition of

iatrochemistry 1: medical science that conceived of the body as a chemical system that must be in balance for good health; initiated by Paracelsus and expanded by Helmont and Sylvius **2:** medicinal chemistry **3:** pharmaceutical chemistry

iatrogenic refers to a disorder caused by a physician's treatment

iatrogenic illness malady or adverse condition that results from the treatment given by a physician

iatrophysical concept of the body as a machine functioning according to mechanical theory

ICD-9 System SEE *International Classification of Diseases System;* SEE ALSO *International Classification of Diseases, Ninth Edition*

icthammol nonprescription chemical of unknown safety and efficacy once used to help resolve furuncles by brining them "to a point"

id in Freudian theory, the part of the personality encompassing instinctual desires; SEE ALSO *ego; superego*

ideal solution SEE *solution*

idio- prefix meaning separate or distinct from

idiopathic refers to an abnormal state of unknown cause

idiosyncrasy an abnormal response or habit that is peculiar to an individual

ileus an obstruction of the bowel due to either motility dysfunction or mechanical blockage

imide chemical compound that contains a nitrogen atom bonded between two carbon atoms, each of which is double-bonded to oxygen atoms

immiscible term to describe two or more liquids that form different layers when placed in the same system; liquids that do not mix easily

immunity ability of the body to resist invasion by foreign organisms or materials and/or to overcome infection

immunity, active type of immunity the body develops by forming its own antibodies against a specific disease

immunity, passive type of immunity in which the antibodies are made in one individual and then transferred to another person to be immunized

immunoglobulin A (IgA) a secretory antibody having an alpha type of heavy globulin and kappa or lambda light chains

immunoglobulin D (IgD) a type of antibody with delta heavy chains and kappa or lambda light chains

immunoglobulin E (IgE) a type of antibody involved in allergies that contains epsilon heavy chains and kappa or lambda light chains

immunoglobulin G (IgG) the most common type of antibody against infectious diseases; contains gamma heavy chains and kappa or lambda light chains

immunoglobulin M (IgM) a macroglobulin type of antibody against infectious diseases that contains mu-type heavy chains and kappa or lambda light chains

immunosuppressive agent a substance that supresses or interferes with the normal immune response

impaction 1: deposition of particles as a result of their lack of momentum in the respiratory tract **2:** a basic mechanism for particle size reduction

impaction, fecal hardened stool caused by failure to ingest sufficient water and/or fiber; stool eventually becomes dessicated and difficult to evacuate

impairment any loss or abnormality of psychological, physiological, or anatomical structure or function

impalpable incapable of being felt by touch; example: finely powdered talc cannot be felt when rubbed between the fingers

impeller mass transfer device that is part of mixing or transporting equipment; examples: propeller, blade, baffle, paddle

impeller humidifier device for increasing humidity in the house or workplace; functions by means of a rapidly rotating hollow spindle immersed in a reservoir of water; water is thrown with force against a screen, breaking it into fine particles that enter room air

impetiginization self-infection of the skin caused by compulsive scratching at the skin with unclean fingernails

impetigo mixed staphylococcal/streptococcal infection of the skin; requires prescription antibiotics for resolution

implant small, sterile, solid masses for placement in the body to provide a continuous release of medicine over time

implant dentistry dental practice involving the replacement of one or more teeth in their natural receptacle (gum and jawbone cavity)

impotence inability of the male to successfully complete sexual intercourse

impulse sales unplanned purchases; purchase decisions made by customers while in the pharmacy in reaction to display items

in situ 1: in the normal place; restricted to an original site without affecting surrounding tissue **2:** chemical term meaning at the time and place of a reaction

in vitro in glass or outside the living body and in an artificial environment

in vivo in the living body of an animal or plant

inborn error of metabolism genetic disease in which there is an absence of a specific enzyme

incidence (epidemiology) measure of the number of new cases of illness or other forms of morbidity over a particular period of time for a given population

incident report written summary of an action taken that was harmful or that did not fulfill a doctor's orders

inclusion compound physical entrapment of molecules of one substance within lattice structures of larger molecules; a type of complexation; synonym: occlusion compound

income statement periodic financial statement that is a summary of revenues (sales), expenses, and net income of a business for a given period of time; synonym: profit and loss statement

incompatible **1:** antagonistic **2:** unsuitable for use together because of undesirable physical, chemical, or physiological effects **3:** incapable of blending into a stable mixture; example: immiscibility of oil and water

incontinence inability to control one's urination or defecation

incontinent unable to contain or retain; example: urinary incontinence

incurred but not reported costs associated with a medical service that has been provided, but for which a claim has not yet been received by the carrier

incurred claims actual carrier liability for a specified period, including all claims with dates of service within a specified period

incurred claims loss ratio the result of incurred claims divided by premiums

indefinite integral SEE *integration*

indemnity an insurance program in which the insured person is reimbursed for covered expenses after services are rendered

independent medical evaluation (IME) an examination carried out by an impartial health care provider, generally board certified, for the purpose of resolving a dispute related to the nature and extent of an illness or injury

independent practice association SEE *individual practice association*

independent practice organization/network a group of independent medical providers that contracts services to managed care plans

independent professional review peer review of medical services by a health team member not directly involved in the services provided to Medicare or Medicaid patients in long-term care facilities

independent variable the part of a mathematical expression that is changed arbitrarily to elicit a response in another variable; CONTRAST *dependent variable*

indeterminate errors random errors that cannot be readily ascertained due to their fluctuation around the true value; errors that lend themselves to statistical methods in that they follow probability laws

Indian Health Service a division of the U.S. Public Health Service; responsible for enhancing and providing health care for native Americans

indigenous native, or not exotic; native to a particular place

indirect costs in pharmacoeconomics, earnings lost because of death or temporary/permanent disability occurring because of illness (as derived from the human capital valuation approach)

indirect dryer drying instrument in which heat is transferred through a separating wall; vapor removal without actual contact with the heat source

indirect expenses expenses (variable or fixed) shared or consumed jointly by both prescription and nonprescription departments; examples: utilities, salaries, advertising

individual practice association a health care model that contracts with physicians and other community health care providers to provide services in return for a negotiated fee

induced dipole–induced dipole interactions SEE *London forces*

inducible gene a gene expressed only under certain conditions

induction 1: enzymatic process by which an inherent part of an enzyme may increase the activity of that enzyme by increasing its biosynthesis **2:** scientific reasoning process in which new concepts are derived by intuition and analogy

induction effect weak attractive forces between molecules involving a dipolar compound that induces polarization in another molecule as it is brought into close proximity to the dipolar compound

inductive effects electronic repulsions or attractions caused by bound atoms and groups within molecules; example: chloroacetic acid is stronger than acetic acid and both lactic acid and alanine are stronger than propionic acid due to electron withdrawing effects by groups substituted adjacent to the carboxyl group

induration being hard or sclerosed; usually in reference to a spot or small area

-ine   **1:** suffix meaning an acetylene or triple-bonded hydrocarbon **2:** ending for alkaloids and the amine compounds

inebriate to intoxicate; to make drunk

inebriation state of being intoxicated or drunk

infarct area of necrosis due to ischemia resulting from a blockage of circulation to that area

infarction formation of an infarct, which is a circumscribed necrosis of tissue due to a deprivation of its blood supply

infectious hepatitis SEE *hepatitis, infectious*

inflammable capable of burning or catching on fire; synonym: flammable

inflammation a generally protective response by body tissues to damage or presence of a foreign material; characterized by pain, redness, a rise in the temperature of the affected part or parts, and swelling; generally initiates the repair process by diluting and opposing the effects of the injury

informed consent rule that patients must be fully informed about the benefits and risks of participating in a clinical trial, taking a medication, or electing to have a medical procedure; a disclosure that is followed by patients' autonomous consent

infra- prefix meaning below or under

infrared dryer instrument or apparatus using radiant heat (in the red light spectrum) for the purpose of removing moisture or dampness

infrared heating heat transferred by thermal waves (thermal radiation) of the infrared spectrum

infrared light electromagnetic radiation emanating from molecular vibrations; wavelengths are in the range of 10^{-6} to 10^{-3} meters (longer than visible light); electromagnetic radiation in the frequency range just below the visible spectrum

infrared spectrophotometer an instrument used to measure the absorbance of varying frequencies of infrared light as it passes through a sample being analyzed

infrared spectrophotometry SEE *spectrophotometry*

infrared spectrum plot of the absorbance (or percent transmittance) of a compound at different wave lengths in the infrared region

infusion 1: an aqueous solution of the active ingredients of vegetable drugs prepared by soaking the drug in hot water and straining (the same procedure used in making hot tea) **2:** process of administering a liquid into the vascular system of the body by allowing it to enter at a rate determined by the force of gravity

inhalant special class of drugs that, by virtue of their high vapor pressure, can be carried by an air current into the nasal passage where they exert their effect; generally administered from a container known as an inhaler

inhalation a drug or a solution of a drug administered by the nasal or oral respiratory route for local or systemic effect; act of breathing in

inhibition the slowing of an enzyme reaction by the interference of a compound known as the inhibitor

inhibition, competitive type of inhibition in which the inhibitor competes with the substrate for the active site of the enzyme; inhibition that can be reversed by increasing the concentration of the substrate

inhibition, noncompetitive type of inhibition in which the inhibitor interacts with the enzyme at a site that is different from the active site, or in a manner that is different from that of the substrate; inhibition that cannot be reversed by increasing the concentration of the substrate

inhibitor substance that slows the rate of an enzyme reaction; a drug that slows an enzyme reaction

inhibitor, competitive substance that slows an enzyme reaction through an interaction with the enzyme that is competitive with substrate binding

inhibitor, noncompetitive substance that slows an enzyme reaction through an interaction with the enzyme in a different site from the active site or by binding in a different manner from that of the substrate

initial dose first dose of a multiple dose regimen of treatment; also called "priming dose" or "loading dose"

initial eligibility period period of time specified in a contract during which eligible persons may enroll themselves and dependents under the health plan, usually without providing evidence of good health

initial enrollment period beginning dates when one may choose to participate in a group insurance plan

initiation the beginning phase of translation

injection 1: sterile solution, suspension, or emulsion suitable for parenteral administration **2:** the act of placing a liquid into a part of the body; example: parenteral administration of a solution into the blood through venous puncture; categorized into five distinct classes, as defined by the *USP*

injection, emulsion a two-phase system in which one liquid is dispersed throughout another liquid in the form of small droplets; consists of a sterile, pyrogen-free preparation intended to be administered parenterally

injection, powder, for solution sterile preparation intended for reconstitution to form a solution for parenteral use

injection, powder, for suspension sterile preparation intended for reconstitution to form a suspension for parenteral use

injection, powder, for suspension, extended release sterile, freeze-dried preparation intended for reconstitution to form a suspension for parenteral use; formulated in a manner to allow at least a reduction in dosing frequency as compared to that drug presented as a conventional dosage form (e.g., as a solution)

injection, powder, lyophilized, for liposomal suspension sterile, freeze-dried preparation intended for reconstitution for parenteral use; formulated in a manner that would allow liposomes (a lipid bilayer vesicle usually composed of phospholipids that is used to encapsulate an active drug substance, either within a lipid bilayer or in an aqueous space) to be formed upon reconstitution

injection, powder, lyophilized, for solution dosage form intended for the solution prepared by lyophilization (freeze-drying), a process that involves the removal of water from products in the frozen state at extremely low pressures; intended for subsequent addition of liquid to create a solution that conforms in all respects to the requirements for injections

injection, powder, lyophilized, for suspension liquid preparation intended for parenteral use that contains solids suspended in a suitable fluid medium and conforms in all respects to the requirements for sterile suspensions; prepared by lyophilization (freeze-drying), a process that involves the removal of water from products in the frozen state at extremely low pressures

injection, powder, lyophilized, for suspension, extended release sterile, freeze-dried preparation intended for reconstitution for parenteral use; formulated in a manner to allow at least a reduction in dosing frequency as compared to that drug presented as a conventional dosage form (e.g., as a solution)

injection, solution liquid preparation containing one or more drug substances dissolved in a suitable solvent or mixture of mutually miscible solvents that is suitable for injection

injection, solution, concentrate sterile preparation for parenteral use that, upon the addition of suitable solvents, yields a solution conforming in all respects to the requirements for injections

injection, suspension liquid preparation, suitable for injection, that consists of solid particles dispersed throughout a liquid phase in which the particles are not soluble; can also consist of an oil phase dispersed throughout an aqueous phase, or vice versa

injection, suspension, extended release sterile preparation intended for parenteral use; formulated in a manner to allow at least a reduction in dosing frequency as compared to that drug presented as a conventional dosage form (e.g., as a solution or a prompt drug-releasing, conventional solid dosage form)

injection, suspension, liposomal liquid preparation, suitable for injection, that consists of an oil phase dispersed throughout an aqueous phase in such a manner that liposomes (a lipid bilayer vesicle usually composed of phospholipids that is used to encapsulate an active drug substance, either within a lipid bilayer or in an aqueous space) are formed

injection, suspension, sonicated liquid preparation, suitable for injection, that consists of solid particles dispersed throughout a liquid phase in which the particles are not soluble; in addition, the product is sonicated while a gas is bubbled through the suspension, resulting in the formation of microspheres by the solid particles

injury physiological damage other than sickness, including all related conditions and recurrent symptoms

inner membrane the innermost membrane of mitochondria

innocuous harmless

inoculation 1: administration of an attenuated or killed pathogen to elicit an immune response by the body **2:** introduction of infectious materials into a culture medium to grow a disease-causing organism for purpose of study or further processing

inophore a substance that transports cations across membranes

inorganic refers to nonliving materials

inosine 1: compound (glycoside) that contains a sugar (ribose) and hypoxanthine **2:** compound formed by removing phosphate from inosinic acid

inotropic to influence the force of muscular contraction

inpatient person who is admitted to a hospital for medical treatment or observation and receives services under the direction of a physician

inscription the main part of the prescription containing the names and quantities of the prescribed drugs; synonym: body of the prescription; SEE ALSO *prescription*

insert vaginal suppository compressed as an oval tablet; used for local vaginal infections or other vaginal disorders

insert, extended release specially formulated and shaped solid preparation (e.g., ring, tablet, or stick) intended to be placed in the vagina by special inserters, where the medication is released, generally for localized effects; designed to allow a reduction in dosing frequency

insoluble soap a calcium, zinc, or magnesium salt of a fatty acid; CONTRAST *soluble soap*

insomnia sleeplessness, insomnolence, or wakefulness

inspection a visual examination to detect errors, contamination, or inappropriate procedures

inspissated juice a semiliquid prepared by expressing fresh plant tissue to remove and then concentrate the juice

institutional ad advertisement that focuses on only the name and prestige of a company, industry, or profession

insufflate fine powder packaged so that it can be blown into a cavity of the body

insufflation the blowing of a powder into a body cavity

insufflator device used to blow a powder, vapor, or gas into a body cavity

insulation a substance that exhibits a low level of conductivity of heat and/or electricity

insulin a peptide hormone (contains 51 amino acids and has a minimum molecular weight of 6,000) that is secreted into the blood by the beta cells of islets of Langerhans of the pancreas and acts to lower blood sugar levels through a variety of mechanisms; a peptide hormone product obtained from porcine pancreas or from *Escherichia coli* by recombinant DNA techniques and administered to diabetics to lower blood sugar level

insulin-like growth factor a protein in humans that mediates the growth-promoting actions of growth hormone; has insulin-like properties (i.e., promotes glucose transport and fat synthesis)

insulinopenic a type of diabetes mellitus in which there is a deficit of insulin levels in the blood; subclasses are juvenile-onset diabetes and brittle-adult diabetes

insulinoplethoric a form of diabetes mellitus in which the blood levels of insulin are either normal or elevated; synonyms: adult-onset diabetes, mild maturity-onset diabetes

integrated behavioral health benefit plan that combines independent managed care services as a seamless delivery system for behavioral health concerns

integrated delivery system a joint effort of physicians and hospitals for a variety of purposes

integrated pharmacologic response a measure of the total pharmacologic response expressed as a product of duration and intensity of drug action over a period of time

integrated provider organization a corporate umbrella for the management of a diversified health care delivery system

integration mathematical operation (calculus) for determination of the summation of the effects of a series of infinitesimal changes or changes between arbitrary limits; examples: the total amount of drug absorbed from time zero to infinity or between time zero and some specified time, the latter, a definite integral, and the former, an indefinite integral

integration rules several respective procedures for integrating specific types of algebraic equations

integrity test scientifically developed questionnaire that provides an employer with an indication of a job applicant's attitude toward theft and other crimes

integumentary relating to the skin; a covering; synonyms: cutaneous, dermal

intein excised peptide segment generated during protein splicing

intensity of segregation a "degree of mixing" expression based on variation in composition of various portions of the mixture

intensive care hospital services prescribed by a physician for individuals with serious medical conditions and delivered under the guidance of a registered nurse

intention tremor tremor that is intensified when a voluntary movement is attempted

inter- prefix meaning between

intercept **1:** usually the y-intercept; that value of the dependent variable (y) when the independent variable (x) equals zero **2:** the intersection of one plot with another plot or one of the axes, or a case in which one of the variables of an equation equals zero

interfacial tension used to express liquid-liquid boundary tension; CONTRAST *surface tension*

interferon one of a group of glycoproteins produced and released by cells in reponse to an invasion of cells by viruses; noninfected cells exposed to interferon become immune to infection by viruses

intermediary letter statement from the Bureau of Insurance to the fiscal administrators (intermediaries) of Medicare regarding policy for the program

intermediate care facility a facility offering a level of care that is less than the degree of care and treatment provided by a hospital or skilled nursing facility (SNF) but greater than that given by an assisted-living facility

internal energy that amount of energy in a system not manifested as "work"

internal medicine medical speciality involving the diagnosis and non-surgical treatment of disorders of internal organs

internal phase the dispersed phase of an emulsion's internal pressure; attractive forces between molecules of gases, liquids, and solids

International Classification of Diseases, **Ninth Revision,** *Clinical Modification* **(ICD-9-CM)** a listing of diagnoses and identifying codes used for reporting diagnoses of health plan enrollees; SEE ALSO *International Classification of Diseases System*

International Classification of Diseases System a diagnosis and procedure coding system for hospital care; SEE ALSO *International Classification of Diseases, Ninth Edition*

International System of Units (SI) accepted international system of basic units of measure; also known as "Le Systéme International d'Unités"

interproximal space between teeth that cannot normally be cleaned by a toothbrush and requires dental flossing

interstitial related to or situated within the space that is within an organ, cell, or crystal

interstitial fluid the fluid containing dissolved salts and protein found in the tissues between the cells; synonym: extracellular fluid

interstitial water water held mechanically in the crevice or lattice of a crystal; CONTRAST *water of crystallization*

intertriginous skin body areas where opposing skin surfaces remain in contact with each other for long periods of time, preventing evaporation of sweat and causing an increased incidence of fungal infection (e.g., athlete's foot between the toes, tinea cruris in the groin)

intra- prefix meaning within

intra-arterial into an artery; example: injection of a drug into an artery

intra-arterial injection administration of a medication by injection directly into an artery using a needle and syringe

intra-articular administration of a drug by injection into a joint

intracardiac administration of a drug by injection into the heart

intracisternal within the caudal region between the cerebellum and the medulla oblongata

intracisternal injection administration of a drug by injection into one of the cisternae of the brain or the enlarged subarachnoid space between the undersurface of the cerebellum and the posterior surface of the medulla oblongata

intracutaneous injection SEE *intradermal injection*

intradermal between the layers of skin

intradermal injection route of administration involving injection between the epidermal layers of the skin

intramuscular into a skeletal muscle

intramuscular injection process of administering a medication by injection into a muscle using a needle and syringe

intraocular into the eye

intraosseous into a bone

intraperitoneal administration of a medication by injection into the peritoneal cavity using a needle and syringe

intraspinal administration injection of substances into the spinal column

intrasynovial into the joint fluid

intrathecal into the cerebral spinal column by way of the subarachnoid space at the base of the spine

intrathecal injection process of administering a medication by injecting it through the theca of the spinal cord into the subarachnoid space using a needle and syringe

intrauterine device device inserted and left in the uterus to prevent conception

intravenous into a vein

intravenous additives therapeutic agents that are added to large-volume intravenous solutions of nutrients or electrolytes for purposes of administering both at the same injection site

intravenous admixture a combination of two parenteral preparations for intravenous administration at the same time using the same device or setup; prepared just before administration to patient

intravenous piggyback small-volume intravenous infusion (usually 25-100 mL), usually administered through a *y*-site on the primary infusion set

intravenous push to inject a medication directly from a syringe into a vein

intrinsic occurring within

intrinsic activity amount or degree of response initiated as a result of a drug-receptor interaction; ability of a drug to initiate a response as a result of a receptor interaction

intrinsic factor substance found in both animal and human intestine that increases absorption of vitamin B_{12}

intro- a prefix meaning in or into

intron the DNA sequence interrupting the protein coding sequence of a gene

inunction SEE *ointment*

inventory **1:** items that a business has available for sale **2:** a determination of the number and value of items in a business available for sale

inventory turnover rate the ratio of cost of goods sold to average inventory; an index of efficiency of purchasing and inventory control

invert sugar an equimolar mixture of glucose and fructose such as that obtained by the hydrolysis of sucrose

investigational drug a compound that is still being researched by the manufacturer and has not been approved by the FDA for use in the general treatment of patients

invoice dating the time during which payment will enable the business to receive a discount; the time when payment of the invoice is due and thereafter any discounts will be nullified

iodide a salt of iodine

iodimetry a procedure used in quantitative chemical analysis in which a standard solution of iodine is used as a titrant in the determination of reducing agents such as thiosulfate and arsenite

iodine dark grayish, volatile, solid element that produces violent, pungent vapors upon heating; one of two solid halogens; compounds used in treating iodine deficiency, and the pure form as a local antiseptic

iodine value number of grams of iodine that reacts with 100 grams of fat or other unsaturated organic material

iodometry procedure used in quantitative chemical analysis of oxidizing agents in which iodine is released from an iodide (such as potassium iodide) by the oxidizing agent, then titrated with a standard sodium thiosulfate solution to a starch test solution end point

iodotherapy use of iodine and iodides as remedies

ion a charged atom or a group of atoms (chemical radical)

ion-dipole interaction attractive forces between an ionic species and a polar solvent in which oppositely charged parts of each become intimately associated; example: dissolving sodium chloride in water

ion exchange chromatography a type of chromatography utilizing anionic and/or cationic exchange resins to remove dissolved ions and/or to separate or purify a particular chemical entity

ion exchange, diffusion controlled a drug delivery system using ionic resins to effect sustained drug release from its dosage form; example: biphetamine resin in capsule form

ionic activity concentration of an ion corrected for interactions between ions in the system; synonym: effective ion concentration; SEE *Debye-Huckel theory*

ionic bond electrostatic holding together of two or more atoms to form a molecule; bond resulting from an attraction of a positive ion for a negative ion

ionic strength SEE *Debye-Huckel theory*

ion–induced dipole interactions attractive forces between homopolar molecules and ions brought about by an ionic species inducing polarization in an otherwise nonpolar molecule; example: the solubilization of iodine in a concentrated solution of potassium iodide

ionization chamber enclosure on which a fixed potential is applied between its electrodes; used to calibrate a radioactive source

ionization constant equilibrium constant for the dissociation of a weak electrolyte; examples: ionization constants for a weak base (Kb) and a weak acid (Ka); SEE *dissociation constant*

ionization potential energy required to remove an electron from an atomic orbital to the point where the atomic nucleus has no influence on its movement or position in space

ion trapping process by which a drug is trapped within a compartment of the body as a result of its high degree of ionization

ipecac the dried rhizomes and roots of *Cephaelis ipecacuanha* that contain the emetic alkaloids emetine and cephaeline, used to induce vomiting

iron a grayish silver, malleable, metallic element

iron deficiency anemia lower than normal red blood cell count due to a lack of iron in the diet or excessive loss of blood

irradiated ergosterol vitamin D_2 or ergocalciferol

irrational numbers numbers that cannot be expressed as integers or as a quotient of two integers

irreversibility (of a dispersion) lack of the ability to easily restore a dispersed system after the dispersion medium has been removed from the dispersed particles, due to the need for extensive processing and considerable energy input

irrigant sterile solution intended to bathe or flush open wounds or body cavities; used topically, never parenterally

irrigating solution a sterile solution, usually aqueous, used to wash sensitive or wounded body tissues

irrigation fluid solution (usually prepared under aseptic conditions) used to wash a body cavity or wound

ischemia lack of blood supply to an area of body tissue, due to a narrowing or obstruction of a blood vessel; example: coronary artery occlusion

-ism suffix meaning condition of or state

iso- prefix meaning equal or alike

isobaric having the same barometric pressure

isobars nuclides having the same mass but different atomic numbers

isoelectric denotes compounds that are similar physically, as well as having the same electrical charge

isoelectric point the pH of an amphoteric molecule at which there are equal positive and negative charges on amino acids, proteins, phospholipids, or other molecules that possess both acidic and basic groups and the pH of an amino acid solution in which zwitterions exist; usually a pH at which an ampholyte has lowered aqueous solubility

isoenzyme an enzyme catalyzing the same biochemical reaction as another enzyme, but has a different electrophoretic mobility; synonym: isozyme

isoionic point condition in a system in which the pH is adjusted to yield (1) an equal number of cations and anions on the side chains of the amino acid protein residues and (2) an equal number of adsorbed cations and anions

isoleucine branched chain amino acid commonly found in proteins; one of the ten essential amino acids; positional isomer of leucine; α-L-amino-3-methylpentanoic acid

isomerase an enzyme that catalyzes the change of one isomer into another; examples: *cis-trans* isomerase, epimerase, D- or L-amino acid racemase and mutase

isomerization the reversible interconversion of isomers

isomers distinctly different compounds that possess the same empirical formula, but different chemical and physical properties; examples: positional (structural) isomers, stereoisomers, *cis-trans* (geometric) isomers, optical (mirror image) isomers, diastereoisomers; SEE *cis-trans isomer; diastereoisomers; optical isomers; positional isomers; stereoisomers*

isometric 1: describes a process occurring at constant pressure **2:** pharmacological measurement using muscle tissue that is maintained at a constant length

isonicotinic acid an isomer of nicotinic acid in which the carboxyl group is substituted on the pyridine ring at a position opposite the ring nitrogen

isoprene hydrocarbon containing five carbon atoms and two double bonds, four of the carbon atoms within a linear chain and the fifth carbon branched off the second carbon of the chain; synonym: 2-methylbutadiene; a molecular component of vitamins D, E, and K

isoquinoline heterocyclic, aromatic, naphthalene-like compound possessing a nitrogen in the 2-position

isostere a molecule that has the same size, shape, and polarity of another molecule; biological—a compound having similar physiological properties to another compound; physical—a compound having similar physical properties to another compound

isosteric group a group or radical on a molecule that has the same size, shape, and polarity as another group

isosterism condition in which two or more molecules possess similar size, shape, and electronic distribution; biological—having similar biological properties; synonym: bioisosterism; physical—having similar physical properties; example: benzene and thiophene

isothermal refers to a process occurring at constant temperature

isotonic refers to a solution that has the same number of dissolved particles as another solution; having the same tone or the same internal pressure; refers to a solution that has the same number of dissolved particles as body fluids (blood, tears, nasal secretions)

isotonicity condition of a solution having the same tone (internal pressure) as body fluids

isotopes two atoms having the same atomic number but different atomic weights

isotropic exhibiting similar physical properties in all directions; examples: cubic crystals, amorphous compounds

isozyme one of two or more forms of the same enzyme activity with different amino acid dequences

-itis suffix meaning inflammation

J

Jakob-Creutzfeldt disease progressive encephalopathy believed caused by a slow virus; synonym: Creutzfeldt-Jakob disease

Jarisch-Herxheimer reaction characteristic response that frequently occurs in a patient being treated for syphilis with penicillin G; commonly involves exacerbation of existing syphilitic lesions, headache, chills, fever, malaise, sore throat, and tachycardia

jaundice an accumulation of bilirubin in the blood with deposition in the skin that imparts a yellow or golden hue; prehepatic—caused by hemolysis; synonym: hemolytic jaundice; hepatic—occurring with liver damage; synonym: hepatitis; posthepatic—occurring as a result of a blocking of the bile ducts; example: gallstones

Jelliffe method a method for determining creatinine clearance

jelly 1: class of gels in which the matrix contains a high proportion of water or other liquid **2:** thick semisolid gelatinous mass intended to be taken orally; used externally or in body orifices

jelly, mineral petroleum jelly petrolatum

Jesuit's bark cinchona bark; source of quinine

jet ejector pump that utilizes a high-velocity stream of fluid to effect mass transfer of a liquid

jet lag condition resulting from crossing time zones rapidly, resulting in time-phase shift

J. Leon Lascoff Memorial Award established in 1944 by the American College of Apothecaries honoring an individual who has made significant contributions to professional pharmacy

John W. Dargavel Medal established by the NARD Foundation to honor sustained contributions on behalf of independent pharmacy

Joint Commission on Accreditation of Health Care Organizations (JCAHO) a private, not-for-profit organization that evaluates and accredits hospitals and other health care organizations providing home, mental health, ambulatory, and long-term care services

journal 1: record of business transactions in order as they occur **2:** periodical publication that contains papers reporting the results of scientific investigations and/or professional innovations and news

jurisprudence system of law

justify 1: to adjust the printing positions of characters on a page so that the lines have the desired length and both the left- and right-hand margins are regular **2:** by extension, to shift the contents of a register so that the most or the least significant digit is at some specified position in the register

Kahler's disease multiple myeloma

kaliuresis increased excretion of potassium

kaolin fine, usually white clay used as an adsorbent and filler; synonym: native hydrated aluminum silicate

karaya gum SEE *sterculia gum*

Kasabach-Merritt syndrome hemangioma-thrombocytopenia syndrome

Kathabar system system of air cleaning in aseptic areas that involves washing the air with an antiseptic solution to remove dirt and microorganisms and to control humidity

Kawasaki's syndrome febrile illness of unknown etiology occurring mainly in children under five years

Kefauver-Harris Amendment 1962 amendment to the Federal Food, Drug, and Cosmetic Act that required drug manufacturers to prove effectiveness (in addition to safety) of their products and to properly advertise prescription drugs

Kelly, Evander Francis (1879-1944) educator at the University of Maryland College of Pharmacy 1903-1926; APhA treasurer from 1918 to 1926 when he was elected the secretary and served until his death; Remington Honor Medal recipient 1933

Keobnerization or Koebner phenomenon phenomenon in which a medical condition occurs anew at the point of injury; example: appearance of new psoriasis lesions or warts in damaged skin

kerato- prefix meaning cornea, or horny tissue

keratolytic agent that loosens keratin and facilitates desquamation; example: salicylic acid in collodion or patch dosage forms

keratoses, solar epidermal lesions in which the upper layer of skin has hypertrophied due to chronic sun exposure

keratosis growth of horny tissue; example: callous

ketal the family of organic compounds with the general formula $RR'C(OR')_2$; formed from reaction of a hemiketal with an alcohol

ketoacidosis acidosis caused by an excessive accumulation of ketone bodies

ketogenesis excess acetyl-CoA molecules are converted to acetoacetate, β-hydroxybutyrate, and acetone, known as the ketone bodies

ketogenic amino acid a molecule whose carbon skeleton is a substrate for synthesizing fatty acids and ketone bodies

ketone carbonyl compound containing a carbon atom double bonded to an oxygen atom and bonded to two other carbon atoms

ketone body acetone, acetoacetate, or β-hydroxybutyrate; produced in the liver from acetyl-CoA

ketosis accumulation of ketone bodies in blood and tissues

kettle large-volume container with an immersion or a jacketed heating source used to heat and/or mix large quantities of liquid or semisolid formulations

Kick's theory quantitative expression for estimating the energy requirement for particle size reduction, which is directly related to the initial and ending diameters of particles being reduced in size

kieselguhr SEE *diatomaceous earth*

kilo- prefix meaning 1,000-fold or 1,000 times a specified basic unit of measure; example: 1 kilogram equals 1,000 grams

Kimmelstiel-Wilson disease glomerulosclerosis (scarring within the kidney glomeruli)

kinase enzyme catalyzing the formation of a phosphate ester; synonyms: phosphotransferase, phosphorylase

kinetic energy energy due to motion; example: molecular vibration causing diffusion and vapor pressure

kinetics the study of reaction rates

kinin endogenous peptide that acts on plasma proteins, blood vessels, smooth muscles, and nerve endings, causing dilation of the blood vessels and inflammation of the surrounding tissue

kit packaged collection of related material

Klein-Levin syndrome periodic attacks of sleep and hunger with amnesia for periods of the attacks; related to narcolepsy

Köhler's disease aseptic necrosis of the navicular bone

Krebs bicycle a biochemical pathway in which the aspartate required in the urea cycle is generated from oxaloacetate, an intermediate in the citric acid cycle

Krebs urea cycle the cyclic pathway that converts waste ammonia molecules along with CO_2 and aspartate into urea; named for its discoverer, Hans Krebs

Kremers, Edward (1865-1941) educator at the University of Wisconsin from 1890 to 1935; credited with the institution of the first four-credit course of study of pharmacy in the United States and the first PhD in pharmacy; an American pharmacy historian; co-author (with George Urdang) of *Kremers and Urdang's History of Pharmacy;* Remington Honor Medal recipient in 1930.

Kremers Award established by the American Institute of the History of Pharmacy in 1961 for original and scholarly publication on the history of pharmacy written by an American

kwashiorkor deficiency of protein that causes stunted growth, retardation, edema, and changes in the liver, hair, and skin; CONTRAST *marasmus*

L- or l- prefix designating stereochemical configuration (Fisher Convention) in which the last asymmetric carbon from the most oxidized (placed at the top of the molecular structure) has the group that is used to designate configuration on the lefthand side of the structure

label 1: usually a piece of paper inscribed with certain information and affixed to a container **2:** written or printed matter accompanying a drug product

label, auxiliary or strip brief warning or special instruction affixed to a prescription container to ensure appropriate use

label contraindication an absolute prohibition to the use of the drug; example: oral contraceptives should not be used in patients with a history of thromboembolytic disorders

label precaution a less-restrictive alert to health professionals; example: with any potent drug, periodic assessment of renal, hepatic, and hematopoietic function should be performed

label warning information used to alert health professionals to certain dangers or restrictions in the use of certain drugs; example: the use of estrogens has been reported to increase the risk of endometrial cancer

labeling written, printed, or graphic material that accompanies an article (drug product) while it is being shipped or held for resale; examples: package insert, information affixed to a container or a dosage unit

labile unstable; example: heat labile (unstable in the presence of heat)

lacerate to tear, rend, or cut

laceration wound

lachrymal pertaining to tears or tear-producing glands

lacrimation tear secretion or the discharge of tears

lactam cyclic amide found in many antibiotics; SEE *beta-lactamase*

lactase persistence term used for individuals who maintain lactase production as adults, and are thus able to ingest dairy products such as milk and cheese

lactate a salt or ester of lactic acid; example: sodium lactate, which has the formula $CH_3H(OH)COONa$

lactated Ringer's injection sterile solution of Ringer's injection and sodium lactate

lactation secretion of milk; breast-feeding

lactic acid a product of the fermentation of milk

lactobionate a salt or an ester that is derived from lactobionic acid

lactone cyclic ester; example: angelica lactone in digitalis glycosides

lactose disaccharide sugar ($C_{12}H_{22}O_{11}$) present in milk that, on hydrolysis, yields glucose and galactose; used as a diluent; synonym: milk sugar

lactose intolerance condition in which the patient cannot ingest lactose without experiencing troubling gastrointestinal symptoms (e.g., diarrhea, bloating); may be primary (due to the natural loss of lactase with aging) or secondary (due to any disease or medication that temporarily or permanently destroys the lactase-producing microvilli of the small intestine)

lag phenomenon occurring in a plot of the time-dependent rise in a measurable parameter such as in a drug plasma concentration curve not passing through the origin; synonym: yield value

lag time time after administration of a drug until its action(s) is (are) manifested; SEE ALSO *latent period; onset time*

lamel or lamella minute glycerol-gelatin discs medicated for use in the eyes

laminar flow 1: streamlined movement of a liquid or air (gas) **2:** the act of moving in a straight path as approximated in a laminar (air) flow hood **3:** liquid movement exhibiting a low Reynolds number; CONTRAST *turbulent flow*

laminar flow hood an enclosure with an open front and streamlined airflow that enters through an absolute filter, providing an environment in which one may perform aseptic techniques in an airflow of 90 ± 20 feet per minute

laminar mixing process of maximizing contact between different substances using straightline or streamline motion; used for combining highly viscous materials such as ointments and creams

laminated coating application of a series of layers of coating to control drug availability and/or site of dissolution in the gastrointestinal tract

lamination separation of a tablet into two or more distinct layers; an undesirable occurrence in the tableting process

lamp black SEE *charcoal*

Langmuir isotherm one of several characteristic plots of the amount of gas adsorbed on a given quantity of material in a unimolecular layer versus pressure (at constant temperature); useful in enzymology and molecular pharmacology

lanolin purified fatlike substance obtained from the wool of sheep; used in hydrophilic ointment bases

laparotomy pack nonabrasive material used to prevent abdominal or other organs from escaping to the area of surgery; synonyms: abdominal pack, tape pack, pack, walling mop, stitching pad, quilted pad, gauze mop

Larsen-Johansson disease osteochondrosis involving the apex of the patella

Lascoff, J. Leon (1867-1943) born in Lithuania; apprenticed in New York City and spent his career in retail practice; an early proponent of a professional pharmacy; one of the founders of the American College of Apothecaries; Remington Honor Award recipient in 1937

laser a source of intensely focused light used in numerous surgical applications

last in—first out accounting technique for assigning a cost to the ending inventory and goods sold, where the most recently purchased goods are assumed to be sold first and the ending inventory is the oldest goods purchased

latent heat of vaporization amount of heat absorbed by one gram of substance as it is changed from the liquid state to the vapor state without a change in temperature

latent period 1: time elapsed between the administration of a drug and the onset of its therapeutic effect **2:** period of time between administration of a stimulus to a nerve and the onset of a spike potential

lateral gene transfer the transfer of genes or gene fragments between unrelated organisms

laughing gas nitrous oxide gas

laurel camphor SEE *camphor*

law of chemical equilibrium after a reversible chemical reaction has reached equilibrium, the product of the concentrations of the reaction products divided by the product of the concentrations of the reactants equals a constant

law of diminishing marginal utility states that the value of any additional goods declines as one consumes more of it

law of mass action the rate of a chemical reaction is proportional to the product of the molar concentrations of the reactants raised to powers equal to their coefficients in the stoichiometric equation

laxative agent that promotes defecation; synonyms: aperient, mild cathartic

lay referral system group of nonprofessional people (usually friends, neighbors, or family) that are used by one for advice concerning health needs

lazy eye SEE *amblyopia*

leaching release or movement of components of a solid into a liquid in contact with the solid; example: plasticizers from a plastic container into its liquid contents; synonym: lixiviation

leaker an incompletely sealed ampule, capsule, or other dosage form that should be sealed (e.g., aerosol, vial); a reject dosage form

leaving group the group displaced during a nucleophilic substitution reaction

Le Chatelier's principle law which states that when a system is at equilibrium and stress is brought to bear on the system, the equilibrium will shift so as to diminish the stress

lecithin phospholipid obtained from egg yolks and soybeans (among other natural sources) and composed of glycerol esterfied to two fatty acids and a phosphate that is also esterified to choline

lectin a carbohydrate-binding protein

legend drug medicinal agent that may not be dispensed without a prescription from a recognized medical practitioner; one that bears the label "Rx only"; synonyms: prescription drug, restricted drug, ethical drug

Legg-Calve-Perthes disease epiphyseal aseptic necrosis of the upper end of the femur

Legionnaire's disease *Legionella pneumophilia* infection

length a measure of distance; examples: cgs unit—centimeter (cm) and SI unit—meter (m)

length of stay the period of time an inpatient remains in a health care institution, usually measured in days

lesion 1: injury or wound **2:** an infected patch as in a skin disease

lethal deadly; capable of causing death

lethargy sluggishness, dullness, or slowness

leucine α-amino acid commonly found in proteins; one of ten essential amino acids; 2-amino-5-methylpentanoic acid

leukocyte white blood cell

leukoderma complete depigmentation of an area treated with an epidermal depigmenting agent (e.g., hydroquinone)

leukopenia a low white blood cell count (below $500/mm^3$)

leukoplakia intraoral lesion, often precarcinogenic, resulting from use of oral tobacco products such as snuff or chewing tobacco

leukotriene a linear derivative of arachidonic acid whose synthesis is initiated by a peroxidation reaction

levigation process of grinding (reducing particle size) a solid in the presence of a small amount of liquid in which the drug is not soluble

levorotatory property of an optically active compound that rotates polarized light to the left

Lewis acid **1:** an oxidizing agent **2:** a substance that accepts electrons in a chemical reaction

Lewis base **1:** a reducing agent **2:** a substance that gives up electrons in a chemical reaction

Lewis electronic theory acid-base concept that defines an acid as a substance capable of accepting a pair of electrons and a base as a substance capable of donating a pair of electrons

Li chemical symbol for lithium

liability **1:** an object, event, or occurrence for which an individual is responsible according to the law **2:** a debt that one incurs or owes

libel written statement of one person that defames the character or reputation of another

lice small parasites (singular: louse) that can infest the skin; characterized by intense itching; wingless blood-sucking insect parasitic on warm-blooded animals

license a credential issued by a governmental body which indicates that the holder is in compliance with minimum mandatory requirements necessary to practice a particular profession

lie detector SEE *polygraph*

lifetime maximum benefit a limitation on financial coverage for health care for an individual stated by an insurer

ligand a group that is complexed (bonded) to the central metallic ion in a sequestered or chelated compound

ligase enzyme catalyzing the joining of two compounds in which an energy source (e.g., ATP) is required; synonym: synthetase

lightheadedness feeling of dizziness and faintness; may be experienced when one abruptly changes positions

light-resistant container SEE *container, light resistant*

light velocity SEE *velocity*

Lilly, Eli (1838-1898) American pharmacist who founded Eli Lilly and Company, a leading U.S.-based pharmaceutical manufacturer

lime, burned calcium oxide; caustic or unslaked lime

limit mathematical expression of the maximum or minimum value of a differential (or derivative) when one variable is a function of another

limited liability the concept whereby a business investor is financially liable only to the extent of his investment in an enterprise

limited partner a person meeting appropriate criteria in a partnership and who incurs only limited liability in place of the usual unlimited liability of a partner

limit of resolution the minimum distance between two separate points that allows for their discrimination

limulus test in vitro test for pyrogens in parenteral preparations; the test is positive with the gelling of a pyrogenic material in the presence of the lysate of the amebocytes of the horseshoe crab, *Limulus polyphemus*

linear regression analysis statistical determination of the degree of linearity in the relationship between two or more variables; example: blood level as a function of time

line of credit a loan arrangement with a bank whereby the borrower is allowed to periodically borrow up to a predetermined maximum amount

liner, dental material applied to the inside of the dental cavity, for protection or insulation of the surface

Lineweaver-Burk plot straight-line plot obtained when the reciprocal of the velocity of an enzyme reaction is plotted against the reciprocal of the substrate concentration; the straight line obtained from the reciprocal of the Michaelis-Menton equation; synonym: doubled reciprocal plot

liniment liquid preparation (usually containing an oil) for external use and to be applied with rubbing; examples: liniment of green soap, Yager's Liniment

Linwood F. Tice Friend of the Academy of Students of Pharmacy Award established by the American Pharmacists Association in 1988 to honor an individual whose long-term services and contributions have benefited students of pharmacy

lipid naturally occurring fatty substance of animal or plant origin; insoluble in water and soluble in organic solvents (e.g., benzene, chloroform, and ether); examples: fat, sphingomylin, spermaceti, vegetable oils, beeswax, carnuba wax

lipid bilayer a biomolecular lipid layer that constitutes the structural framework of the cell membranes

lipo- prefix meaning fat

lipogenesis the biosynthesis of body fat (triacylglycerol)

lipoid lipidlike; fatlike

lipolysis the hydrolysis of fat molecules

lipophilic affinity for lipids (oils and fats)

lipophilizing moiety chemical group that imparts lipid-soluble characteristics to the molecule

lipophobic lack of affinity for lipids (oils and fats)

lipoprotein a conjugated protein in which lipid molecules are the prosthetic groups; a protein-lipid complex that transports water-insoluble lipids in blood

lipoprotein, very low density a type of lipoprotein with a very high relative concentration of lipids; transports lipids to tissues

liposomal drug delivery system dosage form in which the medicament is encased in one or more layers of phospholipids (liposomes) and is designed to be released in the body at or near its site of action; a form of targeted drug delivery system

liposome layer of phospholipids within tissue; cellular organelle that contains lipid

lipstick waxy solid, usually colored cosmetic, in stick form for the lips; may be used as a vehicle for topical medicines

liquid state of substance that is an intermediate one entered into as matter goes from solid to gas; also an intermediate substance in that it has neither the orderliness of a crystal nor the randomness of a gas

liquidation process of settling the affairs of a corporation that is going out of business by selling its assets, paying its debts, and dividing the remainder among the owners

liquid glucose a syrupy liquid consisting primarily of glucose and used as a pill excipient; SEE ALSO *glucose*

liquid-in-glass thermometer SEE *thermometer, liquid-in-glass*

liquid scintillation counter instrument to measure weak beta radiation using a phosphorescing solution, a photoabsorption cell, an electrical amplification system, and a counter to detect and record each energy pulse

liquid scintillator instrument designed to measure weak beta particle emissions from a radioactive nuclide such as C_{14}; utilizes a solution containing the isotope to be measured, a phosphor (chemical that produces minute light flashes in response to a radiating particle), and a photomultiplier, detector-counter system

liquor aqueous solution of a nonvolatile substance

liter-atmosphere (L atm) volume times pressure-energy unit equal to 24.22 calories

lithotripsy procedure utilizing sound waves to disintegrate kidney stones (an alternative to surgical removal)

lithotripter device used to break up kidney stones in situ using projected sound waves; SEE ALSO *lithotripsy*

Little's disease spastic paraplegia

liver of sulfur SEE *sulfurated potash*

lixiviation process for removal of soluble substances from insoluble substances by washing and filtration; SEE ALSO *leaching*

Lloyd, John Uri (1849-1936) prolific researcher and author, especially in the area of plant chemistry; founder of the Lloyd Library and Museum in Cincinnati, Ohio; Remington Honor Medal recipient in 1920

loading dose administration of a drug in a larger initial dose than usual to speed entrance into the blood; synonym: bolus dose

lobe pump SEE *rotary pump*

local anesthetic drug or chemical agent that produces an insensitivity to pain only in the area of administration

locus of control a factor in behavioral change models that refers to whether an individual feels that attainment of a particular outcome is within or outside of his/her control

logarithm numerical expression of a number as an exponent of a standard base number

logarithm, common number expressed as an exponent of the number 10 (Log_{10})

logarithm, natural number expressed as an exponent of the number *e* (*e* = 2.71828, a nonrepetitive number sequence); natural mathematical result of integrating the expression *dx/x*

lollipop lozenge on a stick small disc of medicated sugar intended to be dissolved in the mouth

London forces weak attractive forces between molecules occurring as one molecule induces momentary polarization in another; a type of van der Waal's force; synonyms: induced dipole–induced dipole interactions and dispersion effects; example: attractive forces between molecules of hexane liquid

long-term care assistance and care for persons with chronic disabilities who require help with the activities of daily living or who suffer from cognitive impairment

long-term care insurance insurance coverage designed to help pay some or all of any necessary long-term care costs

long-term liability obligation due longer than one year from the date of classification

loss on drying (LOD) quantitative expression of the decrease in weight of a given quantity of material that has been dried

loss ratio the result of paid claims and incurred claims plus expenses divided by the paid premiums. SEE ALSO *incurred claims loss ratio; net loss ratio, paid claims loss ratio; medical loss ratio*

lot batch or portion of a batch having a specified quality and a specific identifying "lot number"

lotion liquid preparation, suspension, or thixotropic emulsion, for external use, usually applied with little or no rubbing

lotion, emulsion small globules of a liquid dispersed throughout another liquid with which it is immiscible, and stabilized by means of an emulsifying agent; example: hand lotion

lotion, suspension liquid containing finely divided insoluble solids suspended in a liquid medium, usually with the aid of a dispersing or suspending agent; example: calamine lotion

Lou Gehrig's disease SEE *amyotropic lateral sclerosis*

louse SEE *lice*

Lovi's beads glass beads of varying densities used to determine the specific gravity of liquids

low-energy solid or liquid **1:** substance whose molecules are held together by weak attractive forces of the van der Waal type **2:** (pharmacy) nonionic, organic, hydrophobic, or nonpolar substance

lower esophageal sphincter sphincter located at the lower end of the esophagus that normally prevents stomach contents from refluxing back into the esophagus; when not functioning properly can cause gastroesophageal reflux

lozenge solid preparation containing one or more medicaments, usually in a flavored, sweetened base, intended to dissolve or disintegrate slowly in the mouth; synonyms: troche, pastille

lubricant 1: slippery, fine powder mixed with tablet granules to facilitate uniform flow of drug granules into a tablet die and to prevent sticking during compression; example: magnesium stearate **2:** tragacanth jelly; used as a surgical lubricant

Lugol's solution aqueous solution of iodine used (in diluted form) to supply iodine internally; synonym: strong iodine solution

luminescence property of emitting light without heat or external excitation

lunar caustic silver nitrate

luteinizing hormone protein secreted by the pituitary gland that stimulates the corpus luteum to produce progesterone

luteinizing hormone-releasing hormone protein secreted by the hypothalamus that stimulates the pituitary to secrete luteinizing hormone

lyase enzyme catalyzing the removal of a group from a molecule by nonhydrolytic means

Lyman, Rufus (1876-1975) founder of the *American Journal of Pharmaceutical Education;* one of the founders of the Rho Chi Honor Society, founder of pharmacy schools at the University of Nebraska and the University of Arizona

Lyme disease inflammatory disorder caused by *Borrelia burgdorferi* and transmitted by the tick

lymphocyte a type of white blood cells

lyophilic having a strong affinity between a dispersed phase and the liquid in which it is dispersed

lyophilization drying by sublimation; a process of drying a substance under vacuum and in the frozen state; freeze-drying

lyophobic a lack of affinity between a dispersed phase and the liquid in which it is dispersed

lysine basic amino acid commonly found in proteins

lysis destruction of cells

lysogeny the integration of a viral genome into a host genome

lysosome a saclike organelle capable of degrading most biomolecules

lytic cycle a viral life cycle in which a virus destroys its host cell

M **macerate** to extract the constituents from a crude drug by soaking or steeping it in a suitable solvent

macro- prefix meaning large

macrocytic anemia condition in which there is a reduced number of red blood cells accompanied by the presence of red blood cells that are larger than normal; usually seen in folate and vitamin B_{12} deficiencies

macrolides class of antibiotics with large lactones that exert a bacteriostatic effect on gram-positive and gram-negative bacteria by inhibiting protein synthesis; example: erythromycin

macromolecular pertaining to large molecules or polymers; examples: proteins and nucleic acids

macromolecule SEE *polymer*

macrophage large phagocyte that ingests dead tissues and cells

macroscopic large in scope; can be seen with the unaided eye

macula small spot or colored area

magma suspension of a finely divided insoluble, inorganic drug, the particles of which are hydrated; example: milk of magnesia

magnesium salts used as antacids or laxatives; cometal for ATPase; chemical symbol: Mg

magnetic quantum number (Mq) integer describing the magnetic field generated by the momentum of an electron in the atom; for an electron, quantum number where $n = 2$, the magnetic quantum number $= -1$, 0, or $+1$; SEE *quantum number*

mail-order pharmacy a type of pharmacy where prescription medications can be delivered through the postal service to the patient

maintained markup difference between net sales and the total cost of merchandise sold; gross margin minus cash discounts

maintenance dose periodic dose following the "loading dose" given to keep drug plasma concentrations within a therapeutic range

maintenance drug drug prescribed to treat long-term (chronic) disorders

Maisch, John M. (1831-1893) prominent teacher and first permanent secretary of the American Pharmacists Association

maize oil synonym for corn oil

major diagnostic category principal diagnosis or reason for treating a patient; in cases of complicated medical problems, there may be a primary or principal diagnosis and other secondary or preliminary diagnoses; relative to third-party reimbursement, insurers will usually pay providers for services rendered on the basis of the major diagnostic category

major tranquilizer antipsychotic agent

malabsorption syndrome a condition in which essential nutrients are poorly absorbed

malaise general sensation of discomfort, often seen with influenza and, to a lesser extent, the common cold

malignancy denotes a cancerous condition

malignant tendency to become worse until death results; usually refers to a cancerous condition

Mallory-Weiss syndrome hematemesis due to a tear in the esophagus following forceful vomiting

malonate salt or ester of malonic acid; example: diethylmalonate

malonic acid three-carbon dicarboxylic acid; propanedioic acid; methane dicarboxylic acid

malonic ester synthesis alkylation of malonic ester (diethylmalonate) by using alkylhalides and metallic sodium in ethyl alcohol; used to prepare barbiturates, phenylbutazone, and many other drugs

malpractice failure to exercise an acceptable level of professional service

malt preparation containing amylolytic enzymes obtained from the partially germinated grain of various varieties of barley

maltose a degradation product of starch hydrolysis; a disaccharide composed of two glucose molecules linked by an α-(1,4)-glycosidic bond

managed behavioral care mental health or chemical dependency treatment that is screened and monitored for meeting utilization criteria, treatment effectiveness, and/or quality

managed care 1: a system of health care delivery that influences utilization and cost of services and measures performance **2:** a systemized approach that seeks to ensure the provision of the right health care at the right time, place, and cost

managed care organization (MCO) broad term that encompasses various types of health plans, including health maintenance organizations, preferred provider organizations, point-of-service plans, and provider-sponsored organizations

managed health care plan a health care organization that provides managed care (SEE *managed care*) with the following attributes: integration of financing and management with the delivery of health care services to an enrolled population; employment or contracting with an organized provider network which delivers services and which either shares financial risk or has some incentive to deliver quality, cost-effective services; use of an information system capable of monitoring and evaluating patterns of covered persons' use of medical services and the cost of those services

management by objectives leadership and control technique in which subordinates are encouraged by supervisors to set their own objectives and the means whereby achievement of those objectives can be measured

management information system management performed with the aid of automated data processing and a substantially relevant data bank

management service organization organization providing practice management, administrative, and support services to individual physicians or group practices

mandated benefits those benefits that health plans are required by state or federal law to provide to policy holders and eligible dependents

manganese trace mineral element; a brittle, grayish white metal resembling iron; a cometal for various enzymes

Mannich reaction synthetic organic reaction used to prepare intermediates for the synthesis of local anesthetics and narcotic analgesics, among other drug moities; compound with an active alpha-hydrogen (ketone, ketolized phenol) that is reacted with formaldehyde and a primary or secondary amine

mannitol six-carbon polyol that does not ferment; the principal constituent of manna; sugar alcohol from mannose

manual rates rates developed based upon the health plan's average claims data and adjusted for group specific demographic, industry factor, or benefit variations

marasmus retardation of growth and atrophy of muscle due to malnutrition; usually does not affect thought process; CONTRAST *kwashiorkor*

marc residue that remains after extraction of a crude drug (animal, vegetable, or mineral) with a solvent

Marie-Strümpell disease ankylosing spondylitis (arthritis of the spine)

markdown a reduction in price of merchandise by a retailer; used to stimulate sales and reduce inventory

marketable securities stocks, bonds, and other investments expected to be converted to cash or otherwise used in current regular operations during the next year; reported at market value

market pricing prices that are set to meet marketplace conditions, usually a competitive situation in which consumers seek out the lowest price

Maslow's theory hypothesis of motivation, developed by Abraham Maslow, which holds that basic human needs exist in a hierarchy of importance and that lower level needs must be satisfied before higher level needs become important; synonym: Maslow's hierarchy of needs theory

mass expression of an absolute quantity of a substance

mass number the sum of nucleons in an atomic nucleus; for practical purposes, the same as the atomic weight for the atom

mass spectrometry destructive method of analyzing a molecular structure; molecules are subjected to high energy electrons (or protons), breaking them into charged fragments whose spectra are analyzed by their differences in mass

mast- prefix meaning breast; same as masto-

master file collection of information that either is relatively permanent or is treated as an authority in a particular job

master group contract a legal document between the enrolling unit and the carrier, setting forth in detail the rights and obligations of the enrolling unit, covered person, and carrier, as well as terms and conditions of the coverage provided by the contract

mastication chewing

masto- prefix meaning breast; same as mast-

materia medica historical term for the branch of medical study that deals with drugs and their sources, uses, and preparations; modern term: pharmacology

material control quality assurance tests of components that are to become a part of a dosage form; synonym: raw material control

matrix **1:** a groundwork from which something is cast **2:** an insoluble polymer used to entrap a drug in a solid dosage form so that its release can be controlled **3:** (mathematics) a rectangular array of terms or symbols arranged in rows and columns; combination of two vectors (or arrays) in computer science

matrix, extracellular a gelatinous material, containing proteins and carbohydrates, that binds cells and tissue together

maximum allowable cost (MAC) federal cost containment program that limits reimbursement for multisource (generically available) prescription drugs under Medicare, Medicaid, and Public Health Service programs to the lowest cost at which the drug is generally available; some private plans also contain MAC provisions

maximum allowable cost list multisource prescription medications that will be covered at a generic product cost level established by the plan

maximum allowable fee schedule a health care payment system that reimburses up to a specified dollar amount for services rendered

maximum out-of-pocket costs the limit on total member copayments, deductibles, and coinsurance under a benefit contract

maximum permissible body burden the greatest amount of radioactive material that may, on average, be contained within the body before exceeding the maximum permissible radiation dose to the critical organ

McArdle's disease type 5 glycogenosis; accumulation of glycogen in muscle

me-too drug drug product that represents only minor chemical modifications of existing drugs and offers little or no improvement in therapeutic benefit

mean a measure of central tendency of a group of numbers computed by summing a group of numbers and dividing the sum by the total quantity of numbers; average; number obtained by dividing the total of a set of values by the number of values in the set

mean deviation average of the absolute values of the respective errors in a set of data; value obtained by adding the absolute values of the respective differences between the observed data points and the mean and dividing this sum by the number of observations or data points

mean surface diameter that diameter of a group of particles calculated from the square root of the ratio of the sum of the product of the number of particles and the square of their diameters divided by the sum of the particles; best reflects surface area effects

mean volume diameter that diameter of a group of particles calculated from the square root of the ratio of the sum of the product of the number of particles and the cube of their diameter divided by the sum of the particles; best reflects volume effects

mean volume surface diameter that diameter of a group of particles calculated from the ratio of the sum of the products of the number of particles and the cube of their diameters divided by the sum of the products of the number of particles and the square of the diameter of the particles; best reflects combined effects of volume and surface phenomena

median number that lies at the midpoint of a distribution of numbers and hence divides the distribution into two equal halves; a measure of central tendency; that value in a set of values in which the number of values above the number is equal to the number of values below the number (the median itself is not counted)

median effective dose term in molecular pharmacology that refers to the dose of a drug that produces 50 percent of the desired effective dose possible

Medicaid a federal program administered and operated individually by participating state and territorial governments that provides medical benefits to eligible low-income persons needing health care; established under Title XIX of the Social Security Act

Medicaid Management Information System a complex computerized database management system that permits monitoring utilization and cost of services in the Medicaid program; can be used by Medicaid agencies to perform retrospective reviews of drug utilization, physician services, and institutional care as well as the costs of these services

Medicaid Prudent Pharmaceutical Purchasing Act states that Medicaid must receive the best discounted price of any institutional purchaser of pharmaceuticals, enacted as part of OBRA '90

medical expense trend the rate at which medical costs are increasing or decreasing, influenced by a number of factors, such as utilization, new technology, and billed charges

medical loss ratio the cost ratio of health benefits used compared to revenue received; calculated as follows: total medical expenses divided by premium revenue

medically needy under Medicaid, aged, blind, or disabled individuals or families and children who are not otherwise eligible for Medicaid, and whose income resources are above the limits for eligibility as categorically needy but within limits set under the Medicaid state plan

medical necessity the evaluation of health care services to determine if they are medically appropriate and required to meet basic health needs; consistent with the diagnosis or condition and rendered in a cost-effective manner; and consistent with national medical guidelines regarding type, frequency, and duration of treatment

medical service representative field employee of a drug company who "details" or informs physicians and other health professionals of the company's products; synonyms: detail person, manufacturer's representative

Medicare federally administered health insurance program that covers the costs of hospitalization, medical care, and some related services for people age 65 and over and for certain disabled individuals without regard to income; Part A—inpatient costs with Medicare paying for pharmaceuticals provided in hospitals, but not for those provided in outpatient settings; Part B—outpatient costs for Medicare patients; Part C (Medicare + Choice)—managed care (e.g., HMO) option that Medicare patients may choose in lieu of Parts A and B (traditional Medicare)

Medicare beneficiary person designated by the Social Security Administration as entitled to receive Medicare benefits

Medicare supplemental policy a policy guaranteeing that a health plan will pay a policyholder's coinsurance, deductible, and copayments and will provide additional health plan or non-Medicare coverage for services up to a predefined benefit limit; also called "Medigap" or "Medicare wrap"

medication cart movable container that holds (in a systematic way) individual doses of medications from which nurses (or medication technicians) administer drugs to patients

medication history summary of prescription and nonprescription medicines, as well as any illicit medicines and dietary supplements that a patient has taken or is currently taking and the patient's drug idiosyncrasies; usually obtained at the time of one's admission to a hospital or at the first visit to a doctor's office

medication profile record of the medications a patient is taking, the regimen or frequency, and any drug allergies or drug-related diseases that a patient may have; used for effective pharmacy practice; is incomplete if it does not also list patient's use of nonprescription products, herbal preparations, physician samples, etc.; also called "prescription record" or "medication history"

medication therapy management services provided under Medicare Part D (2003) that include patient education and counseling about appropriate medication use; programs designed to increase patient compliance with medication therapy and to detect adverse events due to over- or underutilization of medication

medicinal chemistry area involving study of the chemistry of drugs; involved with the design, synthesis, physical properties, chemical properties, and structure-activity relationships of drugs; synonym: pharmaceutical chemistry

medigap SEE *Medicare supplemental policy*

medium filter microporous, surface filter medium made by fusing synthetic microbeads to produce minute openings of specified size; cellulose esters, nylon, and polyvinyl materials are used to make such filters; filter material to collect particles in the range of 5-25 microns in diameter

mega- 1: prefix meaning large, larger than usual, or larger than normal **2:** prefix meaning one million times a basic unit of measure; same as megalo-

megacolon expansion of the distal colon caused by retention of feces with chronic constipation

megacolon, toxic medical emergency in which megacolon has persisted so long that colonic rupture occurs, with spillage of feces into the peritoneal cavity

megalo- 1: prefix meaning large, larger than usual, or larger than normal **2:** prefix meaning one million times a basic unit of measure; same as mega-

-megaly suffix meaning large or larger than normal; example: hepatomegaly

meiosis method of cell division that occurs in the formation of sex cells whereby, over two successive cell divisions, each daughter cell receives half the number of chromosomes and half the amount of DNA of the parent cell and the two haploid cells develop into gametes—either sperm or ova

melancholia severe form of depression

melanin pigment commonly found in the skin, hair, eye, mucous membrane, and nervous system

melasma condition causing pigmentation of the skin; synonym: chloasma

melena blood in the stools

melting point temperature at which a solid substance begins to change to the liquid state; temperature at which a solid substance exists in equilibrium with its liquid state; CONTRAST *melting range*

melting point lowering constant factor by which 1 mole of a substance will lower the melting point of 1,000 g of another substance; example: 1 mole of a nonelectrolyte (186 g of glucose) decreases the melting point of 1,000 g of water 1.86°C

melting range temperature interval through which a fat or other organic compound begins to melt and the temperature at which it is completely melted; CONTRAST *melting point*

member assistance program a human risk management program that focuses on lowering behavioral and medical health costs by proactively reducing demand on the treatment system

members participants in a health plan who make up the plan's enrollment; also used to describe individuals specified within subscriber contracts who may or may not receive health care services according to the terms of the subscriber policy

members per year the number of members enrolled in the health plan on a yearly basis; calculated as member months divided by 12.

membrane filtration microseparation process using synthetic plastic sheets with minute openings to allow the filtrate to pass while collecting particles larger than the openings

membrane potential potential difference across the membrane of living cells; usually measured in millivolts

menarche first menstrual flow

Ménière's disease endolymphatic hydrops (excessive accumulation of fluid in the inner ear)

meniscus curved upper surface of a liquid in a container (concave when the liquid wets the walls of the container and convex when the liquid does not wet the container wall)

menstruum solvent used to extract the active constituents from animal, vegetable, or mineral drugs

mental confusion when one's mind becomes disoriented with regards to time, place, or person; may also include disordered consciousness

mercurous chloride an insoluble mercury compound once used as a laxative and as a component in the reference electrode of a pH meter; synonym: calomel

mercury silvery metallic liquid element; compounds are used as diuretics and antiseptics and the liquid metal was once used in thermometers

mesh number an expression of the number of openings per linear inch in a sieve made with wires of a specified diameter

messenger RNA (mRNA) an RNA species produced by transcription that specifies the amino acid sequence for a polypeptide

metabolism total chemical and physical processes occurring within an organism or cell in which materials are assimilated and processed to produce intermediates, building material, energy, and waste products

metabolite natural compound (substrate, vitamin, or food material) that reacts in or is formed by a biochemical reaction

metalloporphyro protein cyclic structure composed of pyrrole rings and a central metal combined with a protein; example: hemoglobin

metaloprotein a conjugated protein containing one or more metal ions

metaplasia transformation of one type of adult tissue into another; example: replacement of normal respiratory epithelium composed of columnar cells by stratified squamous epithelium

metastable slight margin of stability of a substance that changes into another substance as conditions change; existing temporarily at a higher energy state than in the most stable form; example: technetium 99m

metastasis transmission of cells or bacteria from one tissue to another, usually involving some distance

metastatic neoplasm SEE *cancer*

metered value aerosol release mechanism that delivers a measured amount of product (one dose)

methionine sulfur-containing amino acid commonly found in proteins; methyl donor in 1-carbon transfer reactions; one of the ten essential amino acids

methylation a type of alkylation reaction in which a methyl group is substituted on an atom of a molecule

methylcobalamin form of vitamin B_{12} in which a methyl group is bound to the central cobalt atom

methyl salicylate volatile oil consisting of an ester formed in a reaction of salicylic acid and methyl alcohol; widely used in liniments; synonym: oil of wintergreen

metrology science of weights and measures

Meyer's disease adenoid disease due to chronic inflammation of the pharyngeal tonsil

micellar solution SEE *solution*

micelle agglomeration of amphiphillic (surfactant) molecules in a dispersion medium (solvent) having a diameter on the order of 50 angstroms (5 nanometers)

Michaelis constant special type of steady-state constant in Michaelis-Menton enzyme kinetics (saturation kinetics) reflecting the formation and breakdown of the enzyme-substrate complex in an enzyme catalyzed reaction

Michaelis-Menton equation mathematical relationship between the velocity of an enzyme and its substrate concentrations in which the overall velocity of the reaction (*V*) equals the product of the maximum velocity (V_{max}) and the substrate concentration (*S*) divided by the sum of the Michaelis constant and the substrate concentration

micro- **1:** prefix meaning small **2:** prefix meaning one-millionth of a basic unit of measure; example: 1 μg = 10^{-6} g

microcrystalline cellulose purified, partially depolymerized cellulose prepared by treating alpha cellulose with mineral acids; used as a tablet disintegrant

microcytic anemia condition in which there is a reduced number of red blood cells accompanied by the presence of smaller than normal red blood cells; usually seen in iron deficiency anemia

microemulsion clear dispersion of oil in water or water in oil in which the dispersed phase has dispersed particles with diameters of 100 Å to 600 Å

microencapsulation process by which solids or liquids are encased in a thin shell as minute particles (globules)

microfilament a component of the cytoskeleton composed of the protein actin

microgram (μg) one-millionth of a gram

microliter (μL) one-millionth of a liter

micrometer (μm) **1:** instrument used to measure small sizes **2:** a micron or 10^{-6} m

micrometrics the study of particle size

micron older term for micrometer

micronization reduction of particles to micrometer diameter sizes

micronize to pulverize a substance into very small particles that are only a few micrometers in size

micronized powders drug particles that are five micrometers or less in diameter

micronizer SEE *fluid energy mill*

microphage small phagocyte that ingests bacteria and protozoa

microscope instrument consisting of lenses enabling minute objects (or their reflections) to be seen; examples: optical microscope, electron microscope

microscopy **1:** examination of objects through the field of a microscope **2:** method of determining particle size distribution by using a microscope **3:** an investigation using a microscope; examples: optical microscopy, electron microscopy

microsomal enzymes biochemical catalysts that are responsible for the biotransformation of drugs in the body; located in small vesicles on the endoplastic reticulum

microvilli minute fingerlike projections found in the intestine; serve to increase the surface area of the intestines enabling the absorption of greater amounts of food or drug; synonym: border brush

microwaves electromagnetic radiation emanating from electron spin transitions

miliaria inflammatory skin disease observed in the summer or in the tropics that consists of vesicles and papules accompanied by a prickly, tingling sensation; synonym: prickly heat

milk acid synonym for lactose

milk-alkali syndrome excessive absorption of calcium caused by alkalosis and resulting in hypercalcemia; occasionally seen with overuse of antacids such as sodium bicarbonate or calcium carbonate

milli- prefix meaning one-thousandth

milliequivalent (mEq or meq) one-thousandth of one gram equivalent weight of a substance

milligram percent one milligram of solute per 100 milliliters of solution

milling process of reducing particle size of a solid by grinding

milling energy energy input requirement for solid particle size reduction; SEE *Kick's theory; Rittinger's theory; Bond's theory; work index for particle size reduction*

mineral acid an inorganic acid; examples: sulfuric acid, phosphoric acid, hydrochloric acid

mineralocorticoid type of adrenal corticosteroid that controls electrolyte balance by regulating sodium and water retention and potassium excretion; effects on electrolyte balance are caused by adrenocorticoids

mineral soap synonym for bentonite

mineral wax SEE *ceresin*

minibag small flexible plastic container that holds 25-100 mL of an intravenous infusion

minim (m or min) a unit of fluid measure in the apothecary system; approximately one-sixteenth of a milliliter

minimum effective concentration concentration of a drug in body fluids (such as the blood) below which an adequate therapeutic response is not obtained

minimum inhibitory concentration blood-level concentration of an antibacterial drug (such as an antibiotic or a sulfa) below which there is no bacteriostatic or bacteriocidal effect

minimum lethal dose the minimum dose of a substance required to produce death of an organism

minor tranquilizer antianxiety agent

miosis constriction of the pupil of the eye

miotic drug used to produce a contraction of the pupil of the eye

mirror image isomers SEE *optical isomers*

misbranding improper and/or illegal labeling of a drug or drug product as a consequence of incomplete, misleading, and/or inaccurate wording

miscible term to describe two or more liquids that combine into a single phase in all proportions

misdemeanor criminal offense that is less serious than a felony and is usually punishable by a fine and/or local incarceration

misrepresentation the act of representing falsely, making an untrue statement, or conveying an untrue idea

mithridate a legendary antidote against poisons

mithridatism acquisition of immunity from the effects of a specific poison by ingesting small amounts at first, followed by increasing amounts over a period of time

mitigate to lessen; to make less severe as in the symptoms of a disease

mitochondria small, rod-shaped organelles in a cell that serve as the major site of metabolism for energy production

mitogen a substance that stimulates cell division

mitosis process of cell division in which each cell forms two daughter cells that normally contain identical chromosomes

mixed anhydride an acid anhydride with two different R groups

mixed terpenoid a biomolecule that is composed of nonterpene components attached to isoprenoid groups

mixing process of combining pharmaceutical materials such that each is distributed in and among the other in the most uniform manner

mixing mechanisms of solids fundamental interactions between particles of drug materials as they are mixed; examples: convective shear, diffusive motion

mixture 1: aqueous liquid containing insoluble solids in suspension and intended for internal use; example: chalk mixture **2:** any combination of substances in varying proportions and in such a manner that they may be separated by nonchemical methods; not a compound or molecule

mobile phase the moving phase in chromatographic methods

modified community rating a separate rating of medical service usage in a given geographic area (community) using age-sex data, etc.

modified fee-for-service a system in which providers are paid on a fee-for-service basis, with certain fee maximums for each procedure

modulator a molecule whose binding to an allosteric site of an enzyme alters the enzyme's activity

Mohr scale of hardness relative index of the hardness characteristic of mineral materials

Mohr-Westphal balance balance used to determine the specific gravity of liquids

moiety term usually used in biochemistry to designate a group or a radical on a compound

moist heat 1: use of heat at a given temperature and the added equivalent of the heat of vaporization of a liquid (usually water) in a process such as sterilization **2:** optional method for use of a heating pad whereby the patient inserts a wet sponge into the cover between the heating pad and the skin

moisture content quantitative expression of the weight of water in a wet sample of material; percent moisture content is equal to the product of the difference of the wet and dry weights of a sample times 100 divided by the weight of the dry sample

molality concentration expression based on the number of moles of solute dissolved in 1,000 grams of solvent

molar elipticity degree to which circular polarized light is converted into an ellipse by its passage through a one molar solution of an optically active substance

molar heat of vaporization the amount of heat absorbed by one mole of substance as it is changed from the liquid into the vapor state at constant temperature

molarity concentration expression based on the number of moles (gram molecular weights) of solute in one liter of solution

molar volume volume occupied by one mole of substance

molded tablets SEE *tablet, compressed*

mole one gram molecular weight of substance; that is, the weight of a substance in grams equal to its molecular weight

molecular biology the science devoted to elucidating the structure and function of genomes

molecular chaperone a molecule that assists in protein folding; most are heat shock proteins

molecular diffusion mixing process brought about by the kinetic motion of molecules of two or more substances in the same system

molecular disease a disease caused by a mutated gene

molecular orbital resultant orbital arising from the overlapping of atomic orbitals of two atoms to form a covalent bond

molecular orbital theory explanation (using wave mechanical theory) of binding forces between atoms resulting from the overlapping of filled molecular orbitals as opposed to simple binding forces between atoms

molecular sieve polymeric layered molecules or groups of molecules with definite pore sizes; used to separate particles or ions by molecular size

molecular weight sum of the atomic weights of atoms that compose a molecule

mole fraction ratio of the moles of one constituent of a solution or mixture to the total moles of all constituents in the solution or mixture

mole percent concentration expression based on the number of moles of one constituent in 100 moles of all substances included in the solution or mixture

Monge's disease mountain sickness

mono mononucleosis or "kissing fever"

mono- prefix meaning single, one, or alone

monogram inscription or trademark placed on units of a dosage form such as tablet or capsule; usually designating the company that produced the product as well as a code number or mark for a specific drug dosage unit

monograph written account concerning a single subject or thing; special treatise on a single subject; example: *USP* monograph about a specific drug

monophase system homogeneous mixture, each component of which is in the same state of matter; examples: a gas, a liquid, a solid

monosaccharide cyclic polyhydroxy derivative of an aldehyde or ketone that cannot be broken down further by acid hydrolysis

monosodium glutamate (MSG) sodium salt of the amino acid, glutamic acid; white or nearly white powder that is very soluble and possesses a meatlike taste; used to flavor meat; may be toxic to children and may be the cause of Chinese restaurant syndrome in adults; synonyms: sodium glutamate

monotropic denotes a polymorphic compound in which crystalline form transitions occur only in one direction from a less stable to a more stable state

monounsaturated fatty acid with a single double bond

mood emotional state; disposition

morbid affected with a disease; diseased

morbidity **1:** term used by epidemiologists that is the ratio of sick persons to well persons in a defined area **2:** the actual state of being diseased

morbidity rate an actuarial determination of the incidence and severity of sicknesses and accidents in a well-defined class or classes of people

mordant agent used to make dyeing more permanent; agent used to fix a dye or colorant

Morgagni's disease SEE *Stokes-Adams syndrome*

Morgan, John (1735-1789) pharmacist and physician; earliest American advocate of splitting the roles of the pharmacist and physician

morphinan parent structure for morphine and its analgesic analogs; example: levorphanol

morphine chief alkaloid of opium *(Papaver somniferum);* present to the extent of 9 percent of the alkaloids of opium; one of the principal drugs used for pain relief

morphology science dealing with the structures and forms of organisms

Morse equation quantitative expression to estimate osmotic pressure based on molarity of a solution

mortality rate ratio of total number of deaths to the total population in a given time

mortar heavy concave vessel usually made of glass or porcelain and used with a pestle for grinding and/or mixing; glass—used mostly for mixing; porcelain—glazed on the outside, but rough and unglazed on the inside; used for grinding and mixing

motivation process of stimulating workers to contribute to the growth and success of the organization

mottled 1: nonuniform colors in a dosage form that may or may not be desired; example: a mixture of different colored granules upon compression will yield a mottled tablet **2:** abnormal stains on teeth, particularly as a result of tetracycline ingestion during tooth formation and due to the excessive use of fluorides

mouthwash an aqueous solution that is most often used for its deodorizing, refreshing, and/or antiseptic effect

moving-bed dryer SEE *agitation dryer*

moxa small cones of combustible material that glow but do not have an open flame when ignited; used to cauterize; also used in unproven pseudo-medical practice referred to as moxibustion

mucilage viscous adhesive preparation made by dissolving or suspending exudates from certain trees and shrubs in water; example: tragacanth mucilage; may also be formed from hydrated synthetic polymers, example: methylcellulose mucilage

mucokinesis process by which cilia located on ciliated cells in the respiratory tract continually move mucus, trapped particles, and infective organisms to the upper respiratory passages

mucus slick, viscid secretion of the mucus membranes

Muldoon, Hugh Cornelius (1898-1956) educator; established the College of Pharmacy at Duquesne in 1925 and served as its dean until 1955; member of the *USP* Committee of Revision for 20 years; also served on the revision committee of the *National Formulary;* Remington Honor Medal recipient in 1953

muller mill apparatus used to reduce particle size of solids by rolling a heavy, wide, "wheel-shaped" device over particles to be reduced in size

multicompartmental model pharmacokinetic model which assumes that the body consists of more than one compartment; example: a two-compartment model consisting of central and peripheral areas

multidose vial SEE *container*

multilayer tablet SEE *tablet, compressed*

multilayer tablet press tabletting machine designed to sequentially feed and compress up to three different layers of granular drug materials in one discretely layered solid dosage unit

multiphase system SEE *polyphase system*

multiple labeling radiolabeling a compound on two or more positions within the same molecule

multiple linear regression statistical computation of the linear relationship between one dependent variable and two or more independent (predictor) variables

multiple option plan a health care plan design that offers employees the option of electing to enroll under one of several types of coverages usually including an HMO, a PPO, or a major indemnity plan

Multistate Pharmacy Jurisprudence Examination computer-adapative assessment that tailors each examination to address the pharmacy law and regulations of the state in which the candidate is seeking licensure

Munchausen syndrome psychiatric condition that causes the patient to pretend to have a medical problem or to self-inflict harm to gain attention from family or health care providers

Munchausen syndrome by proxy form of child abuse where the mother invents symptoms in her child, causing the child painful and unnecessary physical examinations and treatments

murein a complex polymer that contains two sugar derivations: *N*-acetylglucosamine and *N*-acetylmuramic acid and several amino acids; also referred to as peptidoglycan

muscle body tissue that has the properties of irritability, conductivity, and elasticity and can both contract and relax, thereby effecting the movement of the body or its parts

mutagen agent capable of producing genetic mutations in cells or in the body

mutarotation a spontaneous process in which the alpha and beta forms of monosaccharides are readily interconverted

mutation permanent change or modification in the genetic composition of an individual; SEE ALSO *point mutation; transversion mutation*

mute inability to speak

my- prefix meaning muscle; same as myo-

myalgia muscular pain

myasthenia gravis chronic progressive disease characterized by chronic fatigue and muscular weakness

myc- prefix meaning fungus; same as mycet-, myco-

mycet- prefix meaning fungus; same as myc-, myco-

myco- prefix meaning fungus; same as myc-, mycet-

mydriasis dilation of the pupil of the eye

mydriatic drug that produces mydriasis

myel- prefix meaning spinal cord or bone marrow; same as myelo-

myelin lipid sheath surrounding nerves

myelo- prefix meaning spinal chord or bone marrow; same as myel-

myelocyte SEE *granulocyte*

myo- prefix meaning muscle; same as my-

myocardium heart muscle

myoclonus abrupt contractions of part of a muscle or muscle group

myoclonus multiplex ill-defined disorder marked by rapid and widespread muscle contractions

myoglobin muscle hemoglobin

myoneural term describing structures associated with nerve and muscle; synonym: neuromuscular

myoneural junction connection between a nerve and muscle where cholinergic neurotransmission takes place; synonym: motor end plate

myopathy disorder in a muscle

myosin protein that combines with actin to form actomyosin, which is responsible for contraction of muscle tissue myrcia oil; synonym for bay oil

N

name, generic SEE *generic name*

name, proprietary SEE *proprietary name*

narcissism self-love or self-admiration

narcolepsy sleep disorder; characterized by irresistible attacks of daytime sleep

narcotic **1:** a drug or chemical agent obtained from opium, or a synthetic analog of those substances **2:** drug that produces an insensitivity to pain, a stuporlike state, and physical and psychological dependence **3:** any substance included in the Harrison Narcotic Act of 1914

nasal pertaining to the nose

nascent **1:** just born, incipient, or beginning **2:** set free from a compound **3:** usually more chemically reactive than ordinary forms of an element; example: nascent oxygen

naso- prefix meaning the nose or pertaining to the nose

nasolabial fold area of the lip located just below the nostrils

natal pertaining to birth

National Academy of Science/National Research Council an agency of the federal government responsible for advising the Food and Drug Administration concerning the safety and efficacy of drugs

National Association of Boards of Pharmacy organization composed of members of Boards of Pharmacy from each of the United States, the District of Columbia, and Puerto Rico, having the objectives of facilitating license reciprocity, developing uniform licensing examinations, and providing a forum for discussing the legal regulation of the profession; founded in 1904

National Association of Chain Drug Stores organization representing the business interests of chain drug retailers; founded in 1933

National Association of Retail Druggists SEE *National Community Pharmacists Association*

National Catholic Pharmacists Guild of the United States organization of Catholic pharmacists and students with the purpose of promoting and supporting the principles of the Catholic church, especially as they relate to the professional and ethical aspects of pharmacy practice; founded in 1962

National Committee for Quality Assurance (NCQA) an independent, nonprofit HMO accrediting organization composed of independent health care quality experts, employers, labor union officials, and consumer representatives; its accreditation standards focus on (1) quality improvement, (2) credentialing, (3) members' rights and responsibilities, (4) utilization management, (5) preventive health services, and (6) medical records; NCQA uses HEDIS to measure HMO quality

National Community Pharmacists Association organization of independent pharmacy owners with the purpose of protecting the interests of the retail pharmacy owners; founded as the National Association of Retail Druggists in 1898

National Council on Drugs independent organization composed of representatives from public and professional medical associations; serves as an advisory group to government and private sectors on matters of policy and action in drug-related areas; founded in 1976

National Council on Patient Information and Education a national organization dedicated to improving communication between health care professionals and patients

National Drug Code (NDC) a number used for identification of drugs; similar to the Universal Product Code (UPC)

National Drug Code System a coding system used by insurers to pay outpatient pharmaceutical claims

National Formulary compilation of drugs, drug dosage forms, and their standards; originally published by the American Pharmaceutical Association in 1888; currently published by the U.S. Pharmacopeial Convention, Inc.

National Institute for Standards in Pharmacist Credentialing formed by the American Pharmacist Association, the National Association of Boards of Pharmacy, the National Association of Chain Drug Stores, and the National Community Pharmacists Association to promote the value of disease-specific examinations as the consistent and objective means of documenting the ability of pharmacists to provide disease state management services

National Pharmaceutical Association professional organization composed of state and local associations of minority pharmacists; founded in 1947

National Pharmaceutical Council organization of companies engaged primarily in the manufacture of prescription pharmaceutical products; exists to promote optimal professional standards and to ensure quality prescription products; founded in 1953

National Wholesale Druggists Association SEE *Health Distributors Manufacturers Association*

natriuresis abnormal increase in the excretion of sodium

natural immunity immunity that a person or an animal possesses at birth; synonym: inherent immunity

nausea unpleasant feeling in the upper GI tract and in the mind; usually precedes vomiting

NDC System SEE *National Drug Code System*

nebulizer device used to convert a liquid to a mist or fine spray; SEE *atomizer*

necro- prefix meaning death, dead tissue, or dead cells

necrolysis separation or exfoliation of necrotic tissue

necrosis death of individual cells or tissues

negative feedback a mechanism in which a biochemical pathway is regulated by binding a product molecule to a key enzyme in the pathway

negative formulary SEE *formulary*

negatron a negatively charged electron; the same as a beta particle of radiation; CONTRAST *positron;* SEE ALSO *electron, orbital*

negligence failure to exercise the level or quality of care that a reasonable and prudent individual would have used in a similar situation; SEE *malpractice*

nematode classification for roundworms; examples: pinworm, hookworm

neonate newborn up to four weeks of age

neoplasm abnormal, uncontrolled growth of cells and tissue not in coordination with other cells of the body

neoplasm, benign abnormal growth of cells and tissue in a local circumscribed area that neither invades surrounding tissue nor metastasizes to other parts of the body

neoplasm, malignant abnormal growth of cells that invades surrounding tissues and metastasizes to other parts of the body; synonym: cancer

neovascularization stage of wound repair in which capillaries send fresh buds into the healing wound

nephelometer instrument used to determine the degree of turbidity (or conversely the degree of clarity) of a liquid by measuring the "Tyndal effect" (light scattering)

nephr- prefix meaning kidney; same as nephtro-

nephritis inflammation of the kidney

nephro- prefix meaning kindney; same as nephr-

nephrogenic diabetes insipidis an autosomal recessive disease in which the kidneys of affected individuals cannot produce concentrated urine

nephrosclerosis hardening of the kidney or a part of the kidney

neroli oil a source of the terpenic alcohol nerol; synonym: oil of orange flowers

net income excess of revenues over expenses of operation for a business in a specified time period; synonym: net profit

net loss ratio the result of total claims liability and all expenses divided by premiums; the carrier's loss ratio after accounting for all expenses

net profit gross margin minus expenses (not including income tax), for a given period of time; synonym: net income

network model HMO an HMO that contracts with more than one physician group, and may contract with single- and multispecialty groups; physicians may share in utilization savings, but do not necessarily provide care exclusively for HMO members

net worth owner's interest in a business; equal to the assets minus the liabilities of the firm; synonym: owner's equity

neur- prefix pertaining to a nerve or the nervous system; same as neuro-

neuralgia pain that follows the course of a nerve; classified according to the nerve affected

neural mismatch theory theory that a mismatch in input from the proprioceptive, vestibular, and visual systems causes motion sickness

neurasthenia nervous exhaustion; functional neurosis marked by intense nervous irritability and weakness

neuritis inflammation of a nerve

neuro- prefix pertaining to a nerve or the nervous system; same as neur-

neurohormone compound secreted by a gland into the blood that produces neural stimulation in another part of the body

neuroleptic category of drugs that exhibit antipsychotic actions, have the potential to induce extrapyramidal movements, and are generally non-hypnotics

neurologist a physician who has specialized knowledge of the nervous system and treats neurological disorders

neuromuscular blocking agent drug used to relax skeletal muscle during surgery; examples: curare, decamethonium, succinylcholine

neuromuscular blocking agent, polarizing drug that blocks depolarization at the myoneural junction

neuromuscular blocking agent, depolarizing drug that blocks repolarization at the myoneural junction

neuromuscular junction connection between a nerve and a muscle where cholinergic neurotransmission takes place; synonyms: motor end plate, myoneural junction

neurotransmitter compound released by nerve endings in response to a nerve impulse that carries the stimulus across a synapse

neutral fat triacylglycerol molecules

neutral protamine Hagedorn insulin intermediate-acting formulation of insulin consisting of an insulin-protamine zinc complex at neutral pH; synonym: isophane insulin

neutron basic particle of matter; a nucleon, having zero charge and a mass of 1.67×10^{-24} g; a by-product of nuclear fissions; a particle obtained from an atomic pile and used to prepare radioisotopes

neutropenic having an abnormally low number of neutrophils in the blood

new drug (according to the Federal Food, Drug, and Cosmetic Act) any product that is a new chemical entity in whole or part; includes existing approved drugs that have been prepared for a new indication, a new dose, or a new route of administration

New Drug Application (NDA) lengthy documentation (filed with the FDA and required for all new drugs) that fully describes a drug, its manufacture, and the results of all preclinical and clinical tests; approval of a new drug application permits a company to market the drug

Newcomb, Edwin Leigh (1882-1950) leader in the establishment of the American Foundation for Pharmaceutical Education; pharmacy educator, editor, and executive of the National Council of Wholesale Associations; Remington Honor Medal recipient in 1950

Newtonian flow liquid flow characteristic of gases, true solutions, and noncolloidal liquids that exhibits a constant slope when "rate of shear" is plotted against "shearing stress" on a linear graph

Newton's law of viscous flow basic cgs quantitative expression for flow of a moving liquid layer (1 cm^2) past a stationary liquid layer (1 cm^2) separated by 1 cm; measured in a unit called a poise, which is equal to 1 dyne times 1 sec times 1 cm^2

nicotinamide amide of nicotinic acid and a form of the antipellagric factor niacin (nicotinic acid), an essential part of the coenzymes NAD and NADP

nicotinamide adenine dinucleotide (NAD) coenzyme composed of a nucleotide derivative of nicotinic acid and a nucleotide of adenine joined by a pyrophosphate linkage; coenzyme for certain oxidoreductases or dehydrogenases; synonym: diphosphopyridine nucleotide

nicotinamide adenine dinucleotide phosphate (NADP) coenzyme that is the 2'-phosphate ester of nicotinamide adenine dinucleotide; synonym: triphosphopyridine nucleotide

nicotinic acid B-complex vitamin; antipellagral factor; pellegral preventive factor; essential part of the coenzymes NAD and NADP; SEE *nicotinamide*

night cream SEE *cold cream*

nightshade poisonous, solanaceous plant containing several alkaloids, the main one being atropine; synonym: deadly nightshade; SEE *belladonna*

nit egg laid by lice

niter potassium nitrate; synonym: salt peter

nitrocellulose synonym: guncotton; SEE *pyroxylin*

nitrogen mustard chemotherapeutic alkylating agent used in treating cancer; compound consisting of an amino nitrogen substituted with two β-chloroethyl groups that are the so-called "alkylating arms"

nitroglycerin or nitroglycerol trinitrated glycerin; used as a coronary vasodilator in treating angina pectoris; synonyms: glyceryl trinitrate, glonoine

nocturia above normal urination at night

nocturnal occurring during the night or a period of darkness; opposite of diurnal

nocuous harmful; poisonous; CONTRAST *innocuous*

nominal labeling (denoted by "*N*") isotopically labeled compound on which the labeled position is uncertain

nomogram graphic representation consisting of several lines marked off to a scale, arranged in such a way that by using a straight edge to connect known values on two lines an unknown value can be read at the point of intersection with a third line; used to determine drug doses for specific persons

non- prefix denoting lack of, absence of, or negation of

noncontributory a situation in which the plan sponsor pays the entire cost of premium for coverage

nonelectrolyte substance that is not ionized in an aqueous solution; a substance that will not conduct electricity

nonenteral route mode of drug administration that does not directly involve the gastrointestinal tract

nonessential amino acid an amino acid that can be synthesized by the body

nonessential fatty acid a fatty acid that can be synthesized by the body

nonionic refers to a compound that neither ionizes nor is composed of ions

nonionic surfactant surface active agent that does not ionize in solution; exhibits fewer chemical incompatibilities than other surfactants; example: polysorbate 80

nonjudgmental tasks those tasks which do not require professional judgment; example: a pharmacy technician preparing a prescription product in the pharmacy

nonmaleficence a principle of ethics which states that one should avoid harming others

non-Newtonian flow liquid flow characteristic that does not exhibit a constant slope when "rate of shear" is plotted against "shearing stress" on a linear plot; examples: plastic, pseudoplastic, dilatant, and thixotropic flows

nonparenteral glass soda lime glass; not to be used for packaging parenteral products

nonparticipating provider a provider that has not contracted with the carrier or health plan to be a participating provider of health care

nonparticipating provider indemnity benefits health care coverage for services rendered by providers who are not under contract with the health plan; benefits are covered on an indemnity basis, typically carrying high copayment requirements and deductibles

nonpolar molecule a molecule that does not contain a dipole

nonprescription medicines medicines legally available to the general public without the necessity of a prescription; synonyms: proprietary medicine/drug, over-the-counter drug

norm established standard of acceptable behavior in a group; frequency distribution of experimental observations that when plotted exhibits a Gaussian (or bell-shaped) curve

normality concentration expression based on the number of gram equivalent weights of solute per liter of solution; also expressed as the number of milliequivalents (milligram equivalent weights) of solute in one milliliter of solution

normo- prefix meaning normal; examples: normotensive, normocytic

North American Pharmacist Licensure Examination computer-adaptive, competency-based examination that assesses the candidate's ability to apply knowledge gained in pharmacy school to real-life practice situations

nosocomial infection infections acquired during hospitalization

nosology science of the classification of disorders or diseases

Notice of Claimed Investigational Exemption for a New Drug lengthy document required for testing any new drug in human subjects; contains descriptions of its composition, all preclinical studies, and the protocol by which the drug will be tested in humans

NP glass SEE *nonparenteral glass*

nuclear envelope the double membrane that separates the nucleus from the cytoplasm

nuclear magnetic resonance method of spectrometry dependent upon vibrational frequencies generated by a radio frequency signal in the nuclear protons of ^{1}H, ^{13}C, ^{19}F, among others, that are precessing in a magnetic field; synonym: proton magnetic resonance

nuclear pore a channel through the nuclear envelope that allows molecules to pass between the cytoplasm and the nucleus

nucleases enzymes that catalyze the hydrolysis of nucleic acids into nucleotides and other products; examples: RNAase, DNAase

nucleation process of nucleus formation on which further growth occurs; example: crystalline nucleation on which a larger crystal is grown

nucleic acid **1:** polymer composed of ribotide or deoxyribotide units linked together through phosphates **2:** a polynucleotide; examples: DNA, RNA

nucleohistone DNA complexed with histone proteins

nucleoid in prokaryotes, an irregularly shaped region that contains a long circular DNA molecule

nucleolus a structure found in the nucleus when the nucleus is stained with certain dyes; plays a major role in the synthesis of ribosomal RNA

nucleon basic particle of an atomic nucleus; examples: neutron and proton

nucleophile **1:** in organic chemistry, an attracting reagent that has an affinity for electron-sparse or positively charged centers in a molecule **2:** a Lewis base **3:** an electron-rich atom or molecule

nucleophilic substitution chemical reaction in which a nucleophile attacks a molecule, resulting in a new compound; a reaction in which a nucleophile substitutes for an atom or molecular group

nucleoplasm the material within the nucleus that consists of proteins called lamins that form a network of chromatin fibers

nucleoside compound composed of a nitrogenous base and a sugar nucleotidase; enzyme that catalyzes the hydrolysis of a nucleotide into a nucleoside and phosphoric acid

nucleotide compound composed of a purine, pyrimidine, or other nitrogenous base attached to ribose and esterified with phosphate

nucleus 1: the core, kernel, or central mass **2:** the complex central mass in a cell responsible for cellular growth, reproduction, and genetics **3:** the central core containing the protons and neutrons of the atom **4:** a group of nerve cells within the nervous system from which the nerve fibers originate **5:** a central part of a crystal around which other parts of the crystal form **6:** a central part of the structure of an organic chemical molecule; example: an aromatic nucleus

nuclide any atom characterized by a specific number of protons and a specific number of neutrons; examples: carbon-12, carbon-14

nurse one who cares for patients according to accepted practice standards and specific directions of a physician

nursing home long-term care institution that provides minimum care nursing and other health services to the chronically ill and infirm

nutrition sum total of the processes involved in the ingestion and utilization of food substances; imperative to growth, repair, and maintenance of body functions

Nutzche filter porcelain filtration device that has a built-in porous support plate as a filter medium and a false bottom; designed to use vacuum to hasten the filtration process; used for chemicals that are incompatible with metal

nystagmus rapid, jerky, uncontrolled movements (oscillations) of the eye; can be seen on vertical (vertical nystagmus) and horizontal (horizontal nystagmus) meridians

O₂ 1: prescription (or other medication order) notation meaning both eyes **2:** chemical symbol for molecular oxygen

obese excessively overweight; having a BMI greater than 30 percent above normal body weight

objective data data that can be measured; examples: temperature, blood pressure

objectives desired outcomes toward which plans are directed; typically broad and general in scope

obligate aerobe an organism that is highly dependent on oxygen for energy production

obligate anaerobe an organism that grows only in the absence of oxygen

obsession persistent, unwanted idea that cannot be easily eliminated

obstetrician a physician who specializes in treating women during pregnancy and parturition

obstruction blocking of a structure (usually a biological passageway) that prevents it from functioning normally

obtund blunt or dull

occlusion obstruction or closure as in a blood vessel or a pipeline

occlusion compound synonym: clathrate; SEE *inclusion compound*

occlusive refers to a substance or an agent that cuts off or prevents contact with a surface; to shut in or out

occult hidden from view, concealed; example: occult blood

occult blood blood in such minute quantities that it can be recognized only by microscopic or chemical means; hidden blood

octahydronaphthacene parent structure for the tetracyclines

octal 1: a numbering system based on the numbers 0 through 7 **2:** a number system with a base of eight

oculentum eye ointment or salve

oculo- prefix meaning eye

odynophagia pain upon swallowing

office visit provision of health care services in an office setting, usually that of a physician

official drug useful medicine with recognized standards as specified in the *United States Pharmacopeia–National Formulary*

Oguchi's disease hereditary night blindness

OH⁻ chemical symbol for the hydroxyl ion

ohm unit of electrical resistance or impedance; ohm equals voltage divided by amperes (strength of an electrical current)

-oid suffix meaning similar to or like

oil an unctuous, combustible substance that is liquid, or easily liquefiable when warmed, and is soluble in ether but insoluble in water; depending on origin, classified as animal, mineral, or vegetable oil

oil, fixed oil that cannot be distilled without decomposition

oil, infused generally made from drugs containing alkaloids

oil, sugar triturate containing 2 cc of volatile oil and 100 grams of powdered sugar

oil, volatile oil that can be distilled without decomposition

oil-in-water emulsion SEE *emulsion, oil-in-water*

ointment medicated semisolid preparation for external application to the skin or mucous membranes; generally has a greasy base

ointment, ophthalmic specially formulated sterile ointment for application to the eye; usually dispensed in a small applicator tube

-ol suffix meaning alcohol

oleaginous oily, greasy, or fatty

oleate compound of metal or an alkaloid with oleic acid

olefin compound that contains a double bond between two carbon atoms; synonym: alkene

oleoresin extract of a plant containing a resin dissolved in an oil; example: turpentine

oleotherapy an injection or an application of an oil as a form of treatment

oleovitamin preparation of fat-soluble vitamins (A, D, E, and K) in fish liver oil or an edible vegetable oil

olig- prefix meaning few, very little, or scant; same as oligo-

oligo- prefix meaning few, very little, or scant; same as olig-

oligomer a multisubunit protein in which some or all subunits are identical

oligonucleotide a short nucleic acid segment that contains fewer than 50 nucleotides

oligosaccharide sugar polymer, one structured unit of which, on hydrolysis, produces three or more units of monosaccharides

oliguria condition in which there is a small amount of urine being produced

-oma suffix meaning tumor

Omnibus Budget Reconciliation Act of 1990 (OBRA '90) law drafted by the Senate Committee on Aging that requires manufacturers to pay rebates to federal and state governments for projects used by Medicaid recipients; also contains patient counseling and drug utilization review provisions for Medicaid programs; spurred many states to pass regulations requiring pharmacists to counsel *all* patients on the use of their prescriptions

oncogene a mutated version of a proto-oncogene that promotes abnormal cell proliferation

oncologist a physician who specializes in the study and treatment of tumors; a cancer specialist

one-compartmental model SEE *single-compartmental model*

onset time time interval from the administration of a drug until it begins to exert its pharmacological effect(s); the time required to obtain an effective blood level of a drug

opaquant extender substance added to a tablet-film coating process to provide a coating that prevents light exposure to the previously prepared dosage unit or drug particle; substance used to render a clear plastic film opaque

opaquing agent substance added to capsules, capsule vials, or other containers to render them opaque; example: titanium oxide

open access a self-referral arrangement allowing members to see participating providers for specialty care without a referral from another doctor

open enrollment period period during which subscribers in a health benefit program have an opportunity to reenroll or select an alternate health plan being offered to them, usually without evidence of insurability or waiting periods

open formulary SEE *formulary, open*

open-panel HMO organization that contracts with private office physicians and other health care providers to ensure care of their members

open reading frame (ORF) a series of triplet base sequences in mRNA that do not contain a stop codon

open system refers to a process under observation that involves exchanges of heat, work, and matter with its surroundings; CONTRAST *closed system*

operon a set of linked genes that are regulated as a unit

ophthalmic 1: pertaining to the eye **2:** pharmaceutical preparation to be instilled into the eye

ophthalmic solution SEE *solution, opthalmic*

ophthalmoplegia paralysis of the motor nerves of the eye

opiate type of drug obtained from *Papaver somniferum* that has narcotic analgesic effects

opioid analgesic substances derived from opium or endogenous peptides with similar pharmacological effects

opium dried, gummy latex obtained from excised, unripened capsules of the poppy, *Papaver somniferum album*

Oppenheim-Ziehan disease dystonia musculorum deformans

opportunity cost in pharmacoeconomics, the amount that an input could earn in its best alternative use, or the alternative that must be foregone when something is produced

opsin retinal protein that makes up one of the visual pigments

optical isomers type of stereoisomer that contains at least one chiral center, with one molecule being a reflection of the other; examples: D(+)-glyceraldehyde and L(−)-glyceraldehyde; synonyms: mirror image isomers, enantiomorplis and antimers

optical pyrometer SEE *pyrometer*

optical rotation degree and direction of the shifting of polarized light as it passes through a substance; can be clockwise (dextrorotatory) or counterclockwise (levorotatory)

optical rotatory dispersion results of a measurement of the angle of rotation of polarized light at different wavelengths as it passes through a substance or a solution

optometry health care field involving the assessment of visual capability and correction of visual defects with the use of lenses or other optical aids without (or with limited) use of drugs

oral 1: associated with the mouth **2:** route of drug administration in which the drug is placed in the mouth and swallowed

oral administration process of administering a medication by having the patient swallow it

oral release, osmotic mechanism for controlling release of a drug from its dosage form based on the principle of osmosis

orbicules globules of sugar, medicated by dropping a volatile oil on their surface

orbital 1: subshell or probability cloud describing the most likely position of an orbital electron within an atom **2:** s-type—electron orbital for which the quantum numbers l and $m_l = 0$ **3:** p-type—electron orbital for which the quantum number $l =$ and the quantum number $m_l = 1$, 0, or −1 **4:** d-type—electron orbital for which the quantum number $l = 2$ and the quantum number $m_l = 2$, 1, 0, −1, or −2 **5:** f-type—electron orbital for which the quantum number $l = 3$ and the quantum number $m_l = 3$, 2, 1, 0, −1, −2, or −3

order of a reaction/process discrete rate of occurrence; the exponential number to which concentrations of reactants or products must be raised to quantitatively describe a reaction (or process) rate; most described by either a zero-, first-, second-, or third-order rate; examples: chemical and physical degradation rates of drug molecules and absorption, distribution, and elimination rates of drugs in and from the body

organelle a membrane-enclosed structure within a eukaryotic cell

organic refers to living substances or materials derived from a living source; refers to carbon compounds

organification conversion of serum iodide to organic iodine by thyroid cells; an essential process occurring before iodine can be added to tyrosine to form monoiodothyronine, diiodothyronine, triiodothyronine, and ultimately tetraiodothyronine

organization costs costs incurred to legally establish a corporation; an intangible asset

organoclay organic clay compounds; example: bentoquatam (used as a barrier to poison ivy when applied to the skin prior to plant contact)

organoleptic affecting one or more special sense organs

orientation effect SEE *dipole-dipole interactions*

oro- prefix meaning the mouth

orphan drug refers to drug entities that are used to treat certain rare disease states and consequently have limited sales

ortho- 1: prefix meaning normal or straight **2:** prefix in inorganic chemical nomenclature meaning the completely hydrated or hydroxylated form of an acid; example: orthophosphoric acid (H_3PO_4) **3:** prefix in organic chemistry meaning the location of two substituents on adjacent carbon atoms of a benzene ring; example: *o*-aminobenzoic acid

orthodontist a dentist who specializes in the prevention and correction of abnormally positioned or aligned teeth

orthopedic surgeon a physician who specializes in surgical prevention and correction of deformities or injuries to the skeletal structure of the body

orthopnea difficult breathing, especially in the supine position; usually associated with cardiac asthma

orthostatic refers to an event caused by position change or standing erect

Ortner's syndrome left vocal cord paralysis associated with enlarged left atrium in mitral stenosis

-ose suffix meaning sugar

-osis suffix meaning condition of or disease involving

Osler's disease erythremia (increase in size of bone marrow and blood volume)

Osler-Vaquez disease erythemia; polycythemia rubra vera

osmolarity the molar concentration of osmotically active (discrete) particles in a solution

osmolyte an osmotically active substance synthesized by cells to restore osmotic balance

osmosis the passage of a liquid through a semipermeable membrane from a cell of lower concentration of solute to a cell of higher concentration of solute; a natural phenomenon that equalizes the vapor (internal) pressure on each side of a semipermeable membrane

osmotic refers to the process of osmosis; the flow of fluids across a semipermeable membrane

osmotic coefficient correction factor for calculating the osmotic effect of a nonideal solution

osmotic diuresis a process in which solute in the urinary filtrate causes excessive loss of water and electrolytes

osmotic pressure force per unit area exerted on a membrane by dissolved particles that will not diffuse; an important property to be adjusted to that of normal body fluids in parenterals and ophthalmics; one of several colligative properties; pressure required to prevent the flow of water from one side of a semipermeable membrane to the other side; represents the difference in vapor pressure above each of two solutions separated by a semipermeable membrane

osseous bone or bonelike

osteo- prefix meaning bone or bones

osteochrondosis degeneration followed by reossification of one or more ossification centers in children

osteoporosis disease characterized by an increase in porosity of the bone, frequently associated with a loss of calcium ions; abnormal reabsorption of bone structure

ostia small opening into each of the respiratory sinus cavities

ostomy surgical resectioning of the intestine or the ureter to an external opening in the abdominal wall; examples: ileostomy, colostomy, urostomy

Ostwald-Cannon-Fenske viscometer capillary device used to measure viscosity by comparing the flow rate of one liquid with the flow rate of another of known viscosity at a given temperature and pressure

ot- prefix meaning ear; same as oto-

otic pertaining to the ear

otitis inflammation of the ear

oto- prefix meaning ear; same as ot-

otologist a physician who specializes in diseases of the ear; a specialist who is knowledgable in the anatomy, physiology, and pathology of the ear

ounce, apothecary (℥) a unit of weight equal to 8 drams or 480 grains

ounce, avoirdupois (oz or oz av) a unit of weight equal to 28.3495 grams or 437.5 grains

ounce, fluid (fl ℥) an apothecary unit of volume equal to 29.57 mL, 8 fluid drams; or 480 minims; a fluid ounce of water weighs 455 grains

outcome measures assessments including such parameters as the patient's perception of restoration of function, quality of life, and functional status, as well as objective measures of mortality, morbidity, and health status that gauge the effect or results of treatment for a particular disease or condition

outcomes results achieved through a given health care service, including pharmaceutical care, medication, or medical procedure; economic—relating to costs and productivity; humanistic—including patient satisfaction and health status

outcomes management systematically improving health care results by modifying practices in response to data gleaned through outcomes measurement, then remeasuring and remodifying in a formal program of continuous quality improvement

outcomes research studies aimed at measuring the effect of a given product, procedure, or medical technology on health or costs

outer membrane the pourous external membrane of mitochondria

outlier an observation in a distribution that is outside a certain range, often defined as two or three standard deviations from the mean or exceeding a specific percentile

out-of-area coverage health plan benefit for treatment obtained by a covered person outside the network service area

out-of-pocket costs/expenses the portion of payments for health services required to be paid by the enrollee, including copayments, coinsurance, and deductibles

out-of-pocket limit the total payments toward eligible expenses that a covered person funds for himself/herself and/or dependents—i.e., deductibles, copays, and coinsurance—as defined per the contract; once reached, 100 percent coverage for health services received during the rest of that calendar year; some out-of-pocket costs (e.g., mental health, penalties for nonprecertification, etc.) not eligible

outpatient   person who is not admitted to a hospital but receives health care services at a hospital or a dispensary associated with the hospital

over-the-counter medicines   SEE *nonprescription medicines*

owner's equity   that part of a business possessed by the owner including cash, stock, and/or physical items such as a building or land; (accounting) the excess of total assets over total liabilities

oxa-β-lactam   nucleus of the bactericidal antibiotic moxalactam

oxazolidinediones   class of drugs with anticonvulsant activity; used to treat petit mal epilepsy; ineffective for the treatment of grand mal epilepsy; example: trimethadione

oxidase   enzyme that catalyzes a direct reaction of a substrate with oxygen

oxidation   loss of electrons from a substance in a chemical reaction; older definitions include the combination of a substance with oxygen and the loss of hydrogen from a substance

oxidation number   discrete number describing an oxidation state; example: iron may have oxidation numbers of 0, 2, and 3, corresponding to Fe^0, Fe^{++}, and Fe^{+++}

oxidation-reduction   chemical change resulting in an increase in the electronegativity of a molecule (reduction) accompanied by a reduction in electronegativity (oxidation) of another molecule in a system under observation; chemical reaction in which there is an electron donor (reducing agent) and an electron acceptor (oxidizing agent)

oxidation state   level of the positivity or negativity of an element computed by summing the negative atoms and positive atoms in a molecule; the difference of the two sums is the oxidation state; the oxidation state of a free element is zero

oxidative demethylation   metabolic reaction in which a methyl group is removed from a molecule in the form of formaldehyde

oxidative phosphorylation   formation of ATP from ADP and phosphate by using the energy of biological oxidation

oxidative stress   excessive production of reactive oxygen species

oxidize   the removal of electrons

oxidized molecule   a molecule from which one or more electrons have been removed

oxidizing agent substance that accepts electrons from another substance while undergoing a chemical reaction; the oxidizing agent is reduced in the reaction; a compound that is preferentially reduced over another which is being protected from reduction in the system; CONTRAST *antioxidant*

oxidoreductase type of enzyme that catalyzes oxidation-reduction reactions; examples: dehydrogenase, oxidase, oxygenase

oxime chemical compound having the fundamental structure, R-CH = N-O-H or R_2C = N-O-H; chemical compound formed by reaction between a ketone or an aldehyde and hydroxyl amine; synonym: isonitroso compound

oxyanion a negatively charged oxygen atom

oxygenase enzyme that catalyzes a reaction in which oxygen is incorporated into the substrate molecule; SEE *hydroxylase*

ozokerite hard, white, odorless wax resembling spermaceti when purified; occurs naturally in the mountains of Asia Minor; synonyms: earth wax, ceresin

ozone allotropic form of oxygen, the molecule of which is composed of three atoms of oxygen (O_3) rather than two (O_2)

ozonide compound formed upon oxidation of an olefin (alkene) with ozone; ozonides breakdown with water to form aldehydes or ketones

package insert nonpromotional professional labeling information that accompanies a drug product and contains information necessary for safe and effective use

packaging, compliance SEE *unit of use*

packing material, usually covered by or impregnated with a drug, that is inserted into a body cavity or between the tooth enamel and the gingival margin

pack SEE *laparotomy pack*

paddle large surface area blade that rotates slowly to effect large volume mixing of liquids

Paget's disease osteitis deformans (generalized skeletal disorder with thickening and softening of bone)

paid claims amounts paid to providers to satisfy the contractual liability of the carrier or plan sponsor

paid claims loss ratio the result of paid claims divided by premiums

paint liniment applied with a brush

paints, collodion solutions of pyroxylin in ether-alcohol that leave a hard film upon drying

paints, drying liniment medicated mucilages of gums or albumin that leave a thick film upon drying

paints, glycogelatin medicated globules of gelatin with glycerin that are melted at the time of use and applied with a brush

palatable agreeable to the palate; having a pleasant taste

palindrome a sequence that provides the same information whether it is read forward or backward; DNA palindromes contain inverted repeat sequences

pallor unnatural paleness

palmitate refers to a salt or an ester of palmitic acid

palmityl alcohol SEE *cetyl alcohol*

palpate to examine by touching

palpitation rapid, violent, or throbbing pulsation of the heart; usually perceived by the patient as an abnormally rapid fluttering of the heart; an awareness of heartbeat by the patient

palsy paralysis; loss of sensation or ability to move or control movement; examples: Bell's palsy, "shaking palsy" (Parkinson's disease)

***p*-aminobenzoic acid** growth factor for some species of bacteria; part of the structure of folic acid and some local anesthetics; antagonist in sulfonamide therapy; synonym: 4-aminobenzoic acid

pan- prefix meaning all

panacea "cure-all" or a remedy for all diseases

papain proteolytic enzyme obtained from papaya fruit; used both to treat a hematoma and as a meat tenderizer

papers small, folded sheets of paper, each containing a single dose of a powder

papilledema edema (swelling) of the optic papilla

para- 1: prefix meaning beside or parallel with **2:** (in organic chemistry) two groups substituted at opposite points on the benzene ring

para-aminobenzoic acid essential nutrient for many microorganisms; required for the bacterial biosynthesis of folic acid

Paracelsus (1493-1541) Swiss physician who introduced the concept of the human body as a "chemical laboratory" and challenged classical concepts of medicine and drug therapy; also known as "Theophrastus Bombastus von Hohenheim"

parallax apparent movement or displacement of an object resulting when an observer views it from different positions or moves the head or eyes

paralysis partial or total loss of function in a body part due to neural or muscular dysfunction

paramedic individual trained and certified to perform certain emergency procedures by following a treatment protocol under the supervision of health professionals

parametabolite compound that closely resembles a natural substrate (e.g., hormone, vitamin) and can substitute for the natural compound in fulfilling any requirements of an organism for the natural compound

parameter **1:** set of physical properties whose values determine the characteristics or behavior of a substance or process **2:** descriptive numerical measure that is computed from all elements within a given population

paramyoclonus SEE *myoclonus multiplex*

paraprofessional one who carries out a specific task or tasks assigned by or in conjunction with a health professional

parasympatholytic drugs that block the effect of acetylcholine at the muscarinic receptor; synonym: antimuscarinics

parasympathomimetic drug that mimics or copies the effects of the parasympathetic nervous system; action may be directly at the muscarinic receptor or indirectly

parasympathomimetic, direct acting agonist drug acting directly on the muscarinic receptors of acetylcholine; example: pilocarpine

parasympathomimetic, indirect acting drug that inhibits acetylcholine esterase, thus allowing acetylcholine to build up in body and producing an effect; examples: physostigmine, prostigmine, disopropylfluorophosphate

parathyroid one of four small glands responsible for secreting parathyroid hormone; imbedded in the thyroid gland

paravitamin compound that closely resembles a vitamin and may be utilized by an organism as a substitute for the vitamin

paregoric preparation containing opium extract, alcohol, camphor, and other volatile substances; synonym: camphorated opium tincture; used as an antidiarrheal and analgesic

parenteral dosage form usually administered under one or more layers of skin; literally, a dosage form not administered through the alimentary canal; example: normal saline injection

parenteral administration process of administering a medication by a route other than the alimentary canal; introduction of medication into the body using a needle and syringe; examples: intravenous, subcutaneous, and intramuscular injections

paresis partial paralysis

paresthesia burning, prickling, or other abnormal sensation

parkinsonism group of neurological disorders characterized by hypokinesia, tremor, and rigidity; neurological disorder involving fine movement and resulting from a lack of the neurotransmitter dopamine in the pathway from the substantia niger to the globus pallidus (basal ganglia in the brain)

Parkinson's disease shaking/trembling palsy

paroxysm sudden attack or intensification of the symptoms of a disease

Parrish, Edward (1822-1872) pharmacist and early educator at the Philadelphia College of Pharmacy; one of the founders of APhA

Parson's sick role model a model of the social and psychological dynamics of the patient-doctor relationship; describes the patient's responsibilities as seeking competent help and doing all that is necessary to get well, so that, in return, the patient is not held responsible for becoming ill and is temporarily exempt from performing normal social role responsibilities

partial agonist SEE *agonist*

partial differentiation mathematical computation of an infinitesimally small rate of change of one dependent variable in an expression with respect to simultaneous changes of several other independent variables considered individually; other independent variables in the equation are held constant as the effect of each is computed

participating provider provider who has contractually accepted the terms and conditions as set forth by the health plan to deliver medical services to covered persons

particle diameter micrometric expression of particle size of drug materials; quantitatively expressed in many different ways to more accurately reflect its effect with respect to a specific pharmaceutical use; example: volume-surface diameter (dy)

particle size SEE *particle diameter*

particulate matter minute, separate, and distinct particles in a liquid; an undesirable characteristic of a solution dosage form, such as an injection

partition coefficient physical property of a compound that reflects its distribution between two immiscible solvents; the ratio of the concentration of the compound dissolved in one solvent phase to that dissolved in the other solvent phase

partnership form of business arrangement in which two or more persons agree to share in the enterprise

parvules very small sugarcoated pills usually containing potent medicines in small doses

passive absorption SEE *absorption*

passive diffusion movement of drug molecules from a region of higher concentration to a region of lower concentration through a membrane that does not participate in the process; quantitatively expressed by Fick's first law of diffusion

passive immunity development of resistance to a disease as a result of the introduction of antibodies already formed; immunity that occurs naturally (passage from mother to fetus) or by injection of an antitoxin

paste **1:** (pharmaceutical) stiff-drying ointmentlike preparation for external application; example: zinc oxide paste **2:** single-phase gel for external application; example: hydrated pectin gel

paste, dentifrice paste formulation intended to clean and/or polish the teeth; may contain certain additional agents

Pasteur, Louis (1822-1897) French chemist and crystallographer who found microorganisms to be the cause of many diseases; known also for developing the process of "pasteurization" to kill pathogenic microorganisms in milk and for developing several vaccines; laid the foundation for stereochemistry by being the first to separate (resolve) mirror image isomers; disproved the theory of spontaneous generation of living organisms

Pasteur effect the observation that glucose consumption is greater under anaerobic conditions than when O_2 is present

pastille medicated disk used for treating the mucosa of the mouth and throat; synonyms: lozenge, troche

pastille, fumigating small, cone-shaped compounds of balsam and other spices with a combustible substance as a base; used as a fumigator or disinfectant

patch drug delivery system that contains an adhesive backing and that permits its ingredients to diffuse from some portion of it (e.g., the backing itself, a reservoir, the adhesive, or some other component) into the body from the external site where it is applied

patch, extended release drug delivery system in the form of a patch that releases the drug to allow a reduction in dosing frequency compared to that drug presented as a conventional dosage form (e.g., a solution or a prompt drug-releasing, conventional, solid dosage form)

patch, extended release, electrically controlled drug delivery system in the form of a patch which is controlled by an electric current that releases the drug to allow a reduction in dosing frequency compared to that drug presented as a conventional dosage form (e.g., a solution or a prompt drug-releasing, conventional, solid dosage form)

patent legal document extended to the inventor of a product or process that grants the inventor exclusive rights to produce, use, or sell a product for a specified period of time

patent medicine medicines widely sold during the late 1800s and early 1900s that purported to cure a wide range of diseases; ingredients were often secret, unsafe, and ineffective; incorrect synonym for nonprescription medicines

path abbreviation for pathology

-path suffix meaning disease or abnormal condition; same as -pathy

patho- prefix meaning disease

pathogen disease-producing agent or organism

pathogenesis development or the events involved in the production of a disease

pathognomonic characteristic to a specific disease and no other, allowing one to diagnose the disease; example: Auspitz's sign for psoriasis

pathologist a physician who is a specialist in diagnosing the morbid changes in tissues removed during operations and postmortem examinations; a specialist in diseases and disease processes; one who studies diseases

-pathy suffix meaning disease or abnormal condition; same as -path

patient person or animal needing medical advice or treatment

Patient Care Services SEE *pharmaceutical care; cognitive services*

patient-day period of service given to a patient between the census-taking hours on two successive days

patient information leaflets literature distributed to patients by the pharmacist or the physician that pertain to appropriate drug use and precautions to be heeded by the patient

Patient Information Release Form a legal document signed by the patient giving permission to the indicated party to release his/her health information; may be used to allow the pharmacist to obtain a patient's medical records from the physician or hospital in order to provide pharmaceutical care

patient package insert a printed sheet included to provide a person information concerning a drug or a drug product

patient rounds physician or health care team visits to the patients' hospital bedsides to assess treatment progress

patient satisfaction a critical element toward understanding what issues cause patients to select a particular health care system, and what issues are most likely to influence changing their current care affiliation, with either the physician, the hospital, or the health plan; required as an essential component of various accreditation reviews and a growing set of employer standards

Pauli's exclusion principle dictates that no two electrons in an atom may have an identical set of quantum numbers; restricts those electrons occupying the same orbital to those of opposite (antiparallel) spins

payer a public or private organization that pays for or underwrites coverage for health care expenses

pCO$_2$ partial pressure of carbon dioxide usually measured in mm of mercury and used to express CO_2 concentration in the air or in a solution (as in the blood)

peak blood level maximum concentration of a drug in the blood following administration of a single dose; useful parameter in establishing clinical dosing intervals

peanut oil SEE *earth nut oil*

pearlescent having a luster resembling a pearl

pearls soft, rounded, gelatin capsules that usually contain oleaginous liquids

pebble mill SEE *ball mill*

pedia- prefix meaning child

pediatrician a physician who specializes in caring for children

pediculosis infestation with lice

Pediculus humanus var. *capitis* head louse

Pediculus humanus var. *corporis* body louse

pedodontist a dentist who specializes in treating the teeth and mouth conditions of children

peer review the evaluation of quality of total health care provided, carried out by medical staff with equivalent training

peer review organization (PRO) selected panel of health professionals responsible for reviewing diagnosis and treatment (including drug therapy and orders for laboratory tests) of Medicare and Medicaid patients

pellet, coated, extended release solid dosage form in which the drug itself is in the form of granules to which varying amounts of coating have been applied, and which releases a drug (or drugs) in such a manner to allow a reduction in dosing frequency as compared to that drug (or drugs) presented as a conventional dosage form

pellet, implantable small, sterile, solid mass consisting of a highly purified drug (with or without excipients) made by the formation of granules, or by compression and molding; intended for implantation in the body (usually subcutaneously) for the purpose of providing continuous release of the drug over long periods of time

Pelletier, Pierre Joseph (1788-1842) French pharmacist and chemist who, with Caventou, discovered strychnine, brucine, quinine, and other alkaloids

pencil medicinal agents mixed with a stiff mucilage and formed into stick before drying, used mostly as caustics or astringents

pencil, salve medicinal agents mixed with waxes or oils and molded into a stick shape

penetrometer device used to determine the viscosity of semisolids by measuring the depth to which a solid cone of specific dimensions penetrates when dropped a fixed distance; device used to measure the consistency or stiffness in an ointment or a suppository

penicillamine α-amino acid obtained upon degradation of penicillin; used in medicine as a chelating agent for the treatment of poisoning due to excess copper (as in Wilson's disease); chemical names: 2-amino-3-methyl-3-mercaptobutyric acid, 3-mercaptovaline

penicillinase enzyme catalyst for the hydrolysis of the β-lactam ring of various penicillins, forming penicilloic acids that are devoid of antibacterial activity; when produced by certain bacteria (e.g., *Staphylococcus aureus*) leads to penicillin resistance; synonym: β-lactamase

penicillins group of bactericidal antibiotics that block the final stage of cell wall biosynthesis in bacteria by inhibiting transpeptidase

Penicillium notatum mold from which penicillin G was originally isolated

penicilloic acid product resulting from acid, base, or β-lactamase-catalyzed hydrolysis of the β-lactam ring in penicillin

pentose phosphate pathway a biochemical pathway that produces NADPH, ribose, and several other sugars

pep pills central nervous system stimulants, such as amphetamines

pepsin enzyme secreted in the gastric juice; responsible for hydrolysis of proteins; protease secreted by the chief cells of the stomach mucosa

peptic ulcer an inflamed lesion or opening occurring in the lower end of the esophagus, in the stomach, or in the duodenum; usually caused by an oversecretion of pepsin and other gastric juices

peptide polymer that, on hydrolysis, produces amino acids; polymer composed of amino acids held together by peptide bonds; a breakdown product or a building component of a protein

peptide bond chemical linkage of amino acids in which the carboxyl group of one amino acid forms an amide with the amino group of a second amino acid, which in turn may form an amide bond with another amino acid, thus forming chains or polymers of amino acids; SEE *peptide*

peptidyl transferase 1: enzyme that catalyzes the formation of a peptide bond in peptide and protein biosynthesis **2:** γ-peptidyl transferase enzyme in the glutathione metabolic pathway in which a γ-glutamyl group is transferred from one amino acid residue of a γ-glutamyl peptide to any amino acid except proline to form a new γ-glutamyl dipeptide; may be important in amino acid transport and in the diagnosis of obstructive jaundice

percentage part of a whole; expressed in hundredths

percentage error of compounding an estimate of the total error incurred when compounding a dosage form; computed as the square root of the sum of the squared errors in each step of the compounding process; SEE *compounding error*

percentage markup the difference between selling price and cost of an item multiplied by 100 divided by the selling price

percent by volume concentration expression referring to mL of solute per 100 mL of solution

percent by weight concentration expression referring to grams of solute per 100 g of solution

percent weight-in-volume concentration expression referring to grams of solute per 100 mL of solution

per contract per month the dollar amount related to each effective contract holder, subscriber, or member for each month

per diem charge amount charged per day for treatment and/or other services

per member per month the unit of measure (revenue, cost, or utilization) related to each effective member for each month the membership was effective; calculated as number of units divided by member-months

per member per year the same as per member per month but based on a year; SEE *per member per month*

percolate 1: process involving slow passage of a solvent through a permeable drug (powdered vegetable drug) to extract the active constituents **2:** liquid which is collected after it passes through the powdered drug and which contains the extracted constituents

percutaneous absorption movement of a medication (or other substances) from the surface of the skin into layers below the surface and into the blood

perforation the act or process of making a hole through a substance or a body part; example: an ulcer that is advanced to the point that an unnatural opening has resulted (perforated ulcer)

performance evaluation necessary management function that provides an organization feedback regarding the effectiveness of its employees

performance measures a system that aids providers or insurers in making decisions about health care or in enhancing health status and the quality of patient outcomes; a health care network performance matrix, as outlined by the JCAHO, to include clinical performance; health status; satisfaction of patients, practitioners, and purchasers; process effectiveness; and the communication and education of patients, providers, and the public

performance test a measure of mechanical or manipulative ability in which the test closely resembles a real-world task for the job being evaluated; may be an actual sample of the work being evaluated

perfusion model a pharmacokinetic replica based on blood flow to various organs and the rate at which a drug comes to equilibrium between the organs

peri- prefix meaning around

pericranial around the head area

perineal referring to the perineum

perineum tissue that marks externally the approximate boundary of the outlet of the pelvis

periodicity **1:** the fundamental concept (in financial accounting) that involves reporting activities occurring in relatively short periods of time **2:** property of a process or system in which certain observed properties are repeated after regular intervals of time

periodic table systematized arrangement of the basic elements according to atomic weight and generally accepted electronic configuration

periodontal ligament weblike net of living collagen fibers that support teeth in their sockets; they extend from the alveolar bone to the tooth roots

periodontist a dentist who specializes in treating diseases of the periodontium (gums), the tissues investing and supporting the teeth

periodontitis damage to the periodontium that supports the tooth as a result of poor hygiene; tooth mobility and tooth loss result if the problem is not reversed

periorbital around the orbit of the eye

peripheral neuropathy disease or functional disorder of the peripheral nervous system

peristalsis progressive wave of contraction seen in biological tubes such as the intestines and the esophagus

peristaltic pump a type of intravenous fluid pump that moves fluids through flexible tubes by means of a series of rollers sequentially passing over the tubes, imitating intestinal peristaltic movement

peritoneal having reference to the peritoneum

peritoneal dialysis passing of fluids through the peritoneal cavity for the purpose of diffusing solute molecules from the body through the peritoneum into the fluid; used to rid the body of toxic substances

peritoneum the membrane lining of the abdominal and pelvic walls

perlite filter aid made of aluminum silicate

permeable capable of being penetrated; example: cell membranes allowing the passage of molecules

pernicious anemia an illness caused by a deficiency of vitamin B_{12}; symptoms include low red blood cell counts, weakness, and neurological disturbances

peroxisome an organelle that contains oxidative enzymes

perpetual inventory system continuously updated record of the quantity of goods available for sale

persistence the length of time that a patient is adherent (compliant) with therapy recommendations

pertussis whooping cough

pessary an object inserted into the vagina to mechanically support the uterus; synonym: vaginal suppository

pestle oblong-shaped device usually made of glass or porcelain used to grind or mix pharmaceutical preparations in a mortar

petechia small darkened spot due to blood effusion into tissue (plural form: petechiae)

petrolatum gauze SEE *gauze*

petroleum benzin low-boiling distilled fraction of petroleum primarily consisting of pentanes and hexanes; synonym: petroleum ether

petroxolin liquid preparation for external application; usually bases: liquid petrolatum, oleic acid, ammonia, oil of lavender, alcohol

petty cash a monetary fund used to pay for small incidental expenditures

phage 1: particulate, transmissible, ultramicroscopic substance that dissolves or exerts a lytic effect on bacteria; a virus that infects bacteria **2:** a cell type that engulfs and digests bacteria and debris; example: macrophage

-phage 1: suffix referring to a virus that infects bacteria **2:** suffix meaning a cell type that can engulf other cells or cellular debris

phago- prefix meaning to ingest by way of engulfing an object

phagocyte cell capable of ingesting and destroying particulate substances such as bacteria, protozoa, cells, and cellular debris

phagocytosis ingestion and digestion of bacteria and other particles by phagocytes

phantasticant substance capable of inducing fantasy states; synonym: hallucinogen

phantom 1: image or impression not evoked by actual stimuli **2:** device consisting of a mass of material that is approximately equal in radiation absorbing and scattering properties to human tissue; used to simulate the in vivo effects of ionizing radiation

phantom pain pain felt in limb that has been amputated

pharmaceutical alternative drug product that contains the same therapeutic moiety and potency and is administered by the same route but differs in the kind of salt, ester, or dosage form

pharmaceutical care patient-centered, outcome-oriented pharmacy practice that requires the pharmacist work in concert with the patient and the patient's other health care providers to promote health, to prevent disease, and to assess, monitor, initiate, and modify medication use to ensure that drug therapy regimens are safe and effective

pharmaceutical chemist an early pharmacy degree that usually required three years of study; last offered in the early 1930s

pharmaceutical elegance expression of the acceptability of physical appearance and palatability of a drug dosage form; expression used to indicate that a dosage form is pleasing to the normal senses of a patient

pharmaceutical equivalent drug product that contains the same active ingredient(s) and is identical in dosage form and potency to another drug product, but may not be equal in pharmacological or therapeutic response due to dosage-form effects; synonym: generic equivalent

Pharmaceutical Manufacturers Association SEE *Pharmaceutical Research and Manufacturers of America*

Pharmaceutical Research and Manufacturers of America nonprofit, scientific, professional and trade organization representing the major manufacturers of prescription drugs, medical devices, and diagnostic products; formerly Pharmaceutical Manufacturers Association; founded in 1958

pharmaceutical solution SEE *solution*

pharmaceutical substitution act of dispensing a pharmaceutical alternative for the drug product prescribed; examples: the salt form of codeine sulfate for that of codeine phosphate, tetracycline hydrochloride for tetracycline phosphate complex, the ester form of propoxyphene napsylate for propoxyphene hydrochloride, erthromycin ethyl succinate for erythromycin estolate, the dosage form of ampicillin suspension for ampicillin capsules

pharmaceutics that branch of pharmacy involving the study of the chemical, physical, and biological factors that influence formulation, manufacture, stability, and efficacy of dosage forms

pharmacist a health professional who is educated and licensed to dispense medications, provide drug information, and supervise pharmacy technicians

Pharmacist Care Claim Form form for documentation and billing of pharmaceutical care services provided; developed by the National Community Pharmacists Association; typically submitted to an insurance company along with the completed HCFA 1500 form

pharmaco- prefix meaning drug

pharmacodynamics the study of absorption, distribution, metabolism, and excretion of a drug; its mechanism of action; and its biochemical and physiological effects

pharmacogenetics 1: the study of hereditary variations in organisms that are revealed solely by the effects of drugs **2:** variations in the response of an individual to medications due solely to hereditary characteristics

pharmacognosy the study of naturally occurring drugs from plants or animals as well as their sources, nature, and uses

pharmacokinetics the study of the quantitative relationships of the rates of drug absorption, distribution, and elimination processes; data used to establish dosage amount and frequency for desired therapeutic response

pharmacologic effect therapeutic value of, or a result which relates to, a physiologic response to the drug

pharmacologic end point reference point used in recording a physiological response to a drug; example: measurement of beats per minute to determine the effects of a drug used in treating tachycardia

pharmacology study of the action and/or mechanism of action of drugs on living tissue

pharmacopoeia book containing a list of medicinal substances and their standards; selected and established by recognized authorities; examples: *United States Pharmacopeia (USP)* and *British Pharmacopoeia (BP)*

Pharmacopoeia International official drug compendium for many countries

pharmacotherapy use of a drug(s) for treatment or prevention of a disease

pharmacy 1: art and science of preparing, compounding, stabilizing, preserving, and dispensing medications and the provision of information **2:** place where medicines are stored, compounded, and dispensed; synonyms: apothecary, drugstore

Pharmacy and Therapeutics Committee group in a hospital or other institutional setting consisting of physicians and pharmacists who make recommendations on all matters relating to drugs used and establish other drug therapy-related policies

pharmacy benefit manager an organization that specializes in managing the utilization and costs of prescription medications by health plan members

pharmacy-coordinated unit-dose dispensing and drug administration institutionalized (hospital) system in which pharmacy technicians administer medications instead of registered nurses

pharmacy design layout/arrangement of pharmacy; needs to consider how best to support delivery of pharmaceutical care; must include area designated for patient interviews and counseling

pharmacy doctor self-proclaimed title by the membership of some pharmacy associations, without academic or regulatory status

pharmacy extern person engaged in experiential training under the supervision of a registered pharmacist as part of the structured curriculum of a college of pharmacy

pharmacy intern person gaining experiential training outside of the structured education provided by a college of pharmacy by working under the supervision of a registered pharmacist for a specified number of hours as required for licensure by a board of pharmacy

Pharmacy Practice Activity Classification taxonomy of pharmacist activities, covering the domains of dispensing drugs and devices, preventing and resolving drug therapy problems, promoting health and preventing disease, and managing health systems

pharmacy preceptor exemplary practicing pharmacist who is accompanied, observed, and assisted by a student as one facet of the student's education in pharmacy; one who performs as a role model and a supervisor for pharmacy students in an experiential setting

pharmacy services administrative organization a group of pharmacies which have agreed to pool their efforts to compete in the marketplace and which agree upon minimum standards of practice

pharmacy technician an individual who, under the supervision of a licensed pharmacist, assists in pharmacy activities not requiring the professional judgment of a pharmacist

pharmakon Greek word meaning drug; the root word for many pharmacy-related terms

pharynx passageway for air moving from the nasal cavity to the larynx, and for food moving from the mouth to the esophagus; an alternating, discriminatory body valve assembly that directs air and food to their proper locations

phase 1: specific state of matter (solid, liquid, or vapor) which is homogeneous with respect to its composition and which is a part of a system undergoing treatment or study **2:** a particular appearance in a regular cycle of changes; a point on a wave or uniform circular motion; a step in a process of change or a stage of development

phase diagram   plot of temperature and concentrations (usually expressed as percent by weight) of a mixture of two or three substances in order to determine phase composition at equilibrium under various conditions; a diagram giving the conditions of equilibrium between various forms (phases) of a substance

phase I drug metabolism   stage of drug metabolism that involves functionalization reactions, including oxidative, reductive, and hydrolytic biotransformations; includes reactions that introduce polar functional groups into a drug molecule, usually as a first step to facilitate its elimination from the body

phase II drug metabolism   stage of drug metabolism that involves the conjugation of the drug molecule to a small, polar, and ionizable compound (such as glucuronic acid) to form water-soluble conjugated products that are more easily excreted

phenol   chemical compound in which the basic structure consists of a hydroxyl group bound to an sp^2 carbon of a benzene ring; a very potent protein precipitant and sclerosing agent; synonym: carbolic acid

phenylalanine   aromatic amino acid commonly found in proteins; 2-amino-3-phenylpropanoic acid; an essential amino acid

phenylketonuria   congenital deficiency of phenylalanine-4-monooxygenase that may result in severe mental retardation

phenyl salicylate   low melting point phenolic ester of salicylic acid; used as an analgesic and antipyretic and formerly used as an enteric coating for capsules; synonym: salol

pheochromocytoma   tumor of the adrenal medulla, the primary symptoms of which are a result of increased secretion of epinephrine and norepinephrine

-philia   suffix meaning an abnormal attraction to something

phleb-   prefix meaning vein; same as phlebo-

phlebo-   prefix meaning vein; same as phleb-

phlebotomy   drawing of blood from a vein

phonophobia   literally, fear of noise; often applied to medical conditions that cause avoidance of noise, such as migraine headaches

pH optimum the pH at which an enzyme catalyzes a reaction at maximum efficiency

phosphofructokinase enzyme that catalyzes the conversion of fructose-6-phosphate to fructose-1,6-diphosphate in the Emden-Meyerhoff glycolytic pathway

phosphoglyceride a type of lipid molecule found predominately in membrane composed of glycerol linked to two fatty acids, phosphate, and a polar group

phospholipid compound consisting of an amide or ester of a fatty acid and an ester of phosphoric acid with either glycerol, sphingol (sphingosine), choline, or ethanolamine

phosphoprotein a conjugated protein in which phosphate is the prosthetic group

phosphor SEE *liquid scintillation counter; liquid scintillator; phosphorescence*

phosphorescence the ability of a substance to give off visible light after being exposed to electromagnetic radiation

photolabile capable of being destroyed by radiant energy; example: phenothiazines that decompose when exposed to light

photolysis degradation process in a molecule (drug) that is the result of its absorption of light (photons)

photon a quantum of light; energy corpuscles of electromagnetic radiation

photophobia literally, fear of light; often applied to medical conditions that cause avoidance of light, such as migraine headaches

photosensitive a response or a potential response elicited by radiant energy exposure; example: erythema observed in a patient who is taking tetracycline and exposed to sunlight

photostable refers to a compound that is not degraded when exposed to radiant energy; colors not fading upon exposure to light rays

pH scale a measure of hydrogen ion concentration; pH is the negative log of the hydrogen ion concentration in moles per liter

Phthirus pubis pubic louse; a sexually transmitted disease

physical adsorption SEE *adsorption*

physical assessment assessment of the patient's health using physical cues; example: visual review of skin conditions, blood pressure, measurements, etc.; if by a pharmacist looking for drug therapy problems, then different from the physical exam performed by a physician in diagnosing disease

physical inventory an actual counting and listing of all merchandise on hand; typically includes the name, quantity, cost, and/or retail price of all items

physician doctor of medicine and/or doctor of osteopathy who is duly licensed and qualified under the law of jurisdiction in which treatment is received

physician assistant individual trained to perform certain primary care tasks according to a protocol who works under the supervision of a licensed physician; synonym: physician extender

physician associates practice incorporated by two or more physicians

physician contingency reserve "at-risk" portion of a claim deducted and withheld by the health plan before payment is made to a participating physician as an incentive for appropriate utilization and quality of care

physician-hospital organization a legal entity formed to obtain payer contracts; owned by one or more hospitals and physician groups

Physician's Current Procedural Terminology SEE *Current Procedural Terminology System*

physicochemical property a property of a compound which is a measurable characteristic and by which the compound may interact with other systems

physiological antagonism antagonism between two agonists that stimulate action at separate receptors, but cause opposite responses; synonym: functional antagonism

physostigmine alkaloid obtained from *Physostigma venosum* that acts as an indirect cholinergic agent by competitively inhibiting choline esterase

pi bond molecular bond resulting from the parallel overlap of 2p-orbitals; a pi bond and a sigma bond produce a double bond; the pi bond consists of two lobes (electron density areas) on each side of the sigma bond; with conjugated double bonds or in aromatic systems, the pi bonds become delocalized and the pi electrons are free to migrate between the different atoms of the conjugated or aromatic system; SEE ALSO *double bond*

picking adhesion of a part of a tablet to the face or surface of the punch; an undesirable event in the tablet compression process

Pick's disease multiple polyserositis (with ascites, hepatomegaly, peritonitis, and pleural effusion); also cerebral atrophy of frontal and temporal lobes resulting in senile dementia

Pick's syndrome lobar atrophy of the brain; SEE ALSO *Pick's disease*

pill small, rounded, solid body for internal use; consists of a medicinal agent(s) plus other material to make a firm, cohesive mass

pills, concentric consist of successive layers of medicinal matter each having a different action and separated by a coating; used to deliver medicines in the stomach and intestine or to keep ingredients from reacting

pills, enteric-coated coated with a substance that will not dissolve in the stomach but is intended to dissolve in the small intestine

pilocarpine alkaloid obtained from *Pilocarpus microphyllus* or other species; used to produce miosis; a direct-acting parasympathomimetic that exerts its effects by directly stimulating the muscarinic receptor

pilosebaceous unit an anatomical feature of the skin, consisting of a hair follicle and a sebaceous gland; location where acne lesions form

pilot plant an intermediary production laboratory designed to test manufacturing procedures that are being scaled up from small to large batches

pinocytosis engulfing or surrounding of a small amount of an extracellular liquid by a cell membrane and the subsequent formation of a vesicle; the liquid becomes available to the cell when the vesicle is lysed

pint unit of volume equal to 16 fluid ounces, 1/2 quart, 1/8 gallon, or 473.167 mL

pK the negative log (base 10) of the ionization constant of a weak electrolyte; examples: pK_a, pK_b

pK_a the negative log (base 10) of the dissociation constant of a weak acid in aqueous solution

pK_b the negative log (base 10) of the dissociation constant of a weak base in aqueous solution

place of service the location where health services are rendered; examples: office, home, hospital

placebo tablet, capsule, or other dosage form devoid of any active ingredient; sometimes prescribed for a psychological effect or used as a control in drug efficacy testing

plaintiff person who initiates a legal action; synonym: complainant

Planck's constant a discrete radiation energy unit (absorbed or emitted) representing "one quantum," abbreviated by h, where h equals energy (F) divided by the radiation frequency (v); $h = 6.624 \times 10^{-27}$ erg/sec

plan-o-gram blueprint of department locations, sizes and sections, and products; a detailed plan for the use of the available selling space in a retail store

plaque 1: elevated, palpable skin lesion characteristic of certain diseases, such as psoriasis **2:** soft, gel-like mass that begins to grow on the surfaces of the teeth within a few hours of eating

plasma the liquid portion of blood containing all dissolved substances, including all clotting factors, but excluding the formed elements (blood cells)

plasma membrane the membrane that surrounds a cell, separating it from its external environment

plasmas nonfatty, unctuous preparations, used in place of cerates and ointments for local application

plasma water concentration concentration of a drug or metabolite in the plasma ultrafiltrate; synonym: free drug concentration

plasmid small structural units of genetic material containing circular, double-stranded DNA that transmit genetic information from one bacterial cell to another; example: R-factors in bacteria

plaster substance intended for external application, made to adhere to the skin and attach to a dressing; intended to afford protection and support, to furnish an occlusion and macerating action, and/or to bring medication into close contact with the skin

plaster mull thin cloth covered on one side with rubber or gutta-percha upon which a medicine is painted or spread; the impervious backing facilitates absorption

plastic flow characteristic of certain liquids that resist flow with initially low shearing stress and exhibit Newtonian flow (linear flow) when sufficient shearing stress (yield value) has been applied; exhibited by emulsions, creams, and magmas

plasticity capacity for being molded or altered in shape; ability to retain a shape resulting from pressure deformation

plasticizer component of a film-former to give the film more flexibility; films containing a plasticizer do not break or crack easily; examples: castor oil, glycerin, propylene glycol

plastic surgeon a physician who specializes in performing surgery for the restoration, repair, or reconstruction of body structures

plate and frame filter pressure filtration device consisting of a series of metal plates (having large openings) between which the filter pads (filter medium) are placed tightly

platelet-derived growth factor a protein secreted by blood platelets during clotting; stimulates mitosis during wound healing

plateletpheresis SEE *apheresis*

platelets produced in the bone marrow, essential in the clotting process

play-or-pay in any health care reform scheme, a system that would require employers to provide health insurance benefits or pay a tax that government would use to provide coverage

plug 1: a small part of the rubber closure of a vial (or fluid bag) that has been cut or broken and has fallen into the vial (or fluid bag) as a needle was introduced into the rubber closure; an undesirable event for a quality closure of a multidose parenteral **2:** a device to stop flow

Plummer's disease hyperthyroidism with a nodular goiter

pneumato- prefix meaning respiration or air; same as pneumo-

pneumo- prefix meaning respiration or air; same as pneumato-

pod- prefix meaning foot; same as podo-

podiatrist licensed health practitioner engaged in diagnosis, treatment, and prevention of foot problems; synonym: chiropodist

podiatry health care area involving diagnosis, treatment, and prevention of foot problems; synonym: chiropody

podo- prefix meaning foot; same as pod-

-poiesis suffix meaning formation

point mutation genetically inherited change of a single amino acid residue in a protein or polypeptide; may involve mutation of only one purine or pyrimidine base in a DNA strand; SEE ALSO *transversion mutation; mutation*

point-of-service plan a health plan allowing the covered person to choose to receive a service from a participating or nonparticipating provider, with different benefit levels associated with the use of participating providers.

poise basic cgs unit of viscosity; SEE *Newton's law of viscous flow; viscosity*

poison ivy 1: plant belonging to the toxicodendron group; damaged leaves or stems exude urushiol, an oily resin to which many people are violently allergic; cross-sensitizes with poison oak and poison sumac

2: widely used to refer to the allergic reaction arising from contact with urushiols

polarimeter an instrument used to determine the direction and degree of rotation of plane-polarized light as it passes through a solution containing an optically active compound

polarization 1: separation of positive and negative charges in a molecule **2:** filtration of light to produce beams or rays the waves of that vibrate in a single plane and are within a narrow wavelength

polar molecule a chemical compound containing groups that form dipoles; compound with a partial positive atom and a partial negative atom; formal charges not necessarily present

policy and procedure manual a book that describes the manner in which a particular pharmacy is to be operated; a guideline of operational procedures for a specific organization or establishment

polishing pan rounded, canvas lined, rotating vessel used to effect an attractive shiny surface on a batch of coated tablets

political action committee (PAC) nonprofit organization or group that raises funds to support election campaigns of legislators and other officials who have supported or intend to support issues and views compatible with the group

politzer plugs plugs of greased cotton for insert into ear after surgery

poly clinical abbreviation for polymorphonucleocyte; synonyms: seg, neutrophil, granulocyte

polycythemia an increase in the red-cell count per unit volume of blood in the presence of an increased total blood volume

polydipsia excessive thirst

polygraph 1: instrument used to detect lying by a subject while recording the physiological changes assumed to occur when the subject provides false answers to carefully selected questions; synonym: lie detector **2:** instrument used in pharmacology to measure simultaneous physiological changes in several parameters (heart rate, respiration, electrocardiogram)

polymer large molecule composed of repeating subunits chemically bonded together; examples: protein, polypeptide, polysaccharide, polystyrene, polyvinylchloride, polyacrylamide, polyethylene glycol, nylon

polymerase chain reaction a laboratory technique used to synthesize large quantities of specific nucleotide sequences from small amounts of DNA using a heat-stable DNA

polymer drug delivery system dosage form designed for targeted or sustained release using a polymeric carrier matrix

polymorph 1: synonym for segmented neutrophil **2:** a different crystalline form of the same substance

polymorphic capable of existing in more than one crystalline form; exhibiting different physical properties even though the chemical composition is the same

polymorphism existing in many forms; examples: alpha, beta, and gamma crystalline forms of cocoa butter

polymyxins group of bactericidal antibiotics that exert a surfactant effect on the cytoplasmic membrane of bacteria

polynucleotide 1: nucleic acid **2:** polymer consisting of nucelotides

polyol compound having several hydroxy groups; synonyms: polyhydroxyalcohol, polyhydric alcohol

polypeptide a polymer, one unit of which, on hydrolysis, yields a large number of units of amino acids

polypharmacy irrational mixtures or combinations of several drugs in one dose; synonym: "shotgun" therapy

polyphase system quantity of materials, the contents of which exist in two or more states of matter; synonym: multiphase system

polyribosome cluster of ribosomes connected to one another by a strand of mRNA (messenger RNA)

polysaccharide a polymer, one unit of which, on hydrolysis, yields a large number of monosaccharide units; examples: starch, glycogen, cellulose

polyserositis inflammation of serous membranes with serous effusion

polysome an mRNA with several ribosomes bound to it

polyunsaturated refers to a fatty acid with two or more double bonds, usually separated by methylene groups

polyuria excessive urination; a symptom of diabetes insipidus and diabetes mellitus

pomade perfumed, stiff ointment; used especially to treat the hair or the scalp

Pompe's disease type 2 glycogenosis; accumulation of glycogen in the heart, muscle, liver, and nervous system

pooling the process of combining risk for all groups or a number of groups

population statistical term meaning a set representing all objects of interest that have at least one characteristic in common

porcine obtained from or relating to a pig; example: porcine insulin

pore a minute opening in a membrane tissue or other substance permitting passage of large molecules and small particulate colloids; a small opening in a filtration membrane

pore penetration a process by which an infant absorbs large polymeric molecules and fatty globules from the intestinal tract, the wall of which has the ability to convolute and form a minute opening to effect absorption

porous full of pores or minute openings; permeable to liquids or air

porphyria one of a number of diseases involving the excretion of porphyrins in the urine

porphyrin a ring structure composed of four pyrrole rings connected by single carbon atoms (methine groups); parent structure for heme in the hemoglobin molecule, the cytochromes and vitamin B_{12}

portability an individual changing jobs would be guaranteed coverage with the new employer without a waiting period or having to meet additional deductible requirements.

positional isomers compounds that have the same empirical formula, despite having a group, radical, or atom substituted on a different part of their molecular structure; examples: 1-chloropropane and 2-chloropropane, both having the empirical formula, C_3H_7Cl; synonym: structural isomers

positive-displacement flow meter instrument that measures the flow rate of fluid by a direct determination of volume of movement in a specific unit of time

positive-displacement pump/fan/blower/compressor apparatus that functions by entrapping a volume of air or liquid from an inlet post and releasing it through an outlet post for the purpose of mass transfer; SEE *reciprocating pump; rotary pump; lobe pump*

positive formulary SEE *formulary*

positron positively charged electron; CONTRAST *negatron;* SEE ALSO *electron, orbital*

posology the science of dosage or a system of dosage

post- prefix meaning after

postabsorptive the phase in the feeding-fasting cycle in which nutrient levels in blood are low; CONTRAST *postprandial*

postictal the time after a seizure, stroke, or apoplexy

postpartum with reference to the mother, a period of time after childbirth

postprandial the phase in the feeding-fasting cycle immediately after a meal when blood nutrient levels are relatively high; CONTRAST *postabsorptive*

posttranslational modification a set of reactions that alter the structure of newly synthesized polypeptides

posttranslational translocation the transfer of previously synthesized polypeptide across the RER membrane

potable suitable for drinking

potash, sulfurated SEE *sulfurated potash*

potassium monovalent alkali metallic element; electrolyte in the body; important for proper functioning of nerves; the chief intracellular cation

potency **1:** strength of a drug as expressed by dosage amount and biological effect **2:** ability of the male to perform sexual intercourse

potentiate an effect in which two drugs are administered and their combined effect is more than additive, being synergistic or greater than the sum of the individual drug effects

potentiometer device to measure electromotive force; synonym: voltmeter

Pott's disease tuberculous spondylitis (inflammation of the vertebra)

Pott's fracture fracture of the lower end of the fibula with outward displacement of the foot

poultice soft, moist mass of meal, herbs, seed, etc., usually applied hot in cloth that consists of gruel-like consistency

pound, apothecary/troy (lb or lb t) unit of weight equal to 12 ℥

pound, avoirdupois (lb) unit of weight equal to 16 oz

powder a uniform mixture of dry, finely divided drugs and/or chemicals intended for either internal or external use or to make solutions

powder, dentifrice powder formulation intended to clean and/or polish the teeth

powder, for solution an intimate mixture of dry, finely divided drugs and/or chemicals that, upon the addition of suitable vehicles, yields a solution

powder, for suspension an intimate mixture of dry, finely divided drugs and/or chemicals that, upon the addition of suitable vehicles, yields a suspension (a liquid preparation containing the solid particles dispersed in the liquid vehicle)

powder, metered powder dosage form situated inside a container that has a mechanism to deliver a specified quantity

power the rate at which energy is supplied

Power, Frederick B. (1853-1927) organizer and first dean of the school of pharmacy at the University of Wisconsin; became head of the Wellcome Laboratories in England and then the head of the phytochemistry division of the U.S. Department of Agriculture

power number expression of the relationship between the force to drive a mixing impeller and the inertia of the drug material to be mixed

power of attorney a written instrument that authorizes a person to act on behalf of a second party in specified matters; example: a power of attorney given to an employee pharmacist to sign controlled substance order forms

practice guidelines systematically developed statements on medical practice that assist a practitioner and a patient in making decisions about appropriate health care for specific medical conditions

pre- prefix meaning before

preadmission certification review of the need for inpatient hospital care, done prior to the actual admission

preceptor role model professional; contemporary pharmacy practice teacher-mentor in the "real" world of practice

precertification review SEE *utilization review*

precipitated chalk SEE *chalk*

precipitation process of removing from solution one or more constituents in the form of a finely divided solid; the dissolved solid is made insoluble by either physical or chemical means

precision 1: refers to agreement among repeated measurements **2:** quality or state of being exact

preclinical test test of a new drug or device on animal subjects; conducted to gather evidence justifying a clinical trial

precoating preparing a slurry of the filter aid and circulating it through the system to coat the filter medium prior to a filtration process; synonym: body mixing

precursor substance that precedes another; usually an inactive drug that is changed into an active drug or a metabolite that is changed into a physiologically active compound; examples: DOPA as a precursor for dopamine, beta-carotene as a precursor for vitamin A

preeclampsia a toxemia associated with pregnancy and characterized by increasing hypertension, headaches, albuminuria, and edema of the lower extremities; may lead to true eclampsia if left untreated

preexisting condition any medical condition that has been diagnosed or treated within a specified period preceding the covered person's effective date of coverage under the master group contract

preferred provider organization (PPO) a program in which contracts are established with providers of medical care; providers under such contracts referred to as preferred providers; usually provides significantly better benefits (lower copayments) for services received from preferred providers, thus encouraging covered persons to use these providers; covered persons generally allowed benefits for nonparticipating providers' services, usually on an indemnity basis, with significantly higher copayments

preferred providers physicians, hospitals, and other health care providers who contract to provide health services to persons covered by a particular health plan; SEE ALSO *preferred provider organization*

premium the amount paid to a carrier for providing coverage under a contract

prepack container of a drug dosage form prepared in advance for the individual consumer by the hospital, pharmacy, or other pharmacy care provider for dispensing as ordered or required

prepaid expense the situation in which a business pays a bill before it is due; example: prepaid insurance premiums

prepaid group practice plans organized medical groups of full-time physicians in appropriate specialties, as well as other professional and paraprofessional personnel who, for regular compensation, undertake to provide comprehensive care to an enrolled population for premium payments that are made in advance by the consumer and/or their employers

prepaid health plan an agreement by an insurer to provide certain health and medical services to its enrollees for a fixed prepaid premium; very similar to an HMO

preparative ultracentrifuge SEE *ultracentrifuge*

prepared chalk SEE *chalk*

preproprotein an inactive precursor protein with removable signal peptide

presbycusis gradual loss of hearing that occurs with aging, more often in males

Prescott, Albert Benjamin (1832-1905) University of Michigan professor, physician, and pharmacy dean who advocated formal collegiate studies by pharmacy students before they participate in an apprenticeship—a revolutionary concept that led to changes in the nature of pharmacy education; formed the School of Pharmacy at the University of Michigan; was a leading proponent of laboratory work as an integral part of pharmacy education; considered the Father of Phi Delta Chi

prescription medication order for a patient and written (or orally communicated) to a pharmacist by a physician, dentist, podiatrist, or other properly licensed medical practitioner; composed of the superscription, inscription, subscription, and *signatura;* SEE ALSO *superscription; inscription; subscription; signatura, signa, or sig*

prescription balance SEE *balance*

prescription labor expense an expense determined by multiplying each prescription department employee's wage times his/her labor ratio (fraction of time worked in the prescription department) then totaling these products for all employees

prescription medication a drug which has been approved by the FDA and which can, under federal and state law, be dispensed only pursuant to a prescription order from a duly licensed prescriber, usually a physician

presenile dementia SEE *Alzheimer's disease*

presenile psychosis SEE *Alzheimer's disease*

preservative agent added to protect a preparation (dosage form) against decay or spoilage; usually to prevent spoilage by microorganisms; examples: methylparaben, propylparaben

pressure filter device designed to force solid-liquid or solid-air dispersions through one or more filters with forces significantly greater than gravity; pressure filters usually contain a pump or compressor, a series of support plates, and filter pads through which the liquid or air must pass to be clarified or purified

prevalence a measure of the total number of cases of illness or other forms of morbidity present in a given population at a particular point in time; usually measured as the total number of cases per 1,000 persons

preventive care comprehensive care emphasizing priorities for prevention, early detection, and early treatment of conditions, generally including routine physical examinations, immunizations, and well-person care

preventive drug a medication prescribed for a short- or a long-term prophylactic purpose; synonym: prophylactic drug

primary alcohol SEE *alcohol*

primary amine SEE *amine*

primary care provision of medical services directed toward the initial treatment of a patient, including the care of simple or common disorders and preliminary treatment and/or the assessment of more serious disorders that require a specialist

primary care case management managed care arrangements where primary care providers receive a per capita management fee to coordinate a patient's care in addition to reimbursement for the medical services they provide

primary care network a group of primary care physicians who have joined together to share the risk of providing care to their patients who are covered by a given health plan

primary care physician a physician devoted primarily to internal medicine, family/general practice, pediatrics, and obstetrics and gynecology

primary coverage under coordination of benefit rules, the coverage plan that considers and pays its eligible expenses without consideration of any other coverage

primary structure the amino acid sequence of a polypeptide

primase an RNA polymerase that synthesizes short RNA segments, called primers, that are required in DNA synthesis

primer a short RNA segment required to initiate DNA synthesis

prime vendor drug wholesaler through whom a pharmacy centralizes its purchases, thereby reducing time spent on purchase orders, invoices, and purchasing procedures in general

priming dose SEE *initial dose*

principal diagnosis condition determined after study to be mainly responsible for a patient's seeking access to health care services from a provider

principal investigator individual responsible for leading a research project or supported by a grant

principal quantum number primary shell in which an atomic orbital electron is expected to be revolving around the nucleus; SEE *quantum number*

prion proteinaceous infectious particle; believed to be a causative agent of several acquired neurodegenerative diseases (e.g., mad cow disease and Creutzfeld-Jacob disease)

prior authorization process of obtaining prior approval as to the appropriateness of a service or medication; does not guarantee coverage

privileging process by which a health care organization authorizes an individual to perform a specific scope of patient care services within that organization

pro- **1:** prefix meaning before **2:** prefix denoting an advocacy of a particular position on an issue

pro forma income statement projected income statement applicable to the next period

problem-oriented patient record record of patient information organized by drug therapy problem

proct- prefix meaning rectum; same as procto-

Procter, William, Jr. (1817-1874) one of the founders of the American Pharmacists Association; considered the Father of American Pharmacy; practiced as a retail pharmacist and taught at the Philadelphia College of Pharmacy; a staunch supporter of pharmaceutical standards; instrumental in the development of *United States Pharmacopeia* and authored the first pharmacy textbook in the United States

proctitis inflammation of the rectum and/or the anus

procto- prefix meaning rectum; same as proct-

proctologist physician who specializes in diseases and disorders of the colon, rectum, and anus

prodrome a symptom that signals the onset of a medical condition; example: tingling and/or paresthesia of the lip that heralds the onset of herpes simplex lesions

prodrug biologically inactive compound that is converted to an active form in the body by normal metabolic processes

product liability legal obligations of a manufacturer or a distributor for damages caused through the use of their product

proenzyme an inactive precursor of an enzyme

professional associates a practice incorporated by two or more professionals

Professional Pharmacy Service Codes developed by NCPDP to define pharmacy-specific cognitive services; may be used in billing insurers for pharmaceutical care services

professional review organization a physician-sponsored organization charged with reviewing the services provided to patients to determine medical necessity; provided in the appropriate setting in accordance with professional criteria, norms, and standards

Professional Standards Review Organization expert panel established by the U.S. government to monitor health care services paid for through Medicaid, Medicare, and Maternal and Child Health programs to ensure that services provided are medically necessary and economically appropriate

profit target usual income objective for the next period of operation

progestin a type of female sex hormone that maintains pregnancy and functions with estrogen to maintain the menstrual cycle; the naturally occurring progestin is progesterone

prognosis a prediction on the outcome of a disorder; the expected outcome of an illness

Project Impact: Hyperlipidemia APhA demonstration project with 26 pharmacies that proved pharmacist management improved patients' compliance and lipid levels

prokaryotes monocellular organisms that do not contain a nucleus; example: bacteria; SEE *eukaryotes*

prokaryotic cell a living cell that lacks a nucleus

prolapse dropping or falling of a body part (e.g., rectal prolapse)

proline neutral amino acid commonly found in protein, especially in connective tissue protein (collagen); chemical name, pyrrolidine-2-carboxylic acid

prolonged action refers to a dosage form that delivers an initial dose for a rapid therapeutic response, followed by a sufficient dose (or a series of doses) to maintain an effective concentration of the drug for an extended period of time (usually 8 to 12 hours for orally administered medication); contrasts with a single-dose entity that is effective for a shorter time

promoter the sequence of nucleotides immediately before a gene that is recognized by RNA polymerase and signals the starting point and direction of transcription

promotional discount a price reduction extended to a pharmacy as an allowance for advertising and promoting a given product; example: a manufacturer giving a pharmacy a discount if the pharmacy agrees to place the product on a special display or include it in the store's advertisement; synonym: advertising discount

prone 1: lying face down; as in a prone position **2:** tendency to perform an act or behave in a certain way

proof gallon a wine gallon of proof spirit (50 percent alcohol)

proof spirit aqueous solution of alcohol containing 50 percent (v/v) absolute alcohol; aqueous solution that is 100 proof alcohol

propellant compressed or liquefied gas that provides the energy to expel the contents from an aerosol package through the valve-cap assembly

propeller a part of a mixing apparatus designed for a specific material flow pattern; a form of impeller

prophylactic refers to prevention or an agent used to prevent the contracting of a disease or condition; examples: a condom to prevent conception, a vaccine to provide immunity against a disease

prophylaxis the prevention of disease or an unwanted condition

Proprietary Association See *Consumer Healthcare Products Association*

proprietary drug drug product advertised and sold to the public without requiring a prescription; synonym: over-the-counter (OTC) drug; CONTRAST *legend drug*

proprietary hospital a hospital that is operated on a for-profit basis; may be a privately owned or publicly held corporation; synonym: for-profit hospital

proprietary medicine a medicine that is protected against free competition as to name, product composition, or process of manufacture by patent, trademark, and/or copyright

proprietary name drug or drug product title that is a registered name legally established by a particular company (manufacturer or distributor) that may not be used by any other manufacturer; synonyms: brand name, trade name; CONTRAST *chemical name; generic name*

proprioceptive system sensory nerve terminals that provide neural input concerning the movement and position of the body, based on input from muscles, tendons, and other internal tissues

Prospective Payment Assessment Commission federal commission established under the Social Security Act amendments of 1983 to advise and assist Congress and the Department of Health and Human Services in maintaining and updating the Medicare prospective payment system

prospective payment system a standardized payment system that was implemented in 1983 by Medicare to help manage inpatient hospitalization expenditures; payments based on the diagnosis of the patient rather than on the specific products and services consumed in the treatment of the patient

prospective reimbursement method of paying for services in which the amount of payment is established prior to the period in which the services will be used

prostaglandins class of fatty acids derived from arachidonic acid by cyclization to form a five-membered ring near the middle of the fatty acid chain; a class of hormones that possesses a variety of physiological effects, including vasodilation and smooth muscle contraction; examples: PGF_1, PGE_1, and PGA_2

prosthetic group the nonprotein portion of a conjugated protein that is essential to the biological activity of the protein; often a complex organic molecule

protein a polypeptide that contains at least 100 amino acid residues; a polypeptide that has a molecular weight of at least 10,000 daltons (atomic mass units)

protein binding the physical attachment of a drug to plasma protein; a drug-plasma protein complex; a process that renders a drug unavailable for distribution from blood to other body tissues

protein binding, saturation point drug concentration required to occupy the binding sites on plasma protein and beyond which the free (unbound) drug is present in a greater proportion

protein hydrolysate solution containing a mixture of amino acids formed by acid hydrolysis of a protein

protein splicing a posttranslational mechanism in which an intervening peptide sequence is precisely excised from a nascent polypeptide

protein turnover the continuous degradation and resynthesis of proteins in an organism

proteinuria appearance of protein in the urine

proteoglycan a large molecule containing large numbers of glycosaminoglycan chains linked to a core protein molecule

proteolytic enzyme biochemical catalyst that accelerates the hydrolysis of proteins; examples: papain, pepsin, trypsin, thrombin, chymotrypsin

proteome the complete set of proteins produced within a cell

proteomics the analysis of proteomes

proteosome a multienzyme complex that degrades proteins linked to ubiquitin

protogenic solvent a dissolving medium capable of donating protons; an acid medium that is used as a solvent

protolysis an acid-base reaction involving proton transfer and the formation of a new acid and a new base; a protolytic reaction

protomer a subunit of allosteric enzymes

proton a fundamental particle of matter (a nucleon) having a positive charge of 1.6×10^{-19} coulombs and a mass of about 1.67×10^{-24} grams; approximately equal to 1 atomic mass unit (amu)

proton magnetic resonance (PMR or pmr) SEE *nuclear magnetic resonance*

protooncogene a normal gene that promotes carcinogenesis if mutated

protophilic solvent dissolving liquid capable of accepting a proton; a basic medium used as a solvent

protozoacide agent used to kill protozoa and treat their infections; example: amebicide

provider a physician, hospital, group practice, nurse, nursing home, pharmacy, or any individual or group of individuals that provides a health care service

Provider Reimbursement Review Board panel that determines the levels of payment to providers (pharmacies, hospitals, and physicians) for services rendered under a third-party contract

proximal nearer; closer; opposite of distal

pruritus synonym for itching

pseud- prefix meaning false; same as pseudo-

pseudo- prefix meaning false; same as pseud-

pseudodistribution equilibrium a state of drug distribution indicating kinetic homogeneity; an equilibrium during which the plasma concentration can be described by a mono-exponential equation

pseudo–first order rate of a reaction or a process which, for all practical purposes, can be expressed as a function of the concentration of one major component raised to the first power, even through the accurately described process is of a higher order (a function of the concentrations of several reacting species)

pseudomembranous colitis inflammation of the colon caused by a toxin produced by *Clostridium difficile*

pseudoplastic flow characteristic flow of a hydrophilic colloidal solution in which a linear plot of "rate of shear" versus "shearing stress" exhibits a concave shaped curve; example: methylcellulose mucilage exhibits pseudoplastic flow

psychiatric pertaining to psychiatry

psychiatrist a physician who specializes in the study, treatment, and prevention of mental disorders

psychiatry branch of medicine concerned with treating diseases of the mind

psychic 1: reference to the mind 2: a person who claims to possess the ability to read minds or foresee coming events

psychologist one who has studied and is trained in the methods of psychological analysis, therapy, and research

psychology science and study of the functions of the mind

psychosis a major mental disorder of organic or emotional origin in which a person's ability to think, respond emotionally, interpret reality, and behave appropriately is impaired to the point that the individual cannot fulfill the demands of life

psychrometry the measurement of vapor concentration and the carrying capacity of a drying gas such as air or nitrogen; similar to humidity; an expression of water vapor content in air

pull-seal the closing of an ampule by heating its neck in a flame (glass blower's torch) as the ampule is rotated and its upper tip is pulled away

pulmo- prefix meaning lung; same as pulmono-

pulmonary edema a diffuse extravascular accumulation of fluid in the pulmonary tissues and air spaces due to changes in hydrostatic forces in the capillaries or their increased permeability; marked by intense dyspnea

pulmono- prefix meaning lung; same as pulmo-

pulse perceptible expansion of an artery due to the rhythmic contractions of the heart

pumice very finely divided lightweight glass used for smoothing or polishing surfaces

punch metallic piston that is part of a tableting machine; upper and lower punches are used to compress a granular drug mass; punches may be flat, convex, or concave and they may contain monogrammed surfaces for "scoring" and imprinting trademarks on tablets

puncta small openings at the inner corner of the eyelid that allow tears to drain from the eye

purgative agent that causes evacuation of the bowel; classified according to the severity of action; cholagogue—stimulates contractions, watery discharges, and flow of bile resulting in green stools; drastic—produces violent action of the bowels with excessive cramping and griping; saline—produces copious, watery discharges; simple—produces a free discharge from the bowels with some griping (pains)

purification process of freeing, as nearly as possible, a preparation or substance of unwanted components

purified animal charcoal refined charcoal from animal sources used as an adsorbent and decolorizer; synonyms: abasier, purified bone black, spodium

purified bone black SEE *purified animal charcoal*

purified infusorial earth SEE *diatomaceous earth*

purine heterocyclic organic compound in which a pyrimidine ring is fused along its {4,5-d} face to an imidazole ring; the parent structure for adenine and guanine; commonly found as a part of the structures of RNAs, DNAs, coenzymes, nucleotides, and of adenine, guanine, xanthine, hypoxanthine, uric acid, and caffeine

purity state of being pure; absence of dirt, dust, or other pollutants (especially harmful substances)

purity rubric term introduced into the *USP* VIII to limit the quantity of innocuous substances in chemicals by stating in terms of percentage the amount of pure substance that must be present; example: potassium iodide (KI), when dried to constant weight at 100°C, must contain not less than 99 percent KI; a term seldom used today

purpura disorders that cause the skin to appear purple or brownish red due to hemorrhage into the tissue

purpurea glycoside cardiac glycoside from the leaves of *Digitalis purpurea;* example: digitoxin

Purtscher's retinopathy sudden transient blindness following severe trauma or prolonged exposure with exhaustion and shock

purulent containing pus

pus protein-rich fluid composed of leukocytes and microorganisms; an exudate of an infection or abscess

pustule a collection of pus just under the skin

pycnometer standardized volumetric container used for measuring and comparing densities and specific gravities of liquids or solids

pyel- prefix referring to the renal pelvis; same as pyelo-

pyelo- prefix referring to the renal pelvis; same as pyel-

pyelogram X-ray picture of the renal pelvis and ureter

pyo- prefix meaning pus

pyrazole five-membered ring with two nitrogens adjacent to each other; synonym: 1,2-diazole

pyrexia an elevation of body temperature that is caused by a change or disturbance of the heat-regulating mechanism of the body; synonym: fever

pyridine heterocyclic, six-membered, aromatic ring compound containing one nitrogen atom

pyrimidine heterocyclic, aromatic, organic compound composed of a six-membered ring containing two nitrogen atoms separated by one carbon atom; synonym: 1,3-diazine

pyrogen any substance that produces fever; usually organic substances (arising from the growth of microorganisms) that produce fever when injected into the body

pyrogen test determination of the presence of fever-producers (organic fragments, usually of killed microorganisms) in a sterilized product; consult the *USP-NF* for testing methods

pyrometer an instrument to determine very high temperatures by means of radiant energy measurements; optical—determines temperature by measuring radiation intensity at a given wavelength; radiation—can determine a wide range of temperatures using a larger spectrum of radiation wavelengths

pyroxylin cellulose treated with nitric and sulfuric acid to convert it into various nitro compounds; pyroxylin, when dissolved in a mixture of alcohol and ether, yields collodion; the addition of castor oil to collodion produces flexible collodion; synonyms: nitrocellulose, guncotton

pyrrole five-membered ring system that is completely unsaturated and contains one nitrogen atom

quack one who falsely represents himself as a qualified medical practitioner; synonym: charlatan

quackery promotion of medical products, devices, or practices that are not known to be effective and/or safe

qualitative analysis branch of chemistry that involves processes and procedures for substance identification; does not determine the amount of substance present in a system under study; CONTRAST *quantitative analysis*

quality-adjusted life year a measure used in cost-utility analysis; consequences (e.g., life years saved) measured in terms of quality of life, willingness to pay, or preference for one intervention to another

quality assurance methods used to ascertain whether or not a product has been prepared according to required or specified standards; SEE *quality control*

quality control 1: series of tests conducted on components of a drug product, beginning with raw materials, and then on each respective process step; followed by tests on the finished product to ensure purity, potency, uniformity, stability, safety, elegance, and efficacy before a drug product is placed on the market; finally, periodic postmarketing tests for continued assurance **2:** tests conducted to ensure the validity of clinical laboratory analyses

quality improvement a continuous process that identifies problems in health care delivery, tests solutions to those problems, and constantly monitors the solutions for improvement

quality of life in pharmacoeconomics, a measurable health care outcome that assesses an individual's functional status, physiologic status, well-being, and life satisfaction

quality reassurance a formal set of activities to review and affect the quality of services provided; includes quality assessment and corrective actions to remedy any deficiencies identified in the quality of direct patient, administrative, and support services

quanta discrete units of energy; SEE *quantum theory*

quantitative analysis branch of chemistry involving processes by which the amount of a substance is determined; SEE *gravimetric analysis; volumetric analysis;* CONTRAST *qualitative analysis*

quantitative structure-activity relationship a method of drug design in which physical properties such as partition coefficients and quantum calculations, among others, are used to determine the relationship between chemical structure and pharmacological activity of a series of compounds;

enables one to predict the activity of an unknown or new drug in the series; examples: Free-Wilson, Hantsch, and quantum calculations

quantity discount price reduction extended to a buyer for purchasing a certain quantity, usually a large amount, at one time or for purchasing a specified amount over a definite period of time

quantum number any one of four integers used to describe the movement of an electron in an atom: (1) azimuthal—denotes its angular momentum around the atomic nucleus; (2) magnetic field—represents the magnetic field generated by the electron's movement around the nucleus; (3) principal—indicates its primary shell or orbit around the nucleus; (4) spin—denotes its direction of spin on its axis

quantum theory belief that energy absorption or emission into or from an atom, respectively, occurs in discrete units or quanta

quart unit of volume equal to ¼ gallon, 2 pints, 32 fluid ounces, or 946.24 milliliters

quaternary refers to four substitutions on one atom; general example: quaternary ammonium compounds that have four organic radicals substituted for each of the four hydrogens on the ammonium ion; example: benzalkonium chloride

quaternary ammonium salt organic compound in which the four hydrogen molecules of the ammonium ion are substituted with four organic radicals (may be the same or different) to form the positively charged ion which is associated with a negatively charged ion; example: benzalkonium chloride

quaternary structure association of two or more folded polypeptides to form a functional protein

quid plug of chewing tobacco or snuff that is placed in the buccal pouch

Quincke's disease angioneurotic edema; SEE *angioedema*

quinidine diastereo isomer of quinine; alkaloid from cinchona; used as a cardiac depressant and antiarrythmic

quinine major alkaloid from cinchona bark, present to the extent of 5 percent in cinchona; used as an antimalarial and a bitter tonic

quinoline heterocyclic, aromatic, naphthalene-like compound possessing a nitrogen in the 1-position

quintessence 1: the highly concentrated extract of any substance **2:** tincture, extract, or essence containing the most essential components of plant material

racemic mixture equal mixture of both mirror image pairs of optical isomers; SEE *racemization*

racemization transformation of one-half of the molecules of an optically active compound into molecules that are mirror image configurations of each other (the resultant optical rotation becomes zero)

rad basic radiation dosage unit; the absorption of 100 ergs of ionizing radiation energy per gram of substance (tissue)

radiant heat dryer instrument or apparatus that utilizes infrared light rays for the purpose of producing heat to remove moisture

radiation 1: particles and light rays (photons) emitted from atomic nuclei and/or their orbital electrons as a result of internal reductions in energy levels of nucleons or electrons; most common forms of emission in order of particle size: alpha particles (the same as helium nuclei), neutrons, protons, beta particles (the same as electrons or negatrons or positrons, rarely emitted positively charged electrons), X-rays (emanating as a consequence of orbital electron energy level reductions), and gamma rays (emanating as a consequence of intranuclear neutron and proton energy level reductions) **2:** heat or light emanating from hot objects that is transferred as electromagnetic waves traveling in straight lines at the speed of light; examples: infrared heat lamps, heat from the sun

radiation, background radioactivity that can be detected in the absence of the source being studied; consists of cosmic radiation and that from ill-defined sources on earth

radiation pyrometer SEE *pyrometer*

radiation sterilization to render an object devoid of all life forms by using high exposure levels of ionizing radiation (usually gamma rays and beta particles); used primarily to sterilize drug devices

radical 1: extreme **2:** a chemical group (group of atoms) that is a part of a molecule; synonym: moiety **3:** free radicals—a group of atoms separated from a molecule and bearing a single electron; combine with other free radicals by the pairing of their single electrons to form covalent bonds

radioactive denotes an atomic nucleus which does not exist in its most stable state and which emits photons, electrons, neutrons, protons, and/or alpha particles in order to assume a more stable configuration

radioactive concentration activity per unit quantity of any material in which a radionuclide is present; example: microcuries per gram

radioactive contamination pollution of materials or areas with radioactive substances

radioactive tracer radioactive isotope used as a label in a vehicle or on a molecule; used to determine the course of a chemical reaction, a biological process, or the fate of a molecule in the body

radioactivity property of metastable atoms that spontaneously emit particles and/or photons in order to assume a more stable state; examples: X-rays emitted as a result of changes in energy levels of orbital electrons, γ-rays emitted as a result of changes in energy levels of nucleons

radioassay a quantitative procedure utilizing a radiolabeled substance as the basis for its determination

radiographic tracer an isotope of the element being traced; used in medicine for diagnostic purposes

radioisotope form of an element that is unstable and emits rays of energy or subatomic particles; SEE *isotopes*

radiolabel tagging a substance with a radioactive tracer

radiologist a physician who specializes in diagnosing and treating diseases by the use of radiant energy

radionuclide purity the proportion of the total activity that is in the form of the stated radionuclide

radiopaque dye dyes used in radiology to enhance the X-ray pictures of selected internal anatomic structures

radiopharmaceutical drug formulation containing a radioactive isotope used for the diagnosis, mitigation, or treatment of disease

radiowaves electromagnetic radiation emanating from nuclear spin transitions; wavelengths in the range of 10^3 meter

rancid having a rank or offensive smell or taste; example: a vegetable oil that has undergone oxidative degradation

range a measure of variability; computed as the difference between the highest and lowest numbers in a group of related numbers

Raoult's law a quantitative expression of the partial vapor pressure of an "ideal" solution containing volatile solutes (usually liquid pairs); expressed as the mole fraction multiplied by the vapor pressure of the pure volatile substance

Rasmussen's syndrome a type of progressive encephalopathy seen in juveniles

rate the amount of money per enrollment classification paid to a carrier for medical coverage

rate-limiting step one of a series of processes that occurs at a slower rate than all others involved, thereby controlling the rate of occurrence of all other processes; example: the dissolution rate of a slowly dissolving drug that limits absorption, distribution, and elimination processes

rate meter instrument that measures the instantaneous rate of a process; examples: radioactivity exposure, electrical current flow, airflow, water flow

rate of shear an expression of the infinitesimal change in velocity per unit distance of one liquid layer moving past another; directly proportional to revolutions per minute of a spinning-disk viscometer; SEE *Newton's law of viscous flow; viscosity*

rating process process of evaluating a group or individual to determine a premium relative to the type of risk it presents

ratio analysis in financial analysis, a method of using income statement and balance sheet data to detect trends and problems in the business

rational drug therapy prescribing the right drug for the right patient, at the right time, in the right amounts, and with due consideration of relative costs

rational numbers integers (whole numbers) and common fractions; CONTRAST *irrational numbers*

rational therapy medical therapy used in treating diseases based on reasoning and general principles and not on observations alone

raw material specifications series of tests (and corresponding confidence values) conducted on starting materials that are to be used for dosage form production; synonym: material controls

Raynaud's disease idiopathic, paroxysmal, bilateral cyanosis of the digits

reaction kinetics a study of the rate of chemical change and the manner by which the rate of change is influenced by various factors such as the concentrations of reagents and solvents, the temperature and pressure, and the presence of other chemical agents

reactive hyperemia reddening of the skin that occurs after pressure is applied to the area for a time and then removed; thought to be partially responsible for rhinitis medicamentosa

reactive oxygen species a reactive derivative of molecular oxygen, including superoxide radical, hydrogen peroxide, the hydroxyl radical, and singlet oxygen

reading frame a set of contiguous triplet codons in an mRNA molecule

reagent chemical substance with a known reaction; used frequently in clinical testing

real solution SEE *solution, real*

real time pertaining to the actual time during which a physical process transpires

reasonable and customary (R&C) a term used to refer to the commonly charged or prevailing fees for health services within a geographic area; a fee that falls within the parameters of the average or commonly charged fee for a particular service within a specific community

rebate a monetary amount that is returned to a payer from a prescription drug manufacturer based upon utilization by a covered person or purchases by a provider

receptor molecular structure within or on the surface of a cell, and with which a drug or drug metabolite may bind to produce a particular pharmacological response

recidivism the frequency of the same patient returning to the hospital for the same presenting problems; refers to the inpatient hospitalization

recipe formula and method of mixing to prepare a dosage form containing several ingredients

recipient an individual who has been determined eligible for and has used medical services covered under Medicaid

reciprocating pump/compressor apparatus that effects mass transfer of liquids or gases using a piston or plunger and an intake-output valve mechanism; simplex type—one piston; duplex, triplex, or multiplex types—two, three, or more pistons, respectively, in parallel or in stages to decrease pulsation and/or to increase mass transfer rates

reciprocity recognition by one institution, state, or country of the validity of licenses or permits issued by another

recombinant DNA genetic material that has been cleared enzymatically at specific sites and recombined after insertion of a segment of DNA, usually from another species; used pharmaceutically to produce insulin, growth hormone, interferon, and vaccines

recombination a process in which DNA molecules are broken and rejoined in new combinations

recombinational repair a repair mechanism that can eliminate certain types of damaged DNA sequences that are not eliminated before replication; the undamaged parental strands recombine into the gap left after the damaged sequence is removed

reconstitution process of adding a solvent or suspending liquid (usually purified water) to a previously prepared spray-dried or freeze-dried drug formulation intended to be used in a short period of time (usually within two weeks) after the addition (generally refrigerated following reconstitution); example: reconstitution of an antibiotic suspension

recrudescent return of symptoms after remission

recrudescent typhus SEE *Brill's disease*

recumbent supine; lying flat on one's back

red blood cell SEE *erythrocyte*

redox dye chemical compound that changes color when oxidized or reduced; example: methylene blue

redox potential voltage that measures the tendency of a compound to donate or receive electrons; the sum of the voltages of two half cell reactions

reduced molecule a molecule that has gained one or more electrons

reducing agent substance that donates electrons to another substance in a chemical reaction; the reducing agent itself is oxidized in the chemical reaction

reducing sugar a sugar that can be oxidized by weak oxidizing agents

reduction the gain of electrons by a substance in a chemical reaction; older definitions include the combination of a substance with hydrogen and the loss of oxygen by a substance; SEE *oxidation-reduction*

red veterinary petrolatum partially bleached petrolatum, sometimes used as a sunscreen

reengineer modifying the pharmacy layout design and workflow to support delivery of pharmaceutical care

reference standard nationally or internationally recognized unit of measure (or a pure sample of a substance) against which all other units of measure (or analyses) are judged; the United States Pharmacopeial Convention being the major supplier of reference standards for official drugs

referral recommendation by a health care provider and/or health plan for a covered person to receive care from a different health care provider or facility

referral provider a provider that renders a service to a patient who has been sent to him/her by a participating provider in the health plan

reflex stimulant an agent that acts to induce a compensatory physiological change within an organ or tissue that generally opposed the action; examples: cardiovascular compensatory changes produced in response to the administration of sympathomimetics or parasympathomimetics, the use of aromatic spirit of ammonia to awaken a person who has fainted

reflux intermittent reversal of flow

refluxate material refluxed upward into the esophagus with gastroesophageal reflux; consists of partially digested food, acids, and enzymes

reflux distillation SEE *distillation*

reflux esophagitis esophageal damage induced by gastroesophageal reflux

refractive index degree to which polarized light rays are bent as they pass through a substance under study; measured using a refractometer

refractometer an instrument used to measure the purity of solvents (or the concentration of solutions) by determining the refractive indices of samples and comparing them with the indices of standards; examples: Abbe refractometer, Pulfrich refractometer, the immersion or "dipping" refractometer

refractory resistance to stimulation, treatment, or specific drug therapy

registered adjective describing a pharmacist who has met state requirements for licensure and whose name has been entered on a state registry of practitioners who are licensed to practice in that jurisdiction

regression coefficient slope of a linear regression equation line; line that characterizes a set of data points which indicates the relationship between two variables; example: a plot of the amount of drug absorbed versus time

regulation rule developed from authorizing legislation that is written by an administrative agency; example: state board of pharmacy regulation

regulatory agency any federal or state agency charged with enforcement of laws and regulations

regulatory enzyme an enzyme that catalyzes a committed step in a biochemical pathway

regurgitation SEE *vomiting*

reimbursement payment received for services; often received from insurer

reinsurance insurance purchased by an HMO, insurance company, or self-funded employer from another insurance company to protect itself against all or part of the losses that may be incurred in the process of honoring the claims of its participating providers, policy holders, or employees and covered dependents

relative biological equivalent (as in an exposure to radioactivity) a conversion factor to calculate the roentgen equivalent in man (REM) for a given tissue

relative density SEE *density*

relative error statistical value obtained by dividing the true value for a set of determinations into the mean error; the relative error multiplied by 100 produces the percentage error

relative humidity SEE *humidity, relative*

relative value scale **1:** a method of determining the value of a particular service by considering the time and complexity of providing such service **2:** set of parameters that are without dimension; examples: specific gravity, specific conductance

relative viscosity ratio of the viscosity of one liquid to the viscosity of another liquid used as a standard; determined by the capillary method under the same volume, temperature, pressure conditions

releasing factor a protein involved in the termination phase of translation

reliability the extent to which an evaluation is consistent in measure; synonyms: dependability, consistency, stability

Remington, Joseph Price (1847-1918) considered a master teacher; first published *Practice of Pharmacy* in 1885; served in various roles with the United States Pharmacopeial Convention from 1877 until his death; the highest honor of organized pharmacy, the Remington Honor Medal, established following his death

Remington Honor Medal established in 1918 to recognize distinguished service on behalf of American pharmacy during the preceding years; highest honor of the American Pharmacists Association

REM sleep rapid eye movement sleep probably associated with dream states; may be interrupted through the use of certain drugs

renal pertaining to the kidney

renal clearance **1:** removal by the kidney of a solute (or other substance) from a specific volume of blood per unit of time **2:** the ratio of the product of urine concentration of the solute and the rate of urine flow to the plasma concentration of the solute

renal failure a lack of ability of the kidney to perform its essential function; may be acute or chronic

renal insufficiency inability of the kidneys to function properly in removing waste products from the blood

renal plasma flow rate of movement of blood through the glomerular capillaries of the kidney

renewal continuance of coverage under a policy beyond its original term by the acceptance of a premium for a new policy term

renin enzyme produced by the kidney that catalyzes the conversion of angiotensinogen to angiotensin

repeat action a dosage form (usually a tablet) that provides a quick release of part of the active ingredient and then releases the rest at a slower rate

replication the process in which an exact copy of parental DNA is synthesized using the polynucleotide strands of the parental DNA as templates

replication fork the Y-shaped region of a DNA molecule that is undergoing replication; results from separation of two DNA strands

replicon a unit of the genome that contains an origin for initiating replication

repulsive force inherent tendency for the same or different discrete particles of a substance(s) to be repelled from one another when brought together in a system; strong forces exhibited when positively charged nuclei are in close proximity, and weak forces observed between similarly charged particles in the same system or when a "low energy" substance is in contact with a "high energy" substance; can be used to stabilize dispersed pharmaceutical systems

reserves funds for incurred but unreported health services or other financial liabilities

residency postgraduate training in pharmacy, may be general or specific (e.g., pediatric residency, oncology residency) and in hospital, clinic, or community pharmacy-based practice settings

resident care facility health care facility providing hygienic and nonhazardous food and lodging for its residents

residual urine urine remaining in the bladder after voiding

resin naturally occurring brittle, amorphous, solid substance (as an exudate from a plant) that is soluble in alcohol and volatile oils and insoluble in water; example: pine rosin

resistance quantitative expression of the impeded flow of an electrical current through a conductor (expressed in ohms); specific—resistance across 1 cm^3 of a conductor

resistance heating use of electricity as a primary heat source; production of heat by passing an electrical current through an impeded circuit

resistance thermometer SEE *thermometer, resistance*

resolution **1:** separation of mirror image isomers or enantiomorphs **2:** formal statement (usually in writing) of one or more perceived need(s) or action(s) to be addressed by an individual or a group

resonance alternate shifting of electrons in a molecule between two or more possible configurations; a resonance hybrid is the result

resonance energy stability of a resonating molecule over and above that which would be in a molecule with conventional bonding

Resource-Based Relative Value Scale (RBRVS) Medicare fee schedule for health care providers based on the amount of time and resources expended in treating patients, with adjustments for overhead costs and geographical differences

respiration a biochemical process whereby fuel molecules are oxidized and their electrons are used to generate ATP

respiratory burst an oxygen-consuming process in scavenger cells such as macrophages in which reactive oxygen species are generated and used to kill foreign or damaged cells

respiratory control the control of aerobic respiration by ADP concentration

respondeat superior legal doctrine which holds that a superior (employer) may be liable for actions of a subordinate (employee) which are within the subordinate's job-related responsibilities

retention that portion of the cost of a medical benefit program that is kept by the insurance company or health plans to cover internal costs or to return a profit; can also be referred to as "administrative costs"

reticular arousal system center in the brain stem involved with impulses leading to the higher centers of the cerebral cortex

reticuloendothelial system group of organs that contain a network of endothelial cells and macrophages in sinusoids and are used to filter and phagocytize particulate matter in the blood and lymph; composed of the liver, spleen, lymph nodes, and bone marrow

retina innermost portion of the eye that receives images formed by the lens; part of eye primarily responsible for vision

retrospective rate derivation an addendum to insurance coverage that provides for risk sharing, with the employer being responsible for all or part of that risk

retrospective review determination of medical necessity and/or appropriate billing practice for services already rendered

retrovirus one of a group of viruses with RNA genomes that carry the enzyme reverse transcriptase and form a DNA copy of their genome during their reproductive cycle

return on investment (ROI) ratio of net profit to the owners' equity of a business; used as a broad measure of the firm's performance and indicates how effectively the resources of the firm have been employed

revenue inflow of cash or other assets attributable to the sale of goods or services by a business or from interest, rents, and dividends

reversibility of a dispersion the ability to separate a dispersion medium from the dispersed particles in a dispersed system and to subsequently combine them with relative ease (without significant energy input) to form the same dispersion; contrasted with an irreversibility of a dispersion

reversible reaction a reaction that is capable of proceeding in either direction

review of systems methodology used in a patient interview to systematically review the status of each organ system

Reye's syndrome abnormal condition characterized by acute encephalopathy and fatty infiltration of the liver, and possible infiltration of the pancreas, heart, kidney, spleen, and/or lymph nodes; usually seen in children under 18 years of age after they have had an acute viral infection and were given a salicylate

Reynolds number dimensionless ratio that is an index of the degree of turbulence in liquid flow; conversely, an index of the degree of streamlined or laminar flow; value obtained by the product of a geometric length factor (usually the diameter of the pipe), the velocity of the fluid, and its density divided by the fluid viscosity

-rhea suffix meaning to run or flow; example: diarrhea

rheology study (or science) of flow properties of liquids and semisolids (e.g., syrups and ointments); such properties usually measured in viscosity units, which are a function of stress and strain (deformation) on the system

rheometer SEE *viscometer*

rheopexy viscosity-related term that describes a liquid exhibiting reversible shear thickening; example: liquid assuming its original consistency when shearing stress is discontinued; hastened thixotropic thickening by a gentle motion of the sol

rheostat electrical component of a circuit acting to vary the resistance in the circuit

rhesus factor blood factor that causes erythroblastosis fetalis, a hemolytic condition in the newborn

rheumatologist a physician who specializes in the pathology, diagnosis, and treatment of rheumatic disorders (collagen diseases)

rhin- prefix meaning nose; same as rhino-

rhinitis inflammation of the mucous membranes of the nose

rhinitis medicamentosa nasal inflammation caused by overuse of topical nasal decongestants such as oxymetazoline

rhino- prefix meaning nose; same as rhin-

rhinorrhea "runny" nose, usually due to either the common cold or allergic rhinitis

rhodopsin photochemical substance, of a purplish red color, contained in the retina

ribbon blender mixing device used to uniformly distribute wetted, particulate, solid materials for subsequent granulation or other treatment; mixing device consisting of a U-shaped vessel with two or more metallic flat sigmoid blades mounted so that each rotates in opposite directions to effect mixing

riboflavin vitamin involved with oxidative processes associated with flavoproteins; the functional component of the coenzymes FAD and FMN; synonym: vitamin B_2

ribosomal RNA the RNA present in ribosomes; ribosomes contain several types of single-stranded ribosomal RNA that contribute to ribosome structures and are also directly involved in protein synthesis

ribosome a protein-RNA complex where protein is synthesized

ribozyme self-splicing RNA found in several organisms

Rice, Charles (1841-1901) a German immigrant; became the chief apothecary of the Bellevue Hospital in New York; supervised the revision process of the *United States Pharmacopeia* for over 20 years; in 1900, recommended a shift in the *USP* from being a recipe book to one of more official standards

right bundle branch block observed in an EKG as a "slurred" S wave

Ringer's injection sterile solution of sodium chloride, potassium chloride, and calcium chloride in water for injection; used as an electrolyte replenisher; synonym: isotonic solution of three chlorides for injection

rinse liquid used to cleanse by flushing

risk analysis the process of evaluating expected medical care costs for a prospective group and determining what product, benefit level, and price to offer in order to best meet the needs of the group and the carrier

Rittinger's theory quantitative expression for estimation of the energy requirement for particle size reduction, suggesting that it is directly proportional to an increase in surface area and inversely proportional to the product diameter

RNA editing the alteration of the base sequence in a newly synthesized mRNA molecule; bases may be chemically modified, deleted, or added

Roche friabilator a device used to measure chipping tendencies of tablets by rotating them in a half-partitioned cylinder that causes the tablets to fall on each turn of the cylinder

Rochelle salt potassium sodium tartrate; synonym: seignette salt

rod mill SEE *ball mill*

rods cells of the retina that contain rhodopsin and are responsible for vision in dim light

roentgen unit of radiation exposure equivalent to the absorption of 10^{-4} cal per kilogram

roentgen equivalent man (rem) amount of radiation that has the same physiological effectiveness as one rad of X-rays

roentgenography imaging produced by passing X-rays through the internal structures of the body onto sensitized film

Rokitansky's disease postnecrotic cirrhosis of the liver

role pattern of behavior expected of an individual or group in a particular situation; synonyms: social role, professional role

roller mill apparatus consisting of three or more closely spaced cylinders, each rotating alternately clockwise and counterclockwise and between which particles or masses are passed for purposes of reducing particle size and/or blending

room temperature usual temperature in a working or storage area

rose water ointment SEE *cold cream*

rotary drum filter a continuous vacuum filtration system, the contents of which are agitated and separated at various levels on a circulating housing

rotary pump apparatus that uses a chamber with a rotating impeller, lobe, or gear to trap and move discrete quantities of liquid from an inlet to an outlet; synonyms: gear pump, lobe pump

rotary tableting machine SEE *tableting machine*

rotational viscometer spinning-disk instrument used to measure the viscosity of liquids

rough ER a type of endoplasmic reticulum involved in protein synthesis

route of administration method or avenue by which a medication is introduced onto or into the body

route of excretion pathway by which a substance is removed from the body; examples: urinary track, biliary duct, respiratory tract, skin

-rrhage suffix meaning excessive flow; same as -rrhagia

-rrhagia suffix meaning excessive flow; same as -rrhage

-rrhea suffix meaning discharge

rubber closure specially designed resilient sealing stopper for multiple- or continuous-dose sterile drug preparations; must exert enough pressure on the inner side of the container to maintain the seal and include a needle puncture area that reseals, successively, after each puncture

rubefacient substance applied to the skin that elicits a feeling of warmth and reddens the skin

rust disease tuberculous spondylitis of the cervical region

Ruth, Robert J. (1891-1931) pharmacist and teacher; first proposed the idea of a national Pharmacy Week to promote the professional activities of pharmacists to consumers

saccelli prefolded wafer papers used for individual doses of powders

S-adenosyl-methionine coenzyme derived from ATP and methionine; coenzyme involved in methyl transfer reactions; synonym: active methyl

safety closure SEE *child-resistant closure*

Saint Vitus's dance acute disturbance of the central nervous system characterized by involuntary muscular movements of the face and extremities

sales promotion specific activities (e.g., point-of-purchase displays, booklets, and leaflets) that can improve the effectiveness of selling and promotional activities by coordinating and supplementing both effects

salol synonym for phenyl salicylate

sal polychrestum synonym for potassium sulfate

salt product of a reaction between an acid and a base (other than water); strong electrolyte (other than an acid or a base) that is composed of a cation and an anion; crystalline compound that is composed of at least one cation and an anion other than a hydroxyl ion; substance completely ionized, even in the crystalline (solid) form

salt bridge an electrostatic interaction in proteins between ionic groups of opposite charge

salt-polishing process of cleaning and polishing gelatin capsules by rotating them in a container with granular sodium chloride

salvage pathways metabolic pathways in purine and pyrimidine metabolism in which nucleotides may be reformed from the purine or pyrimidine base and phosphoribosylpyrophosphate

salvation sphere a shell of water molecules that clusters around positive and negative ions

salve stiff ointment or cerate applied to wounds or sores

salve mull ointments with high fusing points containing medicinal agents that spread on gauze similar to plaster mulls

salvia synonym for sage leaves; used as a flavoring or condiment

sample 1: a subset of observations or measurements selected from a population of interest; a statistical part of the whole **2:** free product provided by manufacturers for use as trial therapy

sampling 1: the selection of representative units of a drug product or of a component for a drug product, to test for and ensure a reasonable replication of the quality of the entire lot **2:** process of selecting a sample; SEE *sample*

sanction a reprimand, for any number of reasons, of a participating provider

Sanders' disease/syndrome epidemic keratoconjunctivitis

sandwich compound complex group of molecules existing in layers; one molecule superimposed on another and held together by moderately strong binding forces; a type of complex

sanitary pipe fittings stainless steel or glass pipes, pipe joints, cut-off valves, and pumps designed for easy disassembling and cleaning

saponification 1: process of making soap using fats and alkali **2:** alkaline hydrolysis of an ester; example: hydrolysis of glyceryl tristearate with sodium hydroxide yielding sodium stearate (the soap) and glycerin (the by-product)

saponification value   number of milligrams of potassium hydroxide required to neutralize the free acids and saponify the esters contained in one gram of a fat, an oil, or a wax

saponin   a group of amorphous colloidal glycosides that form soapy aqueous solutions

sapotoxin   a poisonous saponin

sarcoidosis   chronic, progressive, generalized granulomatous disease of unknown etiology

satellite DNA   DNA sequences arranged next to each other; form a satellite band when genomic DNA is digested and centrifuges

satellite pharmacy   a small remote pharmacy service unit that is dependent upon the main pharmacy for stock items and other administrative services; a pharmacy unit on a hospital ward to serve patients in that ward

saturated molecule   a molecule that contains no carbon-carbon double or triple bonds

saturation humidity   SEE *humidity, saturation*

saturation temperature   1: temperature at which a vapor will begin to condense to a liquid **2:** temperature at which a liquid and its vapor exist in equilibrium **3:** the "dew point"

Saunders' disease   acute gastritis in infants due to excessive carbohydrates in the diet

scabicide   a drug that kills mites; primarily used against the mite that causes the "seven-year itch" (scabies)

scalar   refers to quantities that have magnitudes, but not directions; examples: speed, mass, volume; CONTRAST *vector quantities*

scale anchor   a point along a scale that defines a level of performance; may be numerical, descriptive, or behavioral in form

scale of segregation   a "degree of mixing" expression based on either diameter or volume of particle(s) being mixed

scaling up   1: extrapolation of a pharmacokinetic or pharmacologic model from animals to humans based on their respective physiologic parameters **2:** the conversion of batch drug manufacturing processes from small laboratory quantities to pilot and then to large-batch production; scale-ups do not usually occur in direct relationships

scanning speech   slow speech, with frequent stops between words or syllables

Schaefer, Hugo H. (1891-1967) educator; served as the dean of the Brooklyn College of Pharmacy from 1937 until his death; APhA treasurer 1941-1967; Remington Honor Medal recipient in 1951

scheduled drug substance classified by the Drug Enforcement Administration (DEA) as having a high potential for abuse by the public; synonyms: controlled drug, controlled substance

Schedule I drug a drug with no accepted medical use and one that has the highest potential for abuse; examples: heroin, LSD

Schedule II drug a drug with accepted medical uses but also has a strong potential for abuse; repeated use may lead to severe physical or psychological dependence; examples: morphine, meperidine, methadone

Schedule III drug a drug with accepted medical uses and a potential for abuse that is less than those substances in Schedules I and II; use may lead to moderate or low psychological dependence or high physical dependence; examples: ketamine, thiopentol

Schedule IV drug a drug with accepted medical use and a lower potential for abuse than those in Schedule III; use may lead to limited physical or psychological dependence; examples: chloral hydrate, meprobamate

Schedule V drug a drug with accepted medical use and a lower potential for abuse than those in Schedule IV; use may lead to limited physical or psychological dependence; includes both legend and OTC drugs; drugs that may be sold without prescription (in some states only) but with a record of sales (formerly known as "Exempt Narcotic Drug"); examples: cough syrups containing no more than one grain of codeine per fluid ounce

Scheele, Carl Wilhelm (1742-1786) Swedish pharmacist-chemist credited with the discovery of chlorine, citric acid, manganese, and barium; codiscoverer (with J. Priestley) of oxygen; first isolated uric acid from urine

schistosomiasis disease resulting from an infestation of man by flukes; *Schistosoma hematobium, Schistosoma mansoini,* and *Schistosoma japonicum* the predominant disease-causing organisms

sciatica pain in the lower back or hip that radiates down the thigh to the lower leg

scientific method generally considered to be an accepted series of steps or procedures designed to solve a problem or enhance understanding of a natural phenomenon; included are the steps of observation, theory (or hypothesis), experimentation, analysis and evaluation, repeated testing and conclusions, and development of laws; other competent researchers should be able to repeat such experiments and observations

scintillation counter an instrument used to measure weak beta radiation that interacts with substances called phosphors and fluors to produce a flash of light that is amplified and recorded

sclero- prefix meaning hard

scleroprotein fibrous protein; insoluble protein; example: keratin (a protein of skin and hair)

sclerosis hardening of tissue, especially due to excessive growth of fibrous tissue

scope of practice boundaries within which a health professional may practice, usually established by the state board

scopine alcohol part of the scopolamine molecule

scopolamine alkaloid found in plants of the Solanaceous family that acts similarly to atropine, but is also used with morphine for analgesia and anesthesia

scored tablet compressed tablet that contains grooves for ease of breaking into halves or quarters (if double scored)

scraped surface heat exchanger a tube-in-a-tube heat transfer device that also contains a rotating shaft with scraping blades in the inner tube; used to continuously prepare and cool emulsions, gels, and creams

screening tests for risk of a disease or condition; patients identified as at risk in the screening process further evaluated for a definitive diagnosis

screw pump apparatus that uses one or more rotating augers to transfer liquids, semisolids, or solids through pipes or tubes from one container to another

scruple 1: apothecary unit of weight equal to 20 grains, or one-third of a dram **2:** moral or ethical principle

scurvy disease usually caused by low amounts of ascorbic acid in the diet; noted by debility and edema and frequently by hemorrhage and ulceration of the gums

SDS polyacrylamide gel electrophoresis a method for separating proteins or determining their molecular weights that employs the negatively charged detergent sodium dodecyl sulfate (SDS)

seal coating the first step of a sugar-coating process for tablets; an initial covering layer that prevents moisture effects on the tablet during subsequent sugar-coating steps

seasonal discount price reduction extended to a customer for ordering or accepting delivery during a period of low activity (an off-season); example: a lower price for an antibiotic during the summer months rather than during the winter months, a time when the demand for antibiotics is expected to be greater

secondary alcohol SEE *alcohol*

secondary amine SEE *amine*

secondary care services provided by medical specialists, such as cardiologists, urologists, and dermatologists, who generally do not have primary contact with patients

secondary coverage a plan that has the responsibility for payment of any eligible charges not covered by the primary coverage

secondary metabolite a molecule derived from a primary metabolite; many serve protective functions

secondary prevention efforts to prevent further worsening of a disease; example: cholesterol management following CABG surgery

secondary structure folding of a polypeptide chain into local patterns such as α-helix and β-pleated sheet; maintained by hydrogen bonds between the amide hydrogen and the carbonyl oxygen of the peptide bond

second genetic code the precision with which amino acids are attached to their cognate tRNAs; catalyzed by the aminoacyl-tRNA synthetases; a principal reason for the accuracy of polypeptide synthesis

second law of thermodynamics SEE *thermodynamics*

second messenger a molecule that mediates the action of some hormones

second opinion an opinion obtained from an additional health care professional prior to the performance of a medical service or a surgical procedure

secretin hormone produced by cells in the jejunum and lower duodenum in response to a lowering of the pH of chyme in these areas; secretin initiates a secretion of bicarbonate

secretion the glandular production of a solution containing hormones, enzymes, electrolytes, lipids, and other substances; fluids may be secreted into a body cavity or outside the body (exocrinic secretion) or they may be secreted into the blood as a hormone that affects the body's physiology (endocrinic secretion); process of passing substances from cells that line the tubules of a nephron into the tubular filtrate to eventually form urine

Section 1115 waivers part of the Social Security Act that grants the Secretary of Health and Human Services broad authority to waive certain laws relating to Medicaid for the purpose of conducting pilot, experimental, or demonstration projects

Section 1915(b) waivers (freedom-of-choice waivers) prior to the passage of the Balanced Budget Act (BBA) of 1997, allowed states to require Medicaid recipients to enroll in HMOs or other managed care plans in an effort to control costs; under the BBA, states can enroll recipients into managed care without applying for these waivers

secured loan one in which the lender's risk is reduced by the borrower pledging something of value as security that the loan will be repaid; synonym: collateral

sedative drug or chemical agent that produces relaxation and/or decreased anxiety, but not necessarily sleep; a central nervous system depressant

sedimentation the aggregation (usually downward) of particles in a suspension due to their size, shape, and density in relation to the density and viscosity of the suspending medium

sedimentation rate erythrocyte sedimentation rate; a test that indicates an inflammatory disease

self-care treating one's own ailments with medicines and/or other health care items, usually without medical advice; a range of behaviors undertaken by individuals to promote or restore health

self-funding, self-insurance a health care program in which employers fund benefit plans from their own resources without purchasing insurance

semiconservative replication DNA synthesis in which each polynucleotide strand serves as a template for the synthesis of a new strand

semipermeable membrane thin film that has theoretical pores or openings so small that only certain substances can pass through; usually passage of a substance depends on its particle size; used for dialysis

sense strand the DNA strand that RNA polymerase copies to produce mRNA, rRNA, or tRNA

sensible heat heat that can be detected by the senses and produces a temperature change

sensitivity 1: (for a prescription balance) the minimum weight required to move its index pointer one scale value; a quantity used in the determination of minimum weighable quantities within a specific error limit **2:** the lowest concentration that is detectable by an instrument

sensitivity requirement (SR) maximum permissible change in load that causes a specified change; usually one subdivision on the index plate, in the position of the indicating element; must not exceed 6 mg for a class A prescription balance

sepsis 1: presence of organisms or their toxins in the blood **2:** contamination

sequential multiple analysis (SMA) method of clinical chemistry in which two or more separate tests are performed sequentially on the same blood or urine sample in a given time period; an Arabic number following the letters SMA designates the number of simultaneous tests performed during a given time period (usually one minute); examples: SMA 12, SMA 16

sequester 1: separation or isolation **2:** a form of complexation in which a molecule is prevented from exerting its usual properties sequestration: complexation of a metallic ion

sequestration complexation of a metallic ion

serendipity discovery of something unexpected and valuable when looking for something else; example: Sir Alexander Fleming's discovery of the antibacterial effects of penicillin while growing a bacteria culture

serous having reference to or resembling serum; producing or containing serum

serum 1: liquid portion of blood containing all dissolved substances, but excluding clotting factors and formed elements (blood cells) **2:** a vaccine **3:** the liquid portion of the blood that separates from a clot by synthesis

serum hepatitis SEE *hepatitis, serum*

service area the geographic area serviced by the health plan as approved by state regulatory agencies and/or as detailed in the certification of authority

sesame oil a fixed oil obtained from sesame seed; used in pharmaceuticals; synonyms: benne oil, teel oil

sesquiterpene hydrocarbon composed of three isoprene units connected in a "head to tail" fashion

severe combined immunodeficiency disease genetic defect in which the body lacks the ability to develop an immune system

sexually transmitted disease infection or ill condition which is contracted almost exclusively by physical sexual interactions; examples: syphilis, AIDS, genital warts, pubic lice, herpes simplex type 2

shampoo liquid soap or detergent used to clean the hair and scalp and often used as a vehicle for dermatologic agents

shampoo, suspension liquid soap or detergent containing one or more solid, insoluble substances dispersed in a liquid vehicle that is used to clean the hair and scalp; often used as a vehicle for dermatologic agents

shearing stress force per unit area applied to one liquid layer flowing past another; SEE *Newton's law of viscous flow*

shear thickening viscosity-related term which indicates that a liquid becomes more viscous as "shearing stress" is applied

shear thinning viscosity-related term indicating that a liquid becomes less viscous as "shearing stress" is applied

shelf life time limit placed on a drug product's original potency and acceptable overall quality; determined by individual chemical and physical properties of the medicinal agents, pharmaceutical adjuncts, and packaging

shell an orbit of an electron or its probable path around the nucleus; designated by K, L, M, N, etc., or 1, 2, 3, 4, etc., where the K or 1 shell is the closest to the nucleus with a principal quantum number of 1 and others in order are progressively farther away from the nucleus

shell freezing process of freezing a liquid mass as it is spinning or rotating in such a manner that a layer of solidified material can be formed against the sides of a partially filled drug container; a process that is usually preliminary to the freeze-drying process

shock 1: sudden disturbance of mental equilibrium **2:** acute peripheral circulatory failure due to derangement of circulatory control or loss of circulating fluid; marked by hypotension, coldness of the skin, usually tachycardia, and often anxiety

short tandem repeat short sequence of DNA, normally a length of two to five base pairs

shotgun cloning a cloning technique in which genomic libraries are created by the random digestion of a genome

shrinkage (management) any process other than normal sales that has the effect of reducing the amount or value of inventories

sial- prefix meaning saliva or the salivary glands; same as sialo-

sialo- prefix meaning saliva or the salivary glands; same as sial-

sialogogue agent that increases the flow of saliva

sialolith small stone occluding a salivary duct

sialometry measurement of salivary flow to determine extent of dry mouth

sickle-cell anemia congenital disease found predominantly in blacks in which the deoxygenated red blood cells assume a sickle or crescent shape and function in an abnormal and detrimental manner

sieve container with a wire (or nylon) mesh bottom, having a specific number of openings per linear inch; used to size drug particles; a series of sieves can be used to ascertain a size-weight distribution of particles in a given batch of material

sieve shaker apparatus designed to accommodate a series of stacked sieves, each with specific size openings and decreasing in size from top to bottom, and that can be vibrated to effect separation of particles by size

signal peptide a short sequence, typically near the amino terminal of a polypeptide, that determines its destination

signal recognition particle a large complex consisting of proteins on a small RNA molecule that mediates the binding of the ribosome to the RER during protein synthesis

signatura, signa, or *sig* directions to be placed on a prescription label to indicate to the patient how to take or use the medication; SEE ALSO *prescription*

signature theory concept that "divine providence" provided plant materials with similar physical characteristics to that of body parts and that these could be used to treat ailments in such body parts; examples: English walnut kernels for brain treatment, ginseng root as a panacea (espoused by Paracelsus)

significant figures numbers that establish magnitude (or quantity) and accuracy by virtue of their location in the numerical expression, with the last significant figure being an approximation; example: 3.00 means accurate to the one-hundredth part and may vary from 2.995 to 3.005

Simmonds' disease hypopituitarism

Simon's disease progressive lipodystrophy; also known as "Barraquer's disease"

simple diffusion a process in which each type of solute, propelled by random molecular motion, moves down a concentration gradient

single-compartmental model for pharmacokinetic purposes, the body is perceived as one compartment throughout which a drug is uniformly distributed; the pharmacokinetics of a specific drug may or may not fit this model; also known as "one-compartmental model"; CONTRAST *two-compartmental model, multicompartmental model*

single-dose container SEE *container, single dose*

single-payer system a health care financing arrangement in which money, usually from a variety of taxes, is funneled to a single entity (usually the government) that then is responsible for the financing and administration of the health system; can be regional, statewide, or nationwide

single-punch tableting machine SEE *tableting machine*

single-source drug a drug available from only one supplier, generally one that is under patent protection

single-unit container SEE *container, single unit*

sintered glass filter SEE *fritted glass filter*

S-isomer method of Cahn, Prelog, and Ingold for designating configuration of optical isomers in which the atom or group of lowest priority (according to atomic number) is placed beneath the molecule and the order of priorities of the remaining groups or atoms is counterclockwise

site-directed mutagenesis technique that introduces specific sequence changes into cloned genes

site of action cell receptors where a biological response is initiated

site-specific recombination recombination of nonhomologous genetic material with a chromosome at a specific site

sitz bath sitting in a lukewarm bath for a time; thought to be helpful in providing palliative treatment for hemorrhoids

sizing of granules separation of granules according to their "effective diameter" using a series of screens of increasing mesh number from top to bottom; sized granules recombined in optimum ratios to facilitate further processing, as in tableting

Sjogren's syndrome group of symptoms associated with rheumatoid arthritis (oral dryness, ophthalmic dryness, vaginal dryness); often seen in menopausal women

skeletal muscle body tissue consisting of elongated cells grouped into bundles that contract when stimulated; alternate contraction and relaxation of muscles produces motion of the body part; synonym: striated muscle; CONTRAST *smooth muscle*

skilled nursing facility a facility, either freestanding or part of a hospital, that accepts patients in need of rehabilitation and medical care that is of a lesser intensity than that received in a hospital

slaked lime synonym for calcium oxide

slander statement of one person that defames the character or reputation of another

sleep efficiency the amount of time in bed one actually spends sleeping

sleep latency the amount of time elapsed between going to bed and falling asleep

slicing cutting fleshy or tuberous parts of plants preparatory to drying

sliding markup a pricing policy in which the percentage or dollar value of markup is decreased as the cost of the product is increased

sling psychrometer device to measure relative humidity using a wet-bulb thermometer and dry-bulb thermometer with an appropriately calibrated chart to convert the temperature differential to relative humidity

slope the rate of change in the relationship of two variables

slug large rough tablet made by compressing finely divided particles of a drug formulation under high pressure; milled and sized to produce a "dry" granulation for subsequent compression into tablets

slugging one step in a process of preparing a dry granulation for tablet compression in which the drug materials are compressed into large rough tablets or slugs and then ground into appropriately sized granules

slugging machine heavy-duty tablet press designed to compress finely divided drug formulations in large, rough, compacted units called "slugs"

slurry 1: a highly concentrated, solid-liquid dispersion; usually a batch of pharmaceutical material to be further processed **2:** dosage form in which activated charcoal is prepared for administration after poisoning

small-group pooling combining all or segments of small group businesses into a pool or pools; expected claims, and therefore premium rates, determined by pool and not on a group-specific basis; SEE ALSO *pooling*

small nuclear ribonuclear particle a complex of proteins and small nuclear RNA molecules that promotes RNA processing

small nuclear RNA a small RNA molecule involved in removing introns from mRNA, rRNA, and tRNA

Smith, Daniel B. (1792-1883) a founder of the Philadelphia College of Pharmacy; one of the founders of the American Pharmacists Association in 1852; also served as its first president

Smoluchowski equation quantitative expression of the flocculation rate of a suspension consisting of discretely dispersed particles

smooth ER a type of endoplasmic reticulum involved in lipid synthesis and biotransformation

smooth muscle a type of muscular tissue arranged in sheets or layers as in the alimentary canal; also found as isolated cells in connective tissue;

muscles are controlled by the autonomic nervous system; synonyms: nonstriated and involuntary muscles; CONTRAST *skeletal muscle*

soap 1: a metallic salt of a fatty acid; example: Castile soap **2:** an anionic surface active agent used to cleanse or wash; SEE ALSO *surfactant* **3:** any compound of one or more fatty acids, or their equivalents, with an alkali; a detergent that is much employed in liniments, enemas, and making pills; also a mild aperient, antacid, antiseptic

SOAP note format used in documenting patient care; records subjective, objective, assessment, and plan; used by pharmacists in documenting pharmaceutical care interventions with patients

social cognitive theory a theory developed by Bandura that attempts to predict behavior based on an individual's expectation or belief that a particular behavior will result in a particular outcome and that the individual has the ability to accomplish this behavior

socialized medicine a health care system that is owned by the government

sodium alkali, metallic, monovalent element; the ion is an important electrolyte in blood plasma and other extracellular fluids; normal blood levels are about 140 mEq/L; the chief extracellular cation

sodium chloride equivalent that weight of sodium chloride that produces a colligative property effect (boiling point elevation, melting point depression, osmotic pressure changes), represented by one gram of a specific drug

sol 1: a colloidal dispersion **2:** the inner layer of respiratory mucus

-sol suffix referring to a colloidal dispersion; example: aerosol

solanaceous related to the nightshade family of plants; examples: belladonna, stramonium, jimsonweed, tomato, and potato plants

solanine poisonous alkaloid obtained from potato sprouts, tomatoes, or other members of the Solanaceae (nightshade) family

sole proprietorship a business entity in which there is a single owner

solidification point that temperature (and pressure) at which a liquid turns to a solid; synonym: freezing point

solubility the maximum amount of solute that may be dissolved in a given amount of a solvent under a specified set of conditions; the concentration of a solute in a solvent at its saturation point

solubility method a means of analyzing complexes by solubility determinations; used in situations where the solubility of one substance in an aqueous medium is increased or decreased by complex formation

solubilization a method used to increase the solubility of a poorly soluble solute by the addition of a third substance such as a soap or another surfactant; example: use of polysorbate 60 to bring more peppermint oil into an aqueous solution

soluble soap sodium or potassium salt of fatty acids; SEE *soap*

solute the substance that is dissolved by a solvent

solution liquid preparation that contains one or more chemical substances dissolved, i.e., molecularly dispersed, in a suitable solvent or mixture of mutually miscible solvents

solution, colloidal a dispersion of minute particles or large polymeric molecules (0.5 to 1.0 nm) in a liquid medium

solution, concentrate liquid preparation (i.e., a substance that flows readily in its natural state) that contains a drug dissolved in a suitable solvent or mixture of mutually miscible solvents; the drug has been strengthened by the evaporation of its nonactive parts

solution, for slush solution for the preparation of an iced saline slush, which is administered by irrigation and used to induce regional hypothermia (in conditions such as certain open heart and kidney surgical procedures) by its direct application

solution, gel forming, extended release solution that forms a gel when it comes in contact with ocular fluid, and which allows at least a reduction in dosing frequency

solution, ideal one in which there are no interacting forces between solute molecules; a very dilute solution may approach ideality

solution, micellar a "clear emulsion" or a liquid system containing micelles (surfactant molecules surrounding minute immiscible droplets)

solution, ophthalmic a sterile solution, essentially free of foreign particles, suitably compounded and packaged for instillation in the eye

solution, real one in which there are interacting forces between molecules of solute; a more concentrated solution

solution, true single-phase (homogeneous) dispersion consisting of atoms, small molecules, or ions (less than 1 nm) as the largest discrete particles

solution tablet SEE *tablet, compressed*

solvate a compound formed by a reaction between the solvent and the solute

solvation process for formation of a solvate

solvent a liquid capable of dissolving other material(s); the substance in which a solute is dissolved

solvolysis a reaction between the solvent and the solute resulting in the cleavage of a chemical bond in the solute molecule; a ring structure may be opened or a molecule may be split into two or more smaller compounds; if the solvent is water, known as hydrolysis

somat- prefix meaning the body

somatomedin a polypeptide that mediates the growth-promoting action of growth hormone

somatostatin a peptide hormone that inhibits the growth hormone, glucagon, and insulin secretion

somnolence sleepiness; drowsiness

soporific a drug or other agent that produces sleep; synonym: narcotic

sorb to take up and hold by either absorption or adsorption

Sorensen pH scale the entire pH spectrum from ultimate acidity through neutrality and to ultimate basicity; a pH scale from 0 to 14 where pH equals the negative log (base 10) of the hydrogen ion concentration in a system

sorptometer instrument used to measure surface area of a particulate sample based on the extent of gas absorbed on the surface in a monomolecular layer and at the temperature of liquid nitrogen

Southern blotting a technique in which radioactively labeled DNA or RNA profiles are used to locate a complementary sequence in a DNA digest

Spalding, Lyman (1775-1821) American physician known as the Father of the *United States Pharmacopeia*

span of control in a given situation, a limit to the number of persons who can be effectively supervised; the limit of supervision depends on the technology involved, the training and knowledge of subordinates, and the clarity of the tasks to be performed

spatial configuration refers to the three-dimensional arrangement of groups around an asymmetric carbon atom, double bond, or ring (the former involves optical isomerism; the latter two involve geometric isomerism)

spatula flat thin blade used for mixing or spreading soft substances (such as ointments and creams) or powders

spatulation a prescription-compounding process of mixing powders on a pill tile or other flat surface by the movement of a spatula through the powder and a turning of the powder; a low-pressure mixing process

species coarsely powdered or bruised drugs intended for the use in the preparation of infusions or decoctions

specific activity **1:** the quantity of radioactivity per unit mass of an element or a compound containing the nuclide; example: 100 millicuries per gram **2:** method of expressing enzyme concentration as units of enzyme per milligram of protein

specific conductance the reciprocal of specific resistance; SEE *conductance*

specific gravity the weight of one body or substance compared to the weight of an equal volume of another body or substance selected as a standard, both bodies being at the same temperature; the most common standard is water (the specific gravity of water is set equal to one)

specific labeling implies that the radionuclide is known to be in the position(s) specified by the numbering and naming of the labeled atom in the compound

specific resistance SEE *resistance*

specific rotation observed optical rotation of a compound corrected for concentration, temperature, wavelength of light, and specific solvent

specific surface surface area per unit weight of substance; example: square meters per gram

spectrometry SEE *spectrophotometry*

spectrophotometry a method of analysis in which electromagnetic radiation is passed through a sample and the absorption of the radiation (due to its interactions with the sample) is measured; determinations conducted either at a fixed wavelength or at varying wavelengths over a specified region; synonym: spectrometry

spectrophotometry, colorimetric SEE *colorimetry*

spectrophotometry, EPR SEE *electron paramagnetic resonance*

spectrophotometry, infrared spectrophotometric measurements made in the infrared region of the electromagnetic spectrum

spectrophotometry, NMR SEE *nuclear magnetic resonance*

spectrophotometry, ultraviolet spectrophotometric measurements made in the ultraviolet region

spend-down under Medicaid, refers to a method by which an individual establishes Medicaid eligibility by reducing gross income through incurring medical expenses until net income (after medical expenses) meets Medicaid financial requirements

spermaceti hard, waxy substance obtained from the head of the sperm whale, *Physeter macrocephalus;* a source of almost pure cetyl palmitate

spherical diameter equivalent a quantitative expression used to estimate the diameter of an irregularly shaped particle of a given volume; the effective diameter of an irregularly shaped particle; used in pharmaceutical micrometric determinations

sphingolipid type of lipid derived from the amino alcohol, sphingol (sphingosine)

sphingomyelin a type of phospholipid that contains sphingosine; the 1-hydroxyl group of ceramide (a fatty acid derivative of sphingosine) is esterified to the phosphate group of phosphorylcholine or phosphorylethanolamine

spike that part of an intravenous fluid container that is connected to an administration set and through which the fluid goes to the patient

spirit an alcoholic or hydroalcoholic solution of a volatile substance; examples: camphor spirit, aromatic ammonia spirit

spirit of camphor SEE *camphor spirit*

splenomegaly abnormal enlargement of the spleen

sponge absorbent pad of folded gauze or cotton

spongiopiline thin cloth with sponge on one side and rubber on the other, intended for the absorption and topical application of hot liquids

spontaneous changes physical or chemical processes that occur with a release of energy

sporadic typhus SEE *Brill's disease*

spore inactive, resting, and resistant state of a bacterium

spray an aqueous or oleaginous solution of medicaments dispensed as coarse or finely divided droplets; may be administered topically or through the nasal-pharyngeal route; liquid minutely divided as by a jet of air or steam

spray, congealing the process of feeding a quantity of a melted semisolid pharmaceutical through an atomizer and exposing the droplets to a stream of cold air, resulting in instantaneous solidification as micron-sized spheres; similar to spray drying except that cold air is used instead of hot air

spray, metered nonpressurized dosage form consisting of valves that allow the dispensing of a specified quantity of spray upon each activation

spray, suspension liquid preparation containing solid particles dispersed in a liquid vehicle and in the form of coarse droplets or finely divided solids to be applied locally, usually to the nasal-pharyngeal tract, or topically to the skin

spray dryer machine that removes moisture from atomized particles almost instantaneously, using a controlled "solution feed" through a high rpm wheel (atomizer) and an upward flow of heated air; particles are dried as they fall through the heated air (fluidized bed) in an enclosed chamber and are collected in a container at the bottom of the chamber; moisture-laden vapor is vented up and out of the chamber

spreading an expression of the ability of a liquid to cover a surface; SEE *wetting; adsorption*

sprue a disease that is the result of malabsorption; marked by sore mouth, indigestion, diarrhea (frothy), and weight loss; synonym: thrush

stab 1: an immature form of polymorphonuclear leukocytes **2:** to pierce with a pointed object

stability an expression of the extent to which the physical and/or chemical nature of dosage forms and/or drug molecules remain the same; the opposite of instability or rapid degradation

stability testing 1: procedures used to determine the time through which a drug or drug product will remain active and acceptable for use under normal handling and storage conditions **2:** accelerated—subjection of drugs and/or dosage forms to exaggerated conditions of temperature, light, and humidity; example: temperature studies conducted at 37°C, 50°C, 60°C, or freezing, refrigerator, and room temperatures

staff model HMO a health care model that employs physicians to provide health care to its members; all premium and other revenues accrue to the HMO, which compensates physicians by salary and incentive programs

staff of Asklepios the rod and serpent symbol of medicine originating in ancient Babylonian and Grecian cultures

stage filtration separation-clarification process that utilizes a series of filter media to remove a wide range of particle sizes, with the larger particles removed first

stakeholders organizations or individuals who are impacted by a specific individual or service; in pharmaceutical care, the patients/recipients, employers, insurers, various health care professionals who refer or receive referrals, and others who have a stake in the success of the service

standard benefit package a set of specific health care benefits that would be offered by delivery systems

standard class rate (SCR) a base revenue requirement on a per member or per employee basis, multiplied by group demographic information to calculate monthly premium rates

standard deviation statistical parameter for a set of data calculated by taking the square root of the mean of the squared errors for large samples; for smaller samples, by taking the square root of the sum of the squared errors divided by the number of determinations, less one, in order to correct for bias; a measure of dispersion in a sample or population

staphylococcal relating to the *Staphylococcus* bacteria

staple product product for which there is a strong demand and is therefore subject to market and administered pricing

starch sugar SEE *dextrose*

stare decisis the legal doctrine of following decisions or principles rendered by previous court actions as long as such decisions do not contradict current principles of law

stasis slowing, stoppage, or decrease in the flow of fluid, usually blood, to an area of the body

statement of financial position SEE *balance sheet*

state of hydration refers to whether or not a drug is in the anhydrous amorphous state or the hydrated crystalline state; expressed as the number of water molecules that are a part of the salt crystal

static-bed dryer device used to remove moisture from a batch of pharmaceutical material by a process in which there is no movement of the particles being dried; example: a tray dryer; CONTRAST *agitation dryer*

stationary phase separable type of matter that does not move in a process; example: the adsorbent in column chromatography

statistic descriptive numerical measure that is computed from all elements within a given sample

statute a law that is enacted by a legislative body

staxis hemorrhage

steady state that point or time interval when a process such as drug absorption is fully initiated and ongoing; a concept used to simplify kinetic data analysis; a dynamic state of equilibrium; a state in a process when the rate of formation and the rate of breakdown of a substance are equal; in pharmacokinetics, the maintenance of a constant blood level of a drug by keeping absorption rate equal to the overall elimination rate

steam distillation a means of purification of a volatile, immiscible organic compound at low temperatures using steam vapors to avoid decomposition of the compound; the volatilization and immediate condensation of a compound using steam vapors; compound volatilized from the distilling flask, and compound and steam collected in the receiver

stearate salt or ester derived from stearic acid and an alkali hydroxide or from stearic acid and an alcohol

steatorrhea very fatty feces, usually due to the malabsorption of fat

Steele-Richardson-Olszewski disease progressive supranuclear paralysis

Stefan-Boltzman law a quantitative expression of the emissive power of a "black body" (a perfect energy radiator); energy per unit time per unit area of a radiating surface of a "black body" proportional to its absolute temperature raised to the fourth power

Stein-Leventhal syndrome hirsutism, amenorrhea, and enlarged polycystic ovary

stenosis narrowing or partial closure of a valve or duct; example: pyloric stenosis

step-care a procedure that requires the use of less expensive interventions in patient treatment before going on to more expensive therapies

stercolith a fecal mass that can tear the intestinal wall; example: activated charcoal given for poisoning in excessive doses

sterculia gum dried gummy exudation from several species of sterculia plants *(Sterculia urens);* synonym: gum karaya

stereoisomers molecules that differ only by the spatial arrangement of their atoms or groups; examples: *cis-trans* (geometric) isomers and optical (mirror image) isomers

sterile 1: free from any living microorganisms or their spores **2:** absence of fertility; unable to bear young in the case of the female and inability to sire an offspring in the case of the male

sterile product pharmaceutical preparation (dosage form) prepared so that its sealed contents are devoid of any life-forms; examples: parenterals, irrigating preparations, ophthalmics

Sterile Water for Injection, USP water that has been sterilized and is packaged in a single-dose container no greater than one liter in size, and which does not contain an antimicrobial agent; used to prepare parenteral medications

sterility test procedures to determine if a preparation contains living organisms or their spores; consult the *USP-NF* for descriptions of official testing methods

sterilization **1:** process for rendering a closed system (such as a parenteral dosage form) void of any life forms such as bacteria, molds, and fungi or their spores **2:** process for making a living organism incapable of reproducing **3:** process by which surfaces of instruments, work, or operating areas are rendered free of microorganisms

Stern's layer SEE *zeta-potential*

steroid cyclic organic compound that contains a cyclopentanoperhydrophenanthrene nucleus and is a part of the structure of adrenal corticol hormones, sex hormones, cardiac glycosides, and cholesterol

sterol an alcohol derivative of a steroid; example: cholesterol

sterol carrier protein a cytoplasmic protein carrier for certain intermediates during cholesterol biosynthesis

Stevens-Johnson syndrome a severe form of erythema multiforme in which the lesions may involve oral and anogenital mucosa, the eyes, and viscera; characterized by headache, malaise, fever, arthralgia, and conjunctivitis

stick dosage form prepared in a relatively long, slender, and often cylindrical form

sticking the adhesion of a tablet or a tablet granulation to the wall of the die or the surface of the punches of a tablet press; an undesirable event in tablet compression

Still's disease juvenile-type rheumatoid arthritis

stimulant a drug that produces a temporary increase in the functional activity of an organ

stock-to-sales ratio ratio calculated by dividing beginning inventory by the amount of sales during a specified time period

Stokes-Adams syndrome slow or absent pulse, vertigo, syncope, and convulsions, usually as the result of heart block

stoma an opening, an orifice, or a mouth

stomatitis inflammation of the mouth

-stomy suffix referring to the artificial formation of an opening into an organ; example: colostomy

stool waste material of defecation; synonym: feces

stool softener a medicinal agent used to facilitate evacuation of the lower bowel by increasing its liquid contents through a surfactant action

stop-loss insurance insurance coverage taken out by a health plan or self-funded employer to provide protection from losses resulting from claims greater than a specific dollar amount per covered person per year

strain gauge device used to measure forces involved in a compression process; example: a tableting strain gauge

straining the passing of a liquid through a woven filter medium or cotton plug to remove large particulate matter; synonym: coarse filtration

strength refers to quantity or amount of active ingredient in a preparation or the degree or extent of an intrinsic property of a substance

streptococcal relating to or caused by streptococci

stretch marks (striae) visual bands or lines that form on the abdominal skin; caused by physical expansion of the abdominal skin; common in pregnant women in the latter stages of pregnancy

stria streak or line

striated muscle SEE *skeletal muscle*

strictness effect the practice of giving consistently low ratings

stridor high-pitched, noisy respiration

strip packaging machine prepackaging device that places unit doses of a drug inside a series of flexible containers

stroke paroxysm or attack usually associated with a cerebral vascular accident caused by either a thrombus or a hemorrhage

structural formula a chemical formula that shows the arrangement of the various atoms in a molecule and the nature of the bonds connecting them

structural gene a gene that codes for the synthesis of a polypeptide or a polynucleotide with a nonregulatory function (e.g., mRNA, rRNA, or tRNA)

structural isomers SEE *positional isomers*

structure-activity relationships relationships between chemical structures of molecules and their pharmacological and/or biological activities

strychnine major alkaloid of *Strychnos nux-vomica,* which is extremely toxic to the central nervous system (CNS) and acts as a powerful CNS stimulant; the classic poisoning symptoms produced by strychnine are an arched back and sardonic grin

styptic 1: refers to the constricting of a blood vessel or the stopping of a hemorrhage by an astringent action **2:** an agent that stops hemorrhage

styptic pencil solid pencil made of fused potassium alum and potassium nitrate; used to stop bleeding from minor cuts

sub- prefix meaning below, under, or less than

subchapter "S" corporation legal form of organization for small businesses that affords the firm the liability protection of a corporation and the tax structure of a sole proprietorship

subcoating application of a series of layers of hydrophilic colloid to round the sharper edges of tablets in preparation for grossing (a subsequent series of coating steps)

subcutaneous the alveolar region beneath the skin

subcutaneous injection the process of administering a medication into the area beneath the surface of the skin (the subcutaneous layer)

subjective data data that cannot be measured or quantified; example: patient's description of pain symptoms

sublimation process in which a solid is converted to a vapor directly from the solid phase without passing through the liquid phase and is subsequently recovered as the solid by condensing the vapor directly on to a cold surface; used primarily as a means of purification; example: sublimed sulfur

sublingual under the tongue

sublingual administration method of drug administration in which a solid dosage form (usually a soluble tablet) is placed under the tongue where the drug is absorbed into the capillaries of the oral mucosa

sublingual tablet SEE *tablet, compressed*

subrogation a procedure under which an insurance company can recover from third parties all or some proportionate part of benefits paid to an insured

subsalt a salt in which oxygen or hydroxide is present; example: bismuth subcarbonate

subscriber the person responsible for payment of premiums or whose employment is the basis for eligibility for membership in an HMO or other health plan

subscriber contract a written agreement describing the individual's health care policy; also called "subscriber certificate" or "member certificate"

subscription prescription directions to the pharmacist, such as to make an ointment or to fill capsules; SEE ALSO *prescription*

subsieve sizer an instrument used to determine the particle size of a particulate solid based on a measure of the ability of a gas to move through the particle bed as compared to a known or standard particle bed

substance abuse inappropriate and deleterious use of any chemical agent or device to produce some desired mental effect; examples: glue sniffing, any form of drug or alcohol misuse

substitution **1:** replacement of a drug by its generic equivalent **2:** dispensing another drug in place of the one prescribed

substrate the reactant in a chemical reaction that binds to an enzyme active site and is converted to a product

subunit a polypeptide component of an oligomeric protein

successive differentiation calculation of the first, second, etc., derivative of an algebraic expression, the second derivative being a means of determining maxima and minima values on a curve; the second derivative of space (distance) versus time is acceleration

sucrose a sweet disaccharide that occurs naturally in most plants; the sugar obtained from sugar cane and sugar beets; hydrolysis forms equal quantities of glucose and fructose; SEE *invert sugar*

sudden infant death syndrome (SIDS) unexplained death of a baby, usually occurring in the first few months of life; synonym: crib death

sudorific an agent that causes sweating

sugar the basic unit of carbohydrates; a class of biomolecule containing hydroxyl groups and an aldehyde group or ketone group

sugarcoated tablet a tablet covered with dried and polished layers of sucrose

sugarcoating the process of applying a series of syrupy coats to a compressed tablet for enhancing appearance and masking an unpleasant taste

sugar starch synonym for powdered dextrose or glucose

sulcus **1:** groove, usually referring to the depressions on the surface of the brain, separated by gyri **2:** crevice between the gum and tooth

sulfanemia anemia that results from use of sulfonamides

sulfonamide **1:** a condensation product of a sulfonic acid with a primary or a secondary amine **2:** a group of bacteriostatic agents that inhibit the biosynthesis of folic acid in microorganisms; examples: an amide of sulfanilic acid (sulfanilamide), derivatives of the amide of *p*-aminosulfonic acid (sulfisoxazole), also nitrogen atoms of urea (used as hypoglycemic agents)

sulfurated potash yellowish-brown lumps containing a mixture of potassium thiosulfate and potassium polysulfides (chiefly trisulfide); synonym: liver of sulfur

summary plan description a description of the entire benefits package available to an employee as required to be given to persons covered by self-funded plans

sun protection factor (SPF) a rating scale for any of several substances that block the harmful ultraviolet rays of the sun and are useful in preventing sunburn

sunscreen product that protects exposed areas of the body from the harmful radiation of the sun

superalimentation to feed excessively; sometimes used to treat patients having a wasting disease

superego in Freudian theory, part of the personality that represents the conscience; SEE ALSO *ego; id*

superheated steam water vapor that is at a higher temperature than that required to saturate with steam a given volume at the same pressure

superinfection infection that can occur during antibiotic therapy as the result of an overgrowth of a micoorganism resistant to the antibiotic

supersaturate to cause a solution to contain more of a solute than it would normally hold at a given temperature; to form a metastable solution

superscription Rx, the symbol for a prescription and generally understood to be a contraction of the Latin verb *recipe,* meaning "take thou"; SEE ALSO *prescription*

supine lying on the back

supplemental services optional services that a health plan may provide in addition to its basis health services

suppository a solid body (dosage form) that is prepared in various weights and shapes and is suitable for insertion into a body cavity (usually the rectum or vagina) where it melts, dissolves, or disintegrates to produce a desired medicinal effect

suppository, extended release drug delivery system in the form of a suppository that allows at least a reduction in dosing frequency

suppuration formation of pus

supra- prefix meaning above or over

surface active agent SEE *surfactant*

surface energy SEE *surface tension*

surface filtration pharmaceutical process of separating a usable solid material called a "cake" from a liquified dispersion medium by use of a flat filter and a support system

surface free energy SEE *surface tension*

surface tension a natural result of unequal attractive forces between molecules near the interface of a substance; used to express air-substance interfacial tension; force per unit length required to break a surface; energy required to expand a surface one area unit; synonym: surface energy

surface-shape factor quantitative expression relating the total surface area(s) of a given quantity of a drug powder to the sum of the products of the frequency (or number) of particles times their projected diameters squared; the more irregular the shape the larger the value of this factor; a measure of irregularity of shape

surfactant surface active agent; substance that reduces surface and interfacial tension in small concentrations; examples: emulsifiers, deflocculants, suspending oils, dispersants, soaps, detergents

surgeon a physician who specializes in surgical treatment of illnesses or malfunctions

surgi-center SEE *freestanding outpatient surgical center*

suspension a preparation of finely divided undissolved drugs dispersed in a liquid medium; used to provide insoluble drugs in a liquid dosage form

suspension, extended release liquid preparation consisting of solid particles dispersed throughout a liquid phase in which the particles are not soluble; formulated in a manner to allow at least a reduction in dosing frequency as compared to that drug presented as a conventional dosage form (e.g., a solution or a prompt drug-releasing, conventional solid dosage form)

sustained action a dosage form designed so that the initial dose of a drug is absorbed rapidly followed by the maintenance of an effective plasma concentration through a continual release of the drug over a period of time

sustained release dosage form (usually a tablet or capsule) in which release of the drug is extended over a period of time; contrasted with a tablet that releases the entire dose at one time

suture 1: act of stitching a wound together **2:** material used to stitch a wound together; strand or fiber used to hold wound edges in apposition during healing **3:** joint that is held very closely together, as in the bones of the skull

swab wad of absorbent material usually wound around one end of a small stick and used for applying medication or for removing material from an area

Swain, Robert L. (1887-1963) editor of *Drug Topics* from 1939-1960; trained as an attorney; served on the Maryland Board of Pharmacy and was the founding chair of the National Conference of Law Enforcement Officials; APhA president from 1933-1934; Remington Honor Medal recipient in 1940

sweating the secretion of fluids from the sweat glands; synonym: perspiring

sweet oil synonym for olive oil

symbiosis the living together or close association of two dissimilar organisms

syrup oral solution containing high concentrations of sucrose or other sugars; also, any other liquid dosage form prepared in a sweet and viscid vehicle, including oral suspensions

system 1: an assembly of methods, procedures, or techniques united by regulated interaction to form an organized whole **2:** an organized collection of people, machines, and methods required to accomplish a set of specific functions

systematic chemical name a name for a compound recognized by the International Union of Pure and Applied Chemistry, Chemical Abstracts Service, or other reference works and derived by using the nomenclature rules of the IUPAC

systematic, totally integrated, individualized, person-centered health care a term referring to total health care provided based on needs of individual consumers; under STIIPCH 2.0, all health care (including preventative care) coordinated with every provider having access to complete electronic records that would list not only medical data but sociologic information

systemic affecting the whole body

SI Le Systéme International d'Unités; SEE *International System of Units*

systole period of contraction, usually refers to contraction of the ventricles of the heart

systolic measurement of the maximum blood pressure in the arteries; top of the two blood pressure numbers

T

T$_4$ SEE *thyroxine*

tablespoonful household measurement equivalent to about 15 ml or 4 fluid drams

tablet solid dosage form containing medicinal substances with or without suitable diluents

tablet, buccal small tablet designed to be placed in the buccal pouch where the drug is absorbed directly through the oral mucosa

tablet, chewable solid dosage form containing medicinal substances with or without suitable diluents that is intended to be chewed, producing a pleasant-tasting residue in the oral cavity that is easily swallowed and does not leave a bitter or unpleasant aftertaste

tablet, coated solid dosage form that contains medicinal substances with or without suitable diluents and is covered with a designated coating

tablet, compressed solid body prepared in various shapes and sizes made by compressing one or more drugs in combination with diluents, excipients, binders, lubricants, and other additives; few tablets consist only of a drug

tablet, delayed release solid dosage form that releases a drug (or drugs) at a time other than promptly after administration; example: enteric-coated articles

tablet, delayed-release particles solid dosage form containing a conglomerate of medicinal particles that have been covered with a coating which releases a drug (or drugs) at a time other than promptly after administration; example: enteric-coated articles

tablet, effervescent solid dosage form containing, in addition to active ingredients, mixtures of acids (e.g., citric acid, tartaric acid) and sodium bicarbonate, which release carbon dioxide when dissolved in water; intended to be dissolved or dispersed in water before administration

tablet, enteric coated a tablet that has a special coating which will not dissolve in the stomach but will dissolve in the intestines; used for drugs that are degraded by gastric juices, for those irritating to the stomach, or for those where absorbtion in the intestines is critical to drug action

tablet, extended release solid dosage form containing a drug that allows at least a reduction in dosing frequency as compared to a drug presented in conventional dosage form

tablet, film coated solid dosage form that contains medicinal substances with or without suitable diluents and is coated with a thin layer of a water-insoluble or water-soluble polymer, utilized to improve appearance, mask unpleasant taste, and/or protect the tablet

tablet, film coated, extended release solid dosage form that contains medicinal substances with or without suitable diluents and is coated with a thin layer of a water-insoluble or water-soluble polymer; formulated in such manner as to make the contained medicament available over an extended period of time following ingestion

tablet, hypodermic very small tablet made of a drug and usually recrystallized lactose under aseptic conditions; used to make a solution that is injected under the skin

tablet, multilayer solid dosage form containing medicinal substances that have been compressed to form a multiple-layered tablet or a tablet-within-a-tablet

tablet, multilayer, extended release solid dosage form containing medicinal substances that have been compressed to form a multiple-layered tablet or a tablet-within-a-tablet (the inner tablet being the core and the outer portion being the shell), which is then covered in a designated coating; formulated in such manner as to allow at least a reduction in dosing frequency as compared to a drug presented as a conventional dosage form

tablet, orally disintegrating solid dosage form containing medicinal substances that disintegrates rapidly, usually within a matter of seconds, when placed upon the tongue

tablet, sintered may be dissolved in mouth or swallowed whole

tablet, soluble solid dosage form that contains medicinal substances with or without suitable diluents and possesses the ability to dissolve in fluids

tablet, solution tablet designed to be added to a given amount of water to produce a solution of fixed concentration; also called "dispensing tablet"

tablet, sublingual small tablet designed to be placed beneath the tongue where the drug is rapidly absorbed directly through the oral mucosa

tablet, sugarcoated solid dosage form that contains medicinal substances with or without suitable diluents and is coated with a colored or an uncolored water-soluble sugar

tablet, vaginal usually a pear-shaped or ovoid tablet made by compression and intended to dissolve in the vaginal cavity for a medicinal effect

tablet coating 1: film or layer of substance that covers the compressed tablet **2:** process of covering a compressed tablet; SEE ALSO *coating; sugarcoated tablet; sugarcoating; enteric coating; film coating; compressed-coated tablet*

tableting machine mechanical apparatus designed to receive granular drug materials and compress discrete amounts into solid doses at a very rapid rate; single punch—one that utilizes only one feeding hopper, one die, and one set of punches (upper and lower); rotary—one that has multiple punches and dies in a circular arrangement for compressing tablets at a fast rate

tablet triturate small, usually cylindrical tablet made by molding or forcing dampened powder under low pressure into a series of plate cavities; also called "molded tablet"

tachy- prefix meaning an increased rate; example: tachycardia

tachycardia unusually rapid heartbeat; typically over 100 beats per minute

tachypnea a state of rapid respiration

take-home medication medicine dispensed by a hospital pharmacy for an inpatient to take home when discharged by the physician; usually a one- or two-day supply

Takeru Higuchi Research Prize established by the American Pharmacists Association in 1981 to honor an international pharmaceutical scientist for sustained accomplishments

talc native, hydrous, magnesium silicate; used in dusting powders and as a filter medium; synonyms: talcum, French chalk

tamper-evident packaging a drug container sealed and/or wrapped in such a manner that it would be readily noticeable by a potential buyer if it had been previously opened; usually double or triple sealed

tamper-resistant packaging a drug container having an indicator or barrier to entry that, if breached or missing, can reasonably be expected to provide visible evidence to consumers that tampering has occurred; to prevent the substitution of the tamper-resistant feature after tampering, the indicator or barrier to entry is required to be distinctive by design or must employ an identifying characteristic

tampon plug made of cotton, sponge, or oakum variously used in surgery to plug the nose, vagina, etc., for the control of hemorrhage or the absorption of secretions

tamponade pathological compression of an organ; example: cardiac tamponade

tangible assets assets that have physical form and qualities; more generally, those items on which a definite value can be placed

tannic acid   substance obtained from the bark and fruit of various trees and shrubs; usually obtained from Turkish or Chinese nutgalls that are produced on the twigs of certain oak trees; used as an astringent and protein precipitant; synonym: tannin

tannin   SEE *tannic acid*

tape   narrow woven fabric, or a narrow extruded synthetic (such as plastic), usually with an adhesive on one or both sides; SEE ALSO *adhesive tape*

tapeworm   parasitic intestinal worm possessing a head and a neck followed by a chain of segments in a ribbon often many feet long; synonyms: cestodes, *Taenia solium, Taenia saginata*

tar camphor   old colloquial name for naphthalene (mothballs)

tardive   a late-appearing disorder; example: tardive dyskinesia (a delayed adverse response caused by certain antipsychotics)

target cell   a cell that responds to the binding of a hormone or growth factor

target drug delivery system   dosage form designed to deliver a drug more accurately into a specific body area or organ where it elicits its therapeutic response; example: red blood cell loading

targeting   process that directs newly synthesized proteins to their correct destinations

target market   technique of identifying specific customer audience for a service or product; used to determine to whom to market a service/product

target marketing   process of segmenting the market into its logical submarkets that differ in their requirements, buying habits, or other critical characteristics

tartar   hardened, rocklike concretions that appear on the teeth if the patient's hygiene is poor and plaque is not removed at least once daily

tartar emetic   antimony potassium tartrate; used in veterinary medicine as an antischistosomal, expectorant, and ruminatoric; also used as a mordant in textile and leather industries; has been used to denature alcohol

tautomer   an isomer that differs from another in the location of a hydrogen atom and a double bond; example: keto-enol tautomers

tautomerism   presence of a molecule in two chemical forms existing in equilibrium and normally not separable

tax credit   a legitimate reduction in the income tax liability of an individual or a firm

Tax Equity and Fiscal Responsibility Act of 1982 the federal law that created the current risk and cost contract provisions under which health plans contract with CMS (formerly HCFA) and which defined the primary and secondary coverage responsibilities of the Medicare program

T cell a T lymphocyte; white blood cell that bears antibody-like molecules on its surface; binds to and destroys foreign cells in cellular immunity

teaching hospital hospital owned by or affiliated with a university that provides an environment for education of health personnel

teaspoonful (tsp or fl ℨ) household measure equivalent to about 5 ml (household approximate) or 1 fluid dram (accurate)

technetium 99m generator device that consists of an alumina column on which molybdenum 99 (a radioactive element) is adsorbed; molybdenum decays to technetium 99m, which is eluted and used to prepare radiolabeled diagnostic preparations

teel oil SEE *sesame oil*

telemedicine the ability to use centralized medical expertise to provide care to patients in rural areas, and for centralized physicians to speak and share images with rural doctors through two-way visual and audio networks

teleradiography process of taking X-rays of a body part with the source of X-rays placed six to seven feet away from the patient

telomere structures at the ends of chromosomes that buffer the loss of critical coding sequences after a round of DNA replication

temperature heat intensity in a given system (or area) expressed in degrees centigrade (Celsius) or degrees Kelvin (absolute), or degrees Fahrenheit and measured by using one of several kinds of thermometers; a property that is independent of the quantity of material in the system

temperature control process of maintaining a reasonably constant environmental temperature by use of heating or cooling elements and thermostatic control devices

temperature control, proportional thermostatic system that supplies heating or cooling to maintain a constant temperature control point with a minimal deviation range; a more infinitesimal differential in temperature is possible with a proportional control system than that obtained with a two-position control

temperature control, two-position thermostatic device that can be set for a narrow range of temperature control with an "on" and an "off" point to switches controlling the heating elements

Temporary Assistance to Needy Families (TANF) federal-state welfare program authorized by the 1996 Welfare Reform Act that replaces Aid to Families with Dependent Children

tendinitis or tendonitis inflammation of the tendon; note: the preferred spelling, rather than tendonitis

tenosynovitis inflammation of a tendon sheath

teratogen an agent that causes congenital defects (an abnormal development of an embryo); usually refers to a chemical, but may be a virus, radiation, or other causes

terminal an individual's clinical condition with a disease state for which the prognosis is death; example: terminal cancer

terminal sterilization sterilization of the finished, sealed product to render it devoid of any life forms

termination phase in translation in which newly synthesized polypeptides are released from the ribosome

termination date the date that a group contract expires; the date that a subscriber and/or covered person ceases to be eligible

terpene a ten-carbon naturally occurring hydrocarbon consisting of two isoprene units connected in "head-to-tail" fashion; terpene derivatives are used in perfumes and flavors

tertiary alcohol SEE *alcohol*

tertiary amine SEE *amine*

tertiary care the highest level of medical care characterized by the availability of specialists and sophisticated diagnostic and treatment facilities; typically given at a university-based hospital

tertiary structure the globular, three-dimensional structure of a polypeptide that results from folding the regions of secondary structure; folding results from interactions of the side chains or R groups of the amino acid residues

tetanus disease caused by *Clostridium tetani* in which affected voluntary muscles are contracted in a painful tonic condition

tetany syndrome characterized by intermittent tonic spasms of muscle groups

tetra- prefix meaning four

tetracyclines a group of broad-spectrum antibiotics that exert their anti-infective action on bacteria by inhibiting protein biosynthesis; composed of four fused rings that bear various phenolic and alcoholic hydroxyl, amide, amine, and alkyl substituents

tetraiodothyronine SEE *thyroxine*

thalidomide sedative marketed in the early 1960s that caused profound deformities in babies when taken by pregnant women; largely responsible for the Kefauver-Harris Amendment to the Food, Drug, and Cosmetic Act

theobroma oil SEE *cocoa butter*

theory of planned behavior an extension of the theory of reasoned action that addresses an individual's degree of control over a behavior; SEE *theory of reasoned action*

theory of reasoned action hypothesizes that two factors lead to an individual's behavioral intentions: (1) the attitude toward performing the behavior and (2) the subjective norm associated with the behavior; behavioral intentions are predictive of behavioral actions

theory X management philosophy which holds that employees inherently dislike work, are not ambitious, have little desire for responsibility, and prefer to be directed

theory Y management philosophy which holds that work efforts are natural behavior if conditions are favorable, that people will learn to accept and even seek responsibility under proper conditions, and that a person's commitment to goals depends upon the rewards associated with his/her achievement

therapeutic 1: pertaining to the medicinal or healing properties of a drug or treatment regimen **2:** an agent or drug used to treat a disease

therapeutic alternate a drug product containing a different therapeutic moiety from the product prescribed, but which is of the same pharmacological class and/or therapeutic class and can be expected to have similar effects when administered to patients in therapeutically equivalent doses

therapeutic duplication patient inappropriately receiving two medications with similar actions; may occur when medications are prescribed by different physicians

therapeutic effect refers to the manner in which a drug acts in the body to influence the process of healing or to treat a disease

therapeutic equivalent a chemical equivalent that, when administered at the same dosage, will provide the same therapeutic effect, as measured by the control of a sign, symptom, or disease

therapeutic goal specific outcome hoped to be achieved from a therapy

therapeutic index refers to the quantitative comparison of a therapeutic effect and an untoward effect of a drug in the body; the ratio of the maximum tolerated dose of a drug to its minimum curative dose

therapeutic relationship the relationship between a health professional and patient that develops when they form a covenant/promise to work together to ensure that the patient achieves positive outcomes from the drug therapy

therapeutic response SEE *biological response*

therapeutics the study of the application of remedies to the treatment of a disease; synonym: therapy

therapeutic substitution the practice of dispensing a therapeutic alternative for the one prescribed; usually requires the prescriber's authorization before the substitution may occur in an outpatient setting

therapeutic systems active drug in a delivery module consisting of a drug reservoir, a rate controller, and an energy source to bring about release of drug molecules

theriaca 1: antidote against poisons **2:** a cure-all

therm- prefix meaning heat; same as thermo-

thermal analysis measurement of physical effects produced by controlled heat changes; examples: differential scanning calorimeter (DSC), differential thermal analysis (DTA), thermogravic analysis, thermochemical analysis

thermal death time time required to kill all spores of a given microorganism under a given set of conditions in a sterilization process

thermo- prefix meaning heat; same as therm-

thermocouple device that converts heat energy into electrical energy; device used to measure temperature by heat-produced changes in electromotive force (emf) through two dissimilar metals welded together; SEE *thermometer*

thermodynamics the science of quantitative relationships between heat and other forms of energy (chemical, electrical, mechanical, radiant) associated with a system under observation and/or experimentation; the study of energy and its interconversion; based upon three laws: (first law) energy can be converted from one form to another, but it cannot be created or destroyed; (second law) the energy of a system will spontaneously move in a direction to accomplish a lower "free energy" state; example: heat moves from a hot body to an adjacent cold body until their temperatures are equal; (third law) the entropy (a measure of molecular disorder) is zero in a substance at absolute zero ($0°$ Kelvin)

thermolabile unstable when heated

thermolabile solution a solution that cannot be thermally sterilized

thermoluminescent dosimeter an instrument that will emit light if it is heated after having been exposed to radiation

thermometer a device for measuring temperature

thermometer, basal device for determining when a female is ovulating

thermometer, bimetallic temperature-measuring device that consists of two dissimilar sheet metals attached to each other, each of which exhibits differential expansion when heat is added, which is then transferred to points on a graduated dial

thermometer, liquid-in-glass device used to measure temperature based on liquid expansion through a capillary in an enclosed calibrated glass bulb

thermometer, otic (tympanic) thermometer that is inserted into the ear, detecting the patient's temperature by reading the patient's tympanic membrane

thermometer, pressure spring pressure-sensitive temperature-measuring device used in constant volume systems; consists of a connecting bulb, capillary, and a coiled spring containing a bimetallic compound that causes the spring to expand or contract with temperature change; may be used for containers that are remote from the graduated pointer

thermometer, resistance an electrical device used to measure temperature based on changes in metallic resistance to the flow of an electrical current with changes in temperature

thermotherapy use of heat to help treat pain, applied to several body parts (e.g., back, sore muscles, abdomen) through the use of any one of several modalities (e.g., therapeutic heat wrap, heating pads, hot water bottles)

thiazide refers to a class of sulfonamide diuretics whose actions occur at the early distal convoluting tubules of the kidney

thin-layer chromatography (TLC) chromatographic method relying on the separation of substances in solution by their differential migrations over an adsorbent that is spread in a thin layer onto glass, plastic, or similar backing

third law of thermodynamics SEE *thermodynamics*

third-party administrator an independent entity that administers group benefits, claims, and administration for a self-insured company/group

third-party payer an organization that pays for or underwrites coverage for health care expenses or another entity, usually an employer

third-party payment reimbursement for health services to a patient paid by an insurance company, governmental agency, or an employer; payment other than directly by the patient

thixotropic flow characteristic flow of certain liquids that form a structured gel when undisturbed and exhibit pseudoplastic flow as "shearing stress" is increased and Newtonian (linear) flow as "shearing stress" is decreased; SEE *thixotropy*

thixotropy the property of a liquid to change into a gel on standing and for the gel to transform into a liquid again on shaking; example: bentonite magma

thoracic surgeon a physician who specializes in performing surgery on the chest

three-compartmental model concept of the body in which a central compartment communicates with two noninterconnected peripheral compartments (shallow and deep); the distribution of a drug into the shallow compartment is at a faster rate than that into the deep compartment

threonine α-amino acid commonly found in proteins; one of ten essential amino acids

thrombo- prefix pertaining to a thrombus or blood clot

thromboangiitis obliterans SEE *Buerger's disease*

thrombocytopenia an abnormal decrease in the number of blood platelets (thrombocytes); synonym: thrombopenia

thrombocytopenia purpura any form of purpura in which the platelet count is decreased, occurring as a primary disease or as a consequence of a primary hematologic disorder

thrombosis the formation of a solid mass (blood clot) in the heart or a blood vessel; such formation may cause a blockade of the vessels and thus produce tissue damage

thromboxanes fatty acid congeners of the prostaglandins that are involved in the aggregation of platelets; aspirin, indomethacin, and related drugs interfere with the formation of both thromboxanes and prostaglandins, thus causing bleeding tendencies

thrombus a blood clot formed within the heart or in a blood vessel; synonym: internal clot

thrush candidiasis of the mouth, as evidenced by white plaques or spots in the mouth; synonym: sprue

thyro- prefix meaning thyroid gland

thyrocalcitonin SEE *calcitonin*

thyrotropin-releasing hormone biochemical secretion from the hypothalamus into the blood that causes the pituitary gland to secrete thyroid-stimulating hormone

thyroxine or thyroxin hormone produced by the thyroid gland that affects the overall metabolic rate of the body; synonyms: tetraiodothyronine, T_4

Tice, Linwood Franklin (1909-1996) proponent of student involvement in the workings of the American Pharmacists Association; Remington Honor Medal recipient in 1971

tight container SEE *container, tight*

time dependence expression indicating that there is an optimum time (or time period) during which a process should take place

tincture an alcoholic or hydroalcoholic solution prepared from vegetable materials or chemical substances; may be prepared by one of several extraction methods or by a dissolution method

tinnitus a ringing or a roaring in the ears

tip seal the closure of an ampule accomplished by melting a bead of glass at the neck of the ampule

tissue localization selective uptake of drugs in a particular body tissue

titration procedure for determining the quantity of substance present by comparing the volume of a standard solution that reacts with the substance

tolerance **1:** ability to withstand higher and higher doses of a medication without suffering ill effects; the decreasing therapeutic effect of a set dose of medication **2:** allowable deviation from a standard

tomography a diagnostic imaging technique in which the shadows of structures behind and before the area under examination are not shown; examples: CAT scan, PET scan

tonicity colligative property involving the osomotic pressure of body fluids; SEE *isotonicity; hypertonic solution; hypotonic solution*

tool for evaluation of documentation tool to evaluate completeness of a pharmacist's documentation and the quality of pharmaceutical care provided

tophus urate deposit found in the joints of patients who have gout

topical local, pertaining to a definite area; usually refers to the surface of the skin

topical administration the process of applying a medication to a localized surface of the body

tort a wrongful civil act committed by one party against another (except in the provisions of a contract)

tortuous twisting, winding, or convoluting

total enteral nutrition a non sequitur, in that virtually every patient receives total enteral nutrition through eating orally

total parenteral nutrition the provision of all the required foods to the body by slowly administering protein hydrolysates and other nutrients through an intra-arterial catheter to the vena cava; differs from hyperalimentation by the presence of a lipid emulsion in the fluid

total pharmacologic activity total area under a pharmacologic response versus time curve

total quality management (TQM) a continuous quality improvement management system directed from the top, but empowering employees and focusing on systemic, not individual, employee problems; SEE *continuous quality improvement*

total system clearance refers to the overall elimination of a drug or a drug metabolite from the body; the sum of all the separate clearances; synonym: whole body clearance

toxemia poisonous bacterial products formed at a local site and absorbed and distributed by the blood throughout the body, thus producing generalized symptoms; the presence of toxic substances in the blood

toxic pertaining to or caused by poison

toxico- prefix meaning poison

toxicology science or study of adverse effects of chemicals on living organisms

toxin poisonous substance; poisonous bacterial product that acts as an antigen and causes the body to develop specific antibodies to combat their presence; toxin injections generally used for diagnostic purposes to determine the susceptibility of the patient to the disease caused by the toxin-containing organism; example: tuberculin

toxin-antitoxin a mixture of toxin and antitoxin in nearly equal portions; example: diphtheria toxin-antitoxin; SEE *toxin; antitoxin*

toxoid a toxin that has been treated by heat or chemical processes to destroy its harmful properties without destroying its ability to stimulate antibody production; example: tetanus toxoid

trace mineral a naturally occurring inorganic ion or compound that may be essential (in very small quantities) for metabolic processes; often provided as a supplement in a multiple vitamin formula

tracer radioactive or stable isotope, the movement or progress of which can be followed with a detector

trade area defined geographic area from which customers are drawn

trade discount price reduction extended to a retailer for performing certain retailing or marketing functions connected with the sale of the product; example: a wholesaler sells to a pharmacy a product below the normal price as compensation for the pharmacy's activities in selling the product; synonym: functional discount

trademark name, symbol, design, work, or device used to distinguish one's product from others; protected by law and may only be used by or with the permission of the owner

trade name 1: name by which an article, process, or service is designated in trade **2:** name given by a manufacturer to designate a proprietary article, sometimes having the status of a trademark or a copyrighted and patented proprietary name; synonym: brand name

traffic flow pathway of least resistance in moving through the pharmacy; typical pathway followed by customers

tragacanth gum vegetable gum used as a suspending agent in some pharmaceutical preparations

tranquilizer a drug capable of calming an animal or a person without sedation and drowsiness; SEE *major tranquilizer; minor tranquilizer*

trans- 1: prefix meaning across or through **2:** (italicized) designation of a geometric isomer in which similar substituents are placed across double bonds or ring systems from one another

transacetylation chemical reaction in which an acetyl radical is transferred from one molecule to another

transactions number of individual activities of a business, usually measured in dollars

transamination a reaction in which an amino group is transferred from one molecule to another

transcription process in which the genetic information in DNA is used to specify the order of bases in the synthesis of mRNA that is complementary but not identical to that of DNA

transcription factor proteins that regulate or initiate RNA synthesis by binding to specific DNA sequences called response elements

transcript localization the binding of mRNAs to certain cellular structures within cytoplasm so that protein gradients can be created within a cell

transdermal delivery system dosage form, usually a patch, designed to deliver a medication through the skin

transduction the transfer of genes between bacteria by bacteriophages

transfection a mechanism by which a bacteriophage inadvertently transfers bacterial chromosome or plasmid sequences to a new host cell

transferase enzyme that catalyzes the transfer of a group from one molecule to another; one of six classes of enzymes recognized by the Enzyme Commission of the International Union of Biochemistry (IUB); examples: aminotransferase, acetyltransferase

transference number that fraction of total current carried by the cation or the anion in electrolysis

transfer RNA a small RNA that binds to an amino acid and delivers it to the ribosome for incorporation into a polypeptide chain during translation

transferrin serum β-globulin that binds and serves to transport iron

transformation occurs when naked DNA fragments enter a bacterial cell and are introduced into the bacterial genome

transfusion clinical procedure in which blood from one individual is transferred to another individual

transgenic animal an animal that results when recombinant DNA sequences are microinjected into a fertilized ovum

transition mutation a mutation that involves the substitution of a different purine base for the purine present at the site of the mutation or the substitution of a different pyrimidine for the normal pyrimidine

transition state theory concept of a chemical reaction based on specific intermediate molecular reactants and product components and their probability of engaging in a reaction; process rate theory; concept in which short-lived reaction intermediates are formed during the course of a reaction; synonym: absolute rate theory

transit time length of time that a drug stays in a part of the GI tract; example: stomach emptying time

translation process whereby the nucleotide sequence in mRNA directs the order of insertion of each amino acid during protein biosynthesis

translocation movement of the ribosome along the mRNA during translation

transmittance extent to which incident light will pass through a solution containing a specific substance; SEE *Beer's law*

transpeptidase enzyme that catalyzes the cross-linking of linear peptidoglycan polymers of the cell wall in bacteria; enzyme that catalyzes the cleaving of a peptide bond to one amino acid and reforms it with another amino acid

transport, facilitated the process by which a solute molecule or ion is transported across a membrane by a carrier, but not against a concentration gradient

transport mechanism, specialized active transport; process by which a solute molecule or ion is moved across a membrane against a concentration gradient (from a solution of lower concentration to one of higher concentration)

transport number SEE *transference number*

transposition the movement of a piece of DNA from one site in a genome to another

transtheoretical model of change theory developed by Prochaska to explain why attempts to change behavior failed or succeeded; theorizes that patients progress through five stages related to changes in behavior: (1) precontemplation, (2) contemplation, (3) preparation, (4) action, and (5) maintenance

transudate fluid that has passed through a membrane; has a low protein and cell content; usually associated with noninflammatory edema

transversion mutation type of point mutation in which a pyrimidine is substituted for a purine or vice versa; SEE ALSO *point mutation, mutation*

trapezoidal rule method for estimating integrals (areas under absorption curves) by adding the respective areas of discrete trapezoids; used for estimating many other pharmacokinetic integrals to determine quantity and/or extent of occurrence of a process

trauma injury that is physical and/or psychological in nature

tray dryer heated chamber designed to remove moisture from particulate pharmaceutical materials (such as granules for subsequent tableting) and accommodating multiple trays on which material to be dried is thinly spread for the moisture removal process; also may be used with circulating air fans or with reduced pressure; synonym: truck dryer

treatment facility a residential or nonresidential facility or program licensed, certified, or otherwise authorized to provide treatment of substance abuse or mental illness pursuant to the law or jurisdiction in which treatment is received

trench mouth SEE *Vincent's angina*

trending a calculation used to predict future utilization of a group based upon past utilization

tri- prefix meaning three; example: triglyceride (three fatty acids esterified on the glycerin molecule)

triacylglycerol an ester formed between glycerol and three fatty acids

triage procedure of sorting or screening patients by their degree of illness or injury and then assigning them a priority for treatment and/or a place or level of treatment

triage, pharmaceutical pharmacist triage for patients who enter the retail pharmacy requesting self-care assistance; the pharmacist may choose to recommend against any treatment or device, to recommend a nonprescription product or device, or to refer the patient to another professional (e.g., physician, dentist, podiatrist)

trichotillomania psychiatric condition that causes the patient to pull compulsively at the hair; may continue until the entire head is denuded of hair

tricyclic antidepressant any of a group of drugs of which the basic chemical structure consists of three fused rings and which potentiate the action of catecholamines; used to treat depression; examples: amitriptyline, imipramine

triphosphopyridine nucleotide SEE *nicotinamide adenine dinucleotide phosphate*

triple bond binding together of two atoms that share three electron pairs, one pair a sigma bond and the other two pi bonds

triple point temperature at which solid, liquid, and vapor phases of a substance exist in equilibrium; a point on many phase diagrams

tritiated refers to a chemical compound labeled with radioactive hydrogen (tritium, ^3H)

trituration **1:** process of reducing the particle size of a substance to a fine powder by grinding it in a mortar with a pestle **2:** process of mixing powders by grinding them in a mortar with a pestle **3:** a dilution of a potent solid substance to a specific concentration by mixing it thoroughly with a suitable diluent

triturator apparatus in which substances can be rubbed or reduced in size by continuous grinding

troche solid body, usually sweetened and flavored, designed to dissolve slowly in the mouth and allow the resulting viscous solution to medicate the mouth and throat; synonym: lozenge

tropanol aminoalcohol portion of atropine and hyoscyamine, synonym: tropine

tropine synonym for tropanol

tropocollagen subunit composed of three polypetide chains; a component of collagen fibrils in connective tissue

truck dryer SEE *tray dryer*

truss device for exerting pressure over the site of a hernia, thus holding in place a part that would otherwise extrude abnormally

trust fund an organization established to control, invest, and otherwise administer moneys, securities, or other property for the benefit of others; operated under the guidance of a trust agreement by trustees whose fiduciary responsibility requires a prudent, successful administration of the fund's purpose

trypanosomicide drug that kills or destroys trypanosomes (parasitic protozoa found in human blood and causing sleeping sickness)

tryptamine decarboxylation product of tryptophan

tryptophan aromatic amino acid commonly found in protein; 3-(3-indolyl)-2-amino propanoic acid; an essential amino acid

t-test a statistical procedure used to compare the means of two groups

tumbling mixer device or machine to mix dry powders (sometimes used to mix slurries) using a specially shaped rotating container; usual types are cyclindrical (mounted on a rotating shaft at an angle); cubical (mounted on a rotating shaft connected at opposite corners); twin shell (a double cylinder joined in a V shape with a rotating shaft connected to the middle of each side)

tumor necrosis factor a protein that suppresses cell division; toxic to tumor cells

tumor promoter a molecule that provides cells a growth advantage over nearby cells

turbid cloudy

turbine a mass-transfer mixing device that uses a blade of varying pitch to effect mixing of very viscous materials; a form of impeller

turbulent flow 1: movement of a liquid or gaseous system with extensive mixing due to formation of eddies or vortexes **2:** act of moving in a zigzag or highly shearing manner **3:** fluid movement exhibiting a high Reynolds number

turbulent mixing process of combining different substances using multi-directional motion to augment or accomplish the desired result; a non-laminar movement of materials being processed (mixed)

turgor feeling or appearance of inflammation or congestion

turista a form of diarrhea that occurs suddenly; synonym: traveler's diarrhea

turnaround time (TAT) the measure of a process cycle from the date a transaction is received to the date completed; for claims processing, the number of calendar days from the date a claim is received to the date paid

turnover 1: the number of times an item is bought and then sold in a specified period of time **2:** term in enzymology for the conversion of substrate into product on the enzyme surface

turnover number term representing the moles of substrate converted to product per mole of enzyme per minute; number of molecules of substrate converted per active enzyme site per minute

turnover rate ratio of cost of goods sold to average inventory

twin shell blender SEE *tumbling mixer*

twin shell mixer also called "twin shell blender"; SEE *tumbling mixer*

two-compartmental model pharmacokinetic model that views the body as two compartments; input and output from the central compartment with mixing occurring between the two compartments; CONTRAST *multicompartmental model; single-compartmental model*

Tyndall effect the scattering of light rays as they pass through a colloidal solution; a result of the reflection of light rays by solid particles

tyramine decarboxylation product of tyrosine that is produced in cheddar cheese and certain other foods and causes a food-drug interaction with monoamine oxidase inhibitors; β-(p-hydroxyphenyl)ethylamine

tyrosine p-hydroxyphenylalanine; an aromatic, phenolic amino acid commonly found in proteins; not an essential amino acid, but can be used to replace part of the phenylalanine requirement of the body

ubiquination the covalent attachment of ubiquitin to proteins; prepares proteins for degradation

ubiquitin a protein that is covalently attached by enzymes to proteins destined to be degraded

ubiquitous existing or found everywhere

UDP-glucuronidyl transferase enzyme located primarily in the liver; catalyzes reactions that couple various functional groups in bile pigments, drugs, or xenobiotics with glucuronic acid

ulceration the act or process of making an ulcer; presence of an ulcer on a body tissue

ulcerative colitis chronic ulceration in the colon causing inflammation; characterized by cramping abdominal pain, rectal bleeding, and discharges of blood, pus, and mucous with scanty fecal matter

ultracentrifuge instrument that operates at extremely high speeds (60,000 rpm or more), producing gravitational forces high enough to cause the sedimentation of large molecules such as proteins, polysaccharides, and nucleic acids; may be used either to separate proteins (preparative ultracentrifuge) or to determine molecular weights of proteins (analytical ultracentrifuge)

ultrafast disposition a biologic half-life that is less than one hour

ultraviolet that region of the electromagnetic spectrum that is above the frequency of violet and below that of X-rays and γ-rays; that region of the electromagnetic spectrum ranging in wavelength from 1 to 400 nanometers

ultraviolet light electromagnetic radiation emanating from valence electron orbitals as electrons fall to lower energy levels; used to aid aseptic technique or to identify and quantify UV-absorbing compounds of clinical (medicinal) importance

ultraviolet spectrophotometry SEE *spectrophotometry*

unbound drug a drug that is not attached (complexed) to a protein in the body; a drug in the blood and available for rapid distribution to other body tissues

unbundling practice of providing separate prices and administrative support for services such as prescription drug benefit management, mental health/substance abuse services, and utilization review

uncoupling agent compound that interferes with the mechanism by which the energy of biological oxidation is used to effect the formation of high-energy phosphates such as ATP; does not inhibit biological oxidation

unction 1: an ointment **2:** the application of an ointment

unctuous fatty, oily; smooth and greasy in feel and appearance

undulant fever SEE *brucellosis*

unguent term for perfumed salves or ointments

Uniform Commercial Code (UCC) consistent set of laws adopted by states to simplify and clarify laws relative to commercial transactions

uniform cost accounting set of accounting methods used by several firms to permit comparisons of financial performance

unilateral on one side only

unit dose system in which each individual dose is prepared (prepackaged) beforehand; provides for a more adequate control of drug dispensing

unit dose container SEE *container, unit dose*

unit dose system medication distribution system in which drugs are prepared and prepackaged in single doses prior to dispensing to the patient or nursing unit

unit of use prepackaged units that provide medication needed for a course of therapy or a specified period of time; example: compliance packaging

United States Adopted Names Council group that provides a new medicinal compound with a nonproprietary or generic name

United States Food and Drug Administration (FDA) agency of the federal government that administers provisions of the Food, Drug, and Cosmetic Act addressing the manufacture and packaging of drug, food, medical devices, and cosmetic products; responsibilities include drug safety, effectiveness, and quality control

United States Pharmacopeia (*USP*) the primary, legally recognized, national, drug-standard compendium for this country; established in 1820 as a joint venture between medicine and pharmacy; revised every five years with interim supplements; since 1985 published in a single volume with the *National Formulary,* known as the *USP-NF*

United States Pharmacopeial Convention an organization of representatives from pharmacy, medicine, government, and certain agencies and organizations that has an interest in drug manufacture and use; responsible for the publication of the *United States Pharmacopeia* and related professional and scientific literature; SEE *United States Pharmacopeia*

United States Pharmacopeial Dispensing Information publication of the United States Pharmacopeial Convention that provides patients and practitioners with information about uses, precautions, side effects, doses, and patient information guidelines for selected drugs; known as the *USP DI*

units, basic SEE *fundamental dimensions*

universal coverage the guaranteed provision of at least basic health care services to every citizen

universal gas constant SEE *gas constant*

unlimited liability a condition whereby a business, investor, or principal may be required to satisfy outstanding debts or judgments from personal assets

unpalatable possessing a disagreeable taste

unsaturated 1: condition in which a solvent does not contain the maximum amount of a solute that can be held in solution at a specific temperature and pressure **2:** organic compound that contains double or triple bonds as a part of its molecular structure

unsaturated fat triglyceride that contains large numbers of double bonds in the esterified fatty acids

unsaturated surface drying period time of a drying process between the appearance of the first surface "dry spots" and the completely dried surface (first decreasing drying rate period); further drying controlled by the diffusion rate of moisture from the solid (second decreasing drying rate period)

upcoding using a higher-level procedure code than the level of service actually provided

uptake absorption of some substance by a tissue, organ, or organism

ur- prefix meaning urine; same as uro-, urono-

URAC accreditation verification that a utilization review organization meets national utilization review standards for prospective and concurrent review services

Urdang, George (1882-1960) co-author of *Kremers and Urdang's History of Pharmacy;* the first director of the American Institute of the History of Pharmacy from 1941-1957

urea diamide of carbonic acid; a waste product of protein metabolism

urea cycle a cyclic pathway in which waste ammonia molecules, CO_2, and aspartate molecules are converted to urea

uremia toxic condition in which excessive amounts of urea and other catabolic products of proteins accumulate in the blood; usually indicates abnormal kidney function

uremic dose the dose of a drug to be administered to a uremic patient; dose of a drug to be administered to a patient who has abnormal kidney function

urgi-center SEE *freestanding emergency medical service center*

-uria suffix meaning urine

uricosuric agent used to promote excretion of uric acid in the urine; used to treat gout

uridine diphosphate nucleotide of uracil, ribose, and phosphate anhydride; ester of uridine with pyrophosphoric acid

uridine monophosphate nucleotide of uracil, ribose, and phosphate; ester of uridine with phosphoric acid

uro- prefix meaning urine; same as ur-, urono-

urologist a physician who specializes in the study and treatment of diseases of the urinary tract in both sexes and the genital tract in males

uronic acid the product formed when the terminal CH_2OH group of a monosaccharide is oxidized

urono- prefix meaning urine; same as ur-, uro-

urticaria a vascular reaction of the skin characterized by transient eruption of slightly elevated patches that are more red or more pale than the surrounding area; associated with severe itching; synonyms: hives, nettle rash

USP Pyrogen Test official biological test in which the presence of pyrogens is determined by measuring the fever response in rabbits following administration of an injectable preparation

USP unit (USP u) a quantitative expression of potency used in the *United States Pharmacopeia* to denote the activity of drugs and other preparations; each specific kind of unit is defined in the *USP*

usual and customary charge method of reimbursement under which the pharmacy is paid the amount normally charged for a given prescription or service

usual, customary, and reasonable a phrase used to refer to the commonly charged or prevailing fees for health services within a geographic area; a fee is considered to be reasonable if it falls within the parameters of the average or commonly charged fee for the particular service within that specific community (e.g., eightieth percentile)

utilization the extent to which the members of a covered group use a program or obtain a particular service, or category of procedures, over a given period of time; usually expressed as the number of services used per year or per 100 or 1,000 persons eligible for the service

utilization management a process of integrating review and case management of services in a cooperative effort with other parties, including patients, employers, providers, and payers

utilization review a formal assessment of the medical necessity, efficiency, and/or appropriateness of health care services and treatment plans on a prospective, concurrent, or retrospective basis

UV-A light ultraviolet light possessing a wavelength of 320 to 400 nm

UV-B light ultraviolet light possessing a wavelength of 290 to 320 nm

UV-C light ultraviolet light possessing a wavelength of 200 to 290 nm; SEE ALSO *UV lamps*

UV lamps lamps used for aseptic techniques that emit radiation at a wavelength of 253.7 nm

UV light SEE *ultraviolet light*

UV spectrophotometry SEE *spectrophotometry*

vaccination the administration of a vaccine

vaccine preparation of killed, attenuated, or fully virulent microorganisms administered to produce or increase immunity (a prophylactic for a particular disease)

vacuum dryer machine used to remove moisture from a batch of pharmaceutical material using a chamber placed under negative (below atmospheric) pressure to hasten vaporization; may be either a moving-bed or a static-bed type

vacuum pump machine used to remove air or vapor from a closed system, resulting in significantly negative (less than atmospheric) pressure; generally a pump of the reciprocating type that is used to remove air or other vapor from a closed system

valence 1: usually the number of electrons in the outer orbit of an atom; an index of the bonding capability of an atom or group of atoms with another atom or group of atoms; combining power of an element or a radical **2:** a designation to indicate the number of diseases or conditions prevented by a vaccine or prevented and treated by an antivenin or an antitoxin **3:** combining power of an antibody for an antigen

valence bond theory concept that the power of atoms to bind together to form molecules is based primarily on the number of orbital electrons in their outer shells

valence electrons electrons in the outer (or valence) shell of an atom

validity extent to which a performance evaluation does the job for which it was designed; relates to the content of the evaluation, its job-relatedness, and the ability of an evaluation to correlate highly with another evaluation method that is designed to measure the same performance characteristic

valine α-amino acid, commonly found in proteins; one of ten essential amino acids; 2-amino-3-methylbutyric acid

valve flow control device designed to enlarge, decrease, or close an opening in a mass transfer system; examples: gate valve, butterfly valve, plug cock, ball valve, globe valve, needle valve, diaphragm valve (each containing the shaped adjustable part to control flow, respectively)

valve, check flow control device designed to permit flow in only one direction

van der Waal's bond bond resulting from electrostatic attractions induced between two neutral atoms that are brought close enough together to produce distortions within their electron clouds; a very weak bond (bond energy of approximately 0.5 kcal/mole)

van der Waal's equation for "real" gases a quantitative expression of pressure, volume, and temperature relationships of gases that do not exhibit "ideal" behavior; correction parameters are included for attractive forces (internal pressures) between molecules and the inherent volume of gas molecules (incompressibility factor)

van der Waal's forces weak attractive forces acting on neutral atoms and molecules that arise from electric polarization, either inherent or induced, in each of the particles by the presence of other particles; SEE *van der Waal's bond; induced dipole–induced dipole interactions*

vanillylmandelic acid urinary test for pheochromocytoma that is based on the metabolic conversion of catechol amines to vanillylmandelic acid

vanishing cream an oil-in-water emulsion formulation for external use; application leaves an almost imperceptible film; a nongreasy cream; SEE ALSO *cream*

van't Hoff equation thermodynamic quantitative expression of the effect of temperature on an equilibrium constant; an analogous expression is used to calculate the effect of temperature on the solubility of a substance

van't Hoff factor an expression of the deviation of a "real" solution from "ideal" behavior; a function of the degree of dissociation and the number of ionic species in a molecule; a correction factor to determine the "effective concentration" of a substance in solution; synonym: i-factor

vaporizer an appliance used in a sick room to fill it with volatile substances (medicated or unmedicated); frequently used to increase room moisture content and relieve respiratory congestions as the patient breathes

vaporizer, steam a device used to increase the level of humidity in the house or workplace, thereby increasing the rate and efficiency of mucokinesis; can include medications in a medication cup located on the top of the vaporizer

vapor lock SEE *air binding*

vapor pressure force per unit area manifested in all directions in the open space above a liquid (or a volatile solid) in a closed container as a result of the kinetic motion of molecules escaping from the surface of the liquid (or volatile solid); also called "equilibrium vapor pressure," indicating a constant pressure exerted by the vapor of a liquid (or volatile solid) in constant volume, temperature, and pressure conditions

Vaquez' disease erythremia; polycythemia rubra vera

variable 1: a part of a mathematical expression that can change; SEE *dependent variable; independent variable* **2:** in an experiment, a parameter that must be controlled (kept constant) to study and/or define a system

variable cost cost of operating a business that fluctuates with changes in sales volume, salaries and wages, cost of goods sold, and income taxes; synonym: variable expense

variable dispensing fee reimbursement method used by third parties in which the fee paid for each prescription dispensed is set for each participating pharmacy depending on that pharmacy's overhead costs

variable expense SEE *variable cost*

variance computed measure of the degree of dispersion (or variability) among a group of numbers

vascular pertaining to blood vessels; indicates abundant blood supply

vascular surgeon a physician who specializes in performing surgery on blood vessels

vaso- prefix pertaining to a vessel or duct

vasoconstrictor drug that acts to reduce the diameter of the lumen of blood vessels

vasodilator compound that acts to increase the diameter of the lumen of blood vessels

vasopressor drug or hormone compound causing an increase in blood pressure by producing a constriction of blood vessels

vector 1: a carrier of an infective agent; example: mosquitoes can carry and transmit vector-borne diseases such as malaria **2:** quantities having magnitude and direction as opposed to scalar quantities; examples: velocity, force **3:** a cloning vehicle into which a segment of foreign DNA can be spliced so it can be introduced and expressed in host cells

vegetative cell bacterial cell capable of multiplication, as opposed to a spore, which cannot multiply

vehicle carrier or inert medium used as a solvent (or diluent) in which a medicinally active agent is formulated and/or administered

velocity 1: the rate of movement of a unit of matter expressed as cm/sec **2:** derivative (differential) of distance traveled with respect to time

velocity of light (in a vacuum) equals 2.99792×10^{10} cm/sec

ven- prefix pertaining to vein; same as vene-, veni-, veno-; synonyms: phleb-, phlebo-

vendor 1: an individual or organization providing health or medical services; a term usually applied to a provider participating in third-party medical programs **2:** a source of goods or services to be purchased

vene- prefix pertaining to vein; same as ven-, veni-, veno-; synonyms: phleb-, phlebo-

venereal disease any of several diseases acquired through sexual contact; examples: syphilis, gonorrhea, herpes simplex type 2 infections; SEE *sexually transmitted disease*

veni- prefix pertaining to vein, same as ven-, vene-, veno-

venipuncture puncture of a vein, usually by a needle to obtain blood

veno- prefix pertaining to vein, same as ven-, vene-, veni-

vented needle needle that permits air to pass to the inside of the injectable fluid container as the liquid is passing through the needle to the injection site

ventri- prefix meaning the front of the body; prefix referring to the abdominal part of an animal as opposed to the dorsal part or the back; same as ventro-

ventricle 1: a cavity in the brain **2:** one of the lower chambers of the heart

ventro- prefix meaning the front of the body; prefix referring to the abdominal part of an animal as opposed to the dorsal part or the back; same as ventri-

veracity a principle of ethics which states that practitioners should always be honest in their dealings with patients

Verified Internet Pharmacy Practice Site Program voluntary program implemented by the National Association of Boards of Pharmacy to certify that participating online pharmacies meet specified rigorous criteria for providing pharmacy services

vermicide agent that will kill intestinal worms

vermifuge medicine that expels worms or intestinal parasites

vermilion border colored part of the lips; often the target of herpes simplex labialis

verruca wart; a benign tumor caused by a virus

verruca vulgaris common warts

vertical strip product placement technique in which the largest sizes are placed at eye level with smaller sizes grouped in descending order beneath them

vertigo feeling that either a patient's surroundings are moving or that the patient is moving; erroneously used as a synonym for dizziness

vesicant agent that produces blisters (less severe in its action than an escharotic)

vial glass container closed with a rubber stopper and an aluminum band; removal of contents requires a needle; may be multidose (with a preservative included) or single dose (lacking a preservative); most often used for parenteral products

Vincent's angina painful pseudomembranous ulceration of the gums, oral mucous membranes, pharynx, and tonsils; synonyms: gingivitis, trench mouth

Vincent's disease necrotizing ulcerative gingivitis (inflammation of the gums)

vinegar acid synonym for glacial acetic acid

vinegars solutions of drugs in dilute acetic acid

virucide an agent that kills viruses

virulence pathogenicity of a microorganism; the ability of a microorganism to invade tissues and produce symptoms of disease or death

virus pathological agent smaller than bacteria and composed mainly of a nucleic acid enclosed in a protein envelope; a minute parasitic organism dependent upon cells for its metabolic and reproductive needs; microorganism that is not visible using an ordinary light microscope and is not filterable through bacterial filters

viscid sticky, glutinous

viscometer instrument or device to measure the viscosity of liquid substances; examples: Brookfield and Ostwald-Cannon-Fenske viscometers; synonym: rheometer

viscosity a measure of resistance of a fluid to flow; the reciprocal of fluidity; the basic cgs unit of viscosity is the poise; synonym: coefficient of viscosity; SEE *Newton's law of viscous flow* for basic quantitative units of flow

visible light electromagnetic radiation emanating from atomic electron shifts to lower energy levels; wavelenghts of electromagnetic radiation that are in the range of 10^{-7} to 10^{-6} meters

visual inventory control any intuitive method of inventory control lacking a formal organization

vitamin 1: any of several so-called growth factors **2:** an essential part of coenzymes, the absence of which causes growth retardation and an a vitaminosis syndrome; cannot be synthesized by the body or are not synthesized in sufficient quantities to fulfill bodily needs (must be in the diet); examples: A, D, E, K, B_1, B_2, B_{12}, C

vitamin B_{12} a complex cobalt-containing molecule that is required for the N^5-methyl THF-dependent conversion of homocysteine to methionine

vitriol a crystalline sulfate; glassy hydrated salt of a metal with sulfuric acid; examples: copper sulfate pentahydrate (blue vitriol) and oil of vitriol (sulfuric acid)

volatile having a high escaping tendency; capable of evaporating or vaporizing rapidly; describes a substance that readily vaporizes at relatively low temperatures

volatile memory information that is erased from a computer when the power is turned off

volatilization the passing of a substance from its liquid or solid form into its vapor form

volume the extent of a measureable space; basic cgs unit is cm^3; SI unit is m^3 or in^3; common units of volume include the fluid dram, fluid ounce, pint, quart, gallon, milliliter, and liter

volume of distribution, apparent biopharmaceutical term expressing the perceived volume (*Vd*) of the body in which a specific amount of unchanged drug (*Ab*) is distributed based on the concentration (*Cb*) of the drug in the blood; $Vd = Ab/Cb$; a characteristic value for a specific drug; an abstract volume that is calculated from the ratio of the amount of drug in the body to its concentration in plasma once partitioning has been stabilized (at steady-state conditions)

volumetric analysis determination of the amount of substance present by using the volume of a standard solution that will exactly react with the substance; requires the use of equipment such as pipets, burets, and volumetric flasks that deliver or contain quantitatively accurate volumes of liquids

vomiting involuntary or voluntary emptying of the contents of the stomach through the mouth; synonyms: emesis, regurgitation

von Gierke's disease type 1 glycogenosis; glycogen accumulation in liver and kidney

vortex cone-shaped formation in a circulating fluidized system that has been subjected to a stirring or mixing process; an impediment to rapid and efficient mixing

Vroom's expectancy theory concept that a person's motivation to perform is determined by his/her expectation that the performance will lead to a desired outcome, such as a promotion or a substantial raise

wafer a thin slice of material containing a medicinal agent

waiver a rider or clause in a health insurance contract excluding an insurer's liability for some sort of preexisting illness or injury; also refers to a plan amendment, such as a CMS (formerly HCFA) waiver or plan modification

Walden inversion chemical reaction in which a nucleophile is substituted on the side opposite the group being replaced, thus inverting the stereo configuration

Warburg respirometer manometric apparatus used to measure oxygen uptake and carbon dioxide release by tissues, tissue homogenates, or isolated enzyme systems

warm temperature any temperature between 30°C and 40°C (86°F and 104°F); a consideration in drug product storage and stability testing

warranty statement or guarantee of the quality and performance of a product or a service and of the seller's responsibility for the quality of the product or service, ranging from any specified period of time to a lifetime

water, aromatic clear, saturated (unless otherwise stated), aqueous solution of a volatile oil or other volatile or aromatic substance

waterbrash phenomenon sudden hypersalivation; signals that an episode of gastroesophageal reflux or vomiting is imminent

Water for Injection, USP pyrogen-free water which has been purified by reverse osmosis or distillation and which contains no more than 1 mg of total solids per 100 ml

water-in-oil emulsion SEE *emulsion, water-in-oil*

water number the number of grams of water that can be physically incorporated into 100 g of fat, ointment base, or other material

water of crystallization water that is in chemical combination with a salt; water that is a part of the crystalline lattice of a compound

water of hydration amount of water necessary for certain substances to crystallize; loss of such water in a drying process exhibits stepwise "equilibrium moisture content" curves depending on the number of water molecules held per molecule of chemical; total loss of water of hydration yields an amorphous powder; SEE *water of crystallization*

waters clear, saturated (unless otherwise stated), aqueous solution of a volatile oil or other volatile or aromatic substance

water sifting SEE *elutriation*

water softener a compound or a mixture of compounds used to remove divalent and trivalent metallic ions from water

wax thick plastic substance used by bees to build hives or any substance with similar properties

wax, paraffin inert, saturated, semisolid, high-molecular-weight hydrocarbon used in ointments and creams; synonyms: mineral wax, ceresin, earthwax, ozokerite, hard paraffin

Wedgwood mortar fine, hard, porcelain-like mortar named for Josiah Wedgwood, a British potter; SEE *mortar*

weight the practical expression of the mass of a substance based on the pull of earth's gravity; its cgs unit is the gram (g); weight equals mass times acceleration of gravity

well-closed container SEE *container, well closed*

well counter scintillation counter with a reentrant hole near the detector; the radioactive sample is placed in that hole when its activity is being measured

wellness a program that encourages physician visits before a condition develops, as well as behavior modifications that reduce the risk for developing a preventable illness

Werner theory of valence refers to covalent bonds formed between two elements in which one element donates both electrons to the shared pair; such bonds are termed dative or coordinate covalent bonds

Westphal balance SEE *Mohr-Westphal balance*

wet-bulb temperature equilibrium temperature of an evaporating surface measured by using a moisture-laden thermometer; air temperature measured with non-moisture-laden thermometer under these conditions is the dry-bulb temperature; humidity computed from the wet-bulb and dry-bulb temperature differential

wet granulation a process of preparing granules in which the tablet materials are wetted and forced through a screen while wet, thereby producing granules that are subsequently dried and sized before compression into tablets

wet-gum method SEE *English method*

wetting phenomenon of a liquid substance (such as water) covering or spreading on the available surface of a solid substance

wetting agent substance that causes a liquid to spread more easily on a solid surface, thus allowing the liquid to be more readily adsorbed or absorbed by the solid; substance that reduces surface tension, thus allowing the liquid (usually water) to wet the solid more easily; SEE *surfactant*

wetting angle SEE *wetting*

wheal slightly raised reddened or pale area on the skin, usually accompanied by itching, due to an allergy

Wheatstone bridge **1:** an instrument used to measure electrical conductance and resistance that forms a part of several kinds of instruments, such as pH meters and spectrophotometers **2:** a diamond-shaped electrical circuit composed of four resistors, each placed on a leg of the diamond; once the resistances are balanced, no current is measured through the middle of the circuit

white blood cell leukocyte; includes lymphocytes, neutrophils, eosinophils, and basophils (the latter three cell types are also known as granulocytes)

white lotion a white drying lotion prepared from sulfurated potash and zinc sulfate and used in the treatment of acne

Whitfield's ointment a semisolid dosage form consisting of benzoic acid and salicylic acid dissolved in an ointment base (PEG); used as a fungistat and keratolytic agent

Whitney, Harvey A.K. (1894-1957) first chairman of the American Society of Health-System Pharmacists and a pioneer in hospital services such as formulary, manufacturing, and the establishment of a specialty literature

whole body clearance SEE *total system clearance*

Wiley, Harvey Washington pioneer in the detection of adulteration in foods and drugs; the moving force behind the Pure Food and Drug Act of 1906

wine gallon SEE *proof gallon*

wines preparations containing medicines dissolved in wine or fortified wine

wintergreen oil synonym for methyl salicylate

withhold SEE *physician contingency reserve*

wobble hypothesis a hypothesis that explains why cells often have fewer tRNAs than expected; freedom in the pairing of the third base of the codon to the first base of the anticodon allows some tRNAs to pair with several codons

wood alcohol methyl alcohol; methanol

work the mechanical equivalent of energy; energy required to move material from one point to another; the unit for work in the cgs system is the erg

workflow flow of work through the pharmacy; must allow both drug-dispensing process and pharmaceutical care service to occur efficiently and effectively; includes assignment of appropriate nonjudgmental tasks to pharmacy technicians

work index for particle size reduction 1: a direct measurement of energy required to reduce particles from a diameter of D_1 to a diameter of D_2 **2:** the number of kilowatt hours required to reduce a finite mass of material from infinite size to a size such that 80 percent of the material will pass through a 100 micron screen

working capital the excess of total current assets over total current liabilities; capital being used to purchase materials, pay wages, etc.

wraparound coverage or plan insurance to cover copays or deductibles not covered by a basic insurance plan

Wurster process a process named for its inventor, Dale Wurster; SEE *air-suspension coating*

xanthene heterocyclic organic compound in which two benzene rings are fused to a central pyran ring; the pyran oxygen bridges the two benzene rings; a parent structure of medicinal agents such as smooth muscle spasmolytics

xanthine purine occurring in plants and animals; a metabolite of adenine and guanine and the parent structure of the xanthine alkaloids such as caffeine, theophylline, and theobromine

xenobiotic drug or other substance not normally found in the body; a foreign substance to the body

xer- prefix meaning dry; same as xero-

xero- prefix meaning dry; same as xer-

xerogenic producing dryness; examples: xerogenic medications, xerogenic environmental conditions

xerophthalmia condition resulting from a deficiency of vitamin A and characterized by a dry, thickened condition of the conjunctiva

xerosis dry skin

xerostomia dry mouth

X-ray electromagnetic radiation emitted from an atom when an orbital electron changes to a lower energy level; wavelengths are longer than gamma rays and shorter than ultraviolet light and in the range of 10^{-8} meter

years-of-profit figure a multiplier factor used with a pharmacy's earnings figure to calculate a purchase price

yeast artificial chromosome a cloning vector that can accommodate up to 100 kb; contains eukaryotic sequences that function as centromeres, telomeres, and a replication origin

yerba santa synonym for eriodictyon

Young's rule method of calculating dosages for children over two years of age; SEE *dosage rules*

Z

Z-DNA a form of DNA that is twisted into a left-handed spiral; named for its zigzag conformation, which is slimmer than B-DNA

zero order reaction/process quantitative expression in which the rate of change is directly proportional to concentration raised to the zero power; one that occurs at a constant rate, and one that is independent of the concentrations of the reactants

zetameter an instrument used to measure the zeta-potential of charged particle surfaces

zeta-potential the effective overall charge on the surface of a particle; a function of the Stern layer (those solvent molecules and counter ionic charges bound to the particle surface) and the "diffuse-double layer" of accompanying solvent molecules and ionic charges in the vicinity of the particle surface (the mobile layer)

zinc grayish white, malleable metal; zinc salts are astringent and antiseptic; zinc ion is a trace mineral and a cometal for several enzymes, including chymotrypsin; zinc metal is useful as a reducing agent in organic chemistry

zinc-eugenol cement a dental paste composed primarily of zinc salts, eugenol, and rosin and that serves as a temporary tooth filling

Zollinger-Ellison syndrome peptic ulceration with gastric hypersecretion

zoonosis disease transmitted from animals to humans

zoopharmacy synonym for veterinary pharmacy

zwitterion molecular ionic species of an ampholyte that exists at a definite pH and as a structure containing equal positive and negative charges, the overall charge being neutral

zymogen the inactive form of a proteolytic enzyme

Abbreviations

A_2	aortic second sound
$A_2>P_2$	aortic second sound greater than pulmonic second sound
AA	amino acid; auto accident; Alcoholics Anonymous
AAA	abdominal aortic aneurysmectomy/aneurysm
AACP	American Association of Colleges of Pharmacy
AAFP	American Academy of Family Physicians
AAHP	American Association of Health Plans
AAL	anterior axillary line
AAN	analgesic-associated nephropathy
AAP	American Academy of Pediatrics
AAPA	American Academy of Physician Assistants
AAPC	antibiotic-acquired pseudomembranous colitis
AARP	American Association of Retired Persons
AAS	atlanto axis subluxation
AAV	adeno-associated virus
AAVV	accumulated alveolar ventilatory volume
Ab	antibody; abortion
A&B	apnea and bradycardia
ABC	absolute band counts; applesauce, banana, cereal (diet); artificial beta cells
abd	abdomen or abdominal
ABDCT	atrial bolus dynamic computer tomography
ABE	acute bacterial endocarditis
ABG	arterial blood gases
ABI	atherothrombotic brain infarction
ABL	allograft bound lymphocytes
ABMT	autologous bone marrow transplantation
abn	abnormal
ABR	absolute bed rest; auditory brain (evoked) responses
ABS	at bedside; admitting blood sugar
ABT	aminopyrine breath test
ABW	actual body weight
abx	antibiotics

AC	before meals; acromio-clavicular; air conduction; abdominal circumference; anchored catheter; antecubital; acetate
ACA	against clinical advice; anterior cerebral artery; acrodermatitis chronicum atrophicans; acute or chronic alcoholism; American College of Apothecaries
ACB	antibody-coated bacteria
ACBE	air contrast barium enema
ACC	adenoid cystic carcinomas; ambulatory care center
ACCP	American College of Clinical Pharmacy
ACD	allergic contact dermatitis; anterior chest diameter; anemia of chronic disease; absolute cardiac dullness; acid citrate dextrose
ACE	angiotensin-converting enzyme
ACEI	angiotensin-converting enzyme inhibitor
ACh	acetylcholine
ACH	adrenocortical hormone
AChE	acetylcholineestrace
AChEI	acetylcholineestrace inhibitor
ACL	anterior cruciate ligament
ACLS	advanced cardiac life support
ACPE	American Council on Pharmaceutical Education
AC-PH	acid phosphate
ACPP-PF	acid phosphatase prostatic fluid
ACR	adjusted community rating
ACS	American Cancer Society; American College of Surgeons; American Chemical Society
ACT	activated clotting time; automated coagulation time; allergen challenge test
ACTH	adrenocorticotropic hormone
ACV	atria/carotid/ventricular
AD	Alzheimer's disease; right ear
A&D	admission and discharge
ADA	American Diabetes Association; American Dental Association
ADCC	antibody-dependent cell-mediated cytotoxicity
ADD	attention deficit disorder
ADEM	acute disseminating encephalomyelitis
ADH	antidiuretic hormone; alcohol dehydrogenase
ADHD	attention deficit hyperactivity disorder
ADL	activities of daily living

ad lib (adlib)	at liberty *(ad libitum);* as desired
adm	admission
ADME	absorption, distribution, metabolism, excretion
adol	adolescent
ADP	adenosine diphosphate
ADR	adverse drug reaction; acute dystonic reaction
ADS	anonymous donor's sperm; anatomical dead space; alternate delivery systems
ADT	anticipate discharge tomorrow
ADX	adrenalectomy
AE	above elbow (amputation); adverse event; air entry
AEC	at earliest convenience
AED	automated external defibrillator
AEG	air encephalogram
AER	acoustic evoked response; auditory evoked response
Aer. M	aerosol mask
AES	antiembolic stocking
AF	atrial fibrillation; acid-fast; amniotic fluid; anterior fontanel
AFB	acid-fast bacilli; aorto-femoral bypass
a fib	atrial fibrillation (A fib; At fib)
A fib	atrial fibrillation (a fib; At Fib)
AFO	ankle-foot orthosis
AFP	alpha-fetoprotein
AFPE	American Foundation for Pharmaceutical Education
AFV	amniotic fluid volume
AFVSS	afebrile, vital signs stable (AVSS)
Ag	silver
AG	antigravity; anion gap; antigen
A/G	albumin-to-globulin ratio
AgNO$_3$	silver nitrate
AGA	appropriate for gestational age
AGD	agar gel diffusion
AGE	angle of greatest extension
AGF	angle of greatest flexion
AGG	agammaglobulinemia
aggl	agglutination
AGL	acute granulocytic leukemia
AGN	acute glomerulonephritis
AGNB	aerobic gram-negative bacilli
AGPT	agar-gel precipitation test
AGS	adrenogenital syndrome

AH	airway hyperresponsiveness; antihyaluronidase
AHA	autoimmune hemolytic anemia; American Heart Association; American Hospital Association
AHC	acute hemorrhagic conjunctivitis; acute hemorrhagic cystitis
AHD	arteriosclerotic heart disease: autoimmune hemolytic disease
AHEC	Area Health Education Center
AHF	antihemophilic factor
AHFS	American Hospital Formulary Service
AHG	antihemophiliac globulin
AHM	ambulatory Holter monitoring
AHRQ	Agency for Health Care Research and Quality
AI	allergy index; aortic insufficiency; artificial insemination; artificial intelligence
AI-Ab	anti-insulin antibody
AICA	anterior inferior communicating artery; anterior inferior cerebellar artery
AICD	automatic implantable cardioverter/defibrillator
AID	artificial insemination donor; automatic implantable defibrillator
AIDS	acquired immunodeficiency syndrome
AIF	aortic-iliac-femoral
AIH	artificial insemination with husband's sperm
AIHA	autoimmune hemolytic anemia
AIHP	American Institute of the History of Pharmacy
AIMS	abnormal involuntary movement scale; arthritis impact measure scale
AIN	acute interstitial nephritis
AION	anterior ischemic optic neuropathy
AIP	acute intermittent porphyria
AIR	accelerated idioventricular rhythm
AJ	ankle jerk
AK	above knee
AKA	also known as; above knee amputation; alcoholic ketoacidosis
ALA	aminolevulinic acid; alpha linolenic acid
ALAT	alanine transaminase (alanine aminotransferase; SGPT)
alb	albumin
ALC	acute lethal catatonia; alcohol
ALD	alcoholic liver disease; aldolase; adrenoleukodystrophy

aldost	aldosterone
ALFT	abnormal liver function tests
ALG	antilymphocytic globulin
alk	alkaline
alk-p	alkaline phosphatase
ALL	acute lymphocytic leukemia
ALMI	anterolateral myocardial infarction
ALOS	average length of stay
ALP	alkaline phosphatase
ALS	amyotrophic lateral sclerosis; acute lateral sclerosis
ALT	alanine aminotransferase (SGPT)
AM	adult male; amalgam; morning *(ante meridiem);* myopic astigmatism (AsM)
AMA	against medical advice; antimitochondrial antibody; American Medical Association
AMAP	as much as possible
A-MAT	amorphous material
amb	ambulate; ambulatory
AMC	arm muscle circumference
AMCS	automated medical coding system
AMD	age-related macular degeneration
AMegL	acute megokaryoblastic leukemia
AMG	acoustic myography
AMHO	Association of Managed Healthcare Organizations
AMI	acute myocardial infarction
AML	acute myelogenous leukemia; acute mylocytic leukemia
AMMOL	acute myelomonoblastic leukemia
amnio	amniocentesis
AMOL	acute monoblastic leukemia
amp	amputation; ampule
AMP	adenosine monophosphate
AMR	alternating motor rates
AMS	acute mountain sickness; altered mental state; amylase
AMSIT	appearance; mood; sensorium; intelligence; thought process (portion of the mental status examination)
amt	amount
AMV	assisted mechanical ventilation
amy	amylase
ANA	antinuclear antibody; American Neurological Association; American Nurses Association

ANAD	anorexia nervosa and associated disorders
ANC	absolute neutrophil count
ANDA	Abbreviated New Drug Application
anes	anesthesia
ANF	antinuclear factor; atrial natriuretic factor
ang	angiogram
ang II	angiotensin II
ANLL	acute nonlymphoblastic leukemia
ANOVA	analysis of variance
ANP	atrial natriuretic peptide
ANS	autonomic nervous system; answer
ant	anterior
AO	atypical odontalgia
A&O	alert and oriented
A&O × 3	awake and oriented to person, place, and time
A&O × 4	awake and oriented to person, place, time, and date
AoA	Agency on Aging
AOA	American Optometric Association; American Osteopathic Association
AOAP	as often as possible
AOB	alcohol on breath
AOC	area of concern
AODM	adult-onset diabetes mellitus
ao-il	aorta-iliac
AOM	acute otitis media
AOP	aortic pressure
AOSD	adult-onset Still's disease
AP	anterior-posterior; antepartum; apical pulse; abdominalperitoneal; appendicitis
A&P	anterior and posterior; auscultation and percussion; assessment and plans
APB	atrial premature beat; abductor pollicis brevis
APC	arterial premature contraction
APCD	adult polycystic disease
APD	automated peritoneal dialysis; atrial premature depolarization
APE	acute psychotic episode
APhA	American Pharmacists (formerly Pharmaceutical) Association
APHA	American Public Health Association
APKD	adult onset polycystic kidney disease

APL	acute promyelocytic leukemia; abductor pollicis longus; anterior pituitary lobe; accelerated painless labor
APN	advanced practice nurse
APPM	Academy of Pharmacy Practice and Management of the American Pharmacists Association
approx	approximate
appt	appointment
APR	abdominoperineal resection
APRS	Academy of Pharmaceutical Research and Sciences of the American Pharmacists Association
aPTT	activated partial thromboplastin time
aq	water *(aqua)*
aq dest	distilled water *(aqua destillata)*
AR	airway resistance; allergic rhinitis; aortic regurgitation
A-R	apical-radial (pulse)
ARB	angiotensin receptor blocker
ARC	abnormal retinal correspondence; AIDS-related complex; American Red Cross
ARD	acute respiratory disease
ARDS	adult respiratory distress syndrome; acute respiratory distress syndrome
ARF	acute renal failure; acute rheumatic fever; acute respiratory failure
ARLD	alcohol-related liver disease
ARM	artificial rupture of membranes
ARMD	age-related macular degeneration
AROM	active range of motion; artificial rupture of membranes
ARS	antirabies serum
ART	arterial; automated reagin test (for syphilis)
ARV	AIDS-related virus
AS	aortic stenosis; arteriosclerosis; anal sphincter; left ear; ankylosing spondylitis
ASA I	healthy patient with localized pathological process (American Society of Anesthesiologists classification system)
ASA II	patient with mild to moderate systemic disease (American Society of Anesthesiologists classification system)

ASA III	patient with severe systemic disease limiting activity but not incapacitating (American Society of Anesthesiologists classification system)
ASA IV	patient with incapacitating systemic disease (American Society of Anesthesiologists classification system)
ASA V	moribund patient not expected to live (American Society of Anesthesiologists classification system)
ASAP	as soon as possible
ASAT	aspartate transaminase (aspartate aminotransferase) (SGOT)
ASB	anesthesia standby; asymptomatic bacteriuria
ASC	altered state of consciousness; ambulatory surgery center
ASCP	American Society of Consultant Pharmacists; American Society of Clinical Pathologists; American Society of Clinical Pharmacology
ASCVD	arteriosclerotic cardiovascular disease
ASD	atrial septal defect
ASE	acute stress erosion
ASH	asymmetric septal hypertrophy
ASHD	atherosclerotic heart disease
ASHP	American Society of Health-System Pharmacists (formerly American Society of Hospital Pharmacists)
ASIS	anterior superior iliac spine
ASK	antistreptokinase
ASL	antistreptolysin (titer); airway surface liquid; American sign language
AsM	myopic astigmatism (AM)
ASO	administrative services organization; administrative services only; arteriosclerosis obliterans; automatic stop order
ASOT	antistreptolysin-O titer
ASP	Academy of Students of Pharmacy of the American Pharmacists Association; American Society of Pharmacognosy; acute suppurative parotitis
ASPL	American Society of Pharmacy Law
ASS	anterior superior supine
ast	astigmatism
AST	aspartate transaminase (SGOT); aspartic acid transaminase; accelerated stability testing
ASVD	arteriosclerotic vessel disease

AT	applanation tonometry; atraumatic; antithrombin
ATD	autoimmune thyroid disease; antithyroid drug
At Fib	atrial fibrillation (a fib; A fib)
ATG	antithymocyte globulin
ATgA	antithyroglobulin antibodies
ATHR	angina threshold heart rate
ATL	Achilles tendon lengthening; atypical lymphocytes; adult T cell leukemia
ATLS	advanced trauma life support
ATN	acute tubular necrosis
ATNC	atraumatic normocephalic
ATNR	asymmetrical tonic neck reflux
ATP	adenosine triphosphate
ATPase	adenosine triphosphatase
ATPS	ambient temperature and pressure, saturated
ATR	Achilles tendon reflex; atrial
ATT	arginine tolerance test
AU	both ears; gold
AUC	area under the curve
AU HAA	Australia antigen (hepatitis-associated antigen)
Aur Fib	auricular fibrillation
Av	avoirdupois system of weights and measures
AV	arteriovenous; atrioventricular; auditory-visual
AVA	arteriovenous anastomosis
AVD	apparent volume of distribution
AVF	arteriovenous fistula
AVH	acute viral hepatitis
AVM	atriovenous malformation
AVN	atrioventricular node; arteriovenous nicking; avascular necrosis
avoir	avoirdupois
AVR	aortic valve replacement
AVS	atriovenous shunt
AVSS	afebrile, vital signs stable (AFVSS)
AVT	atypical ventricular tachycardia
A&W	alive and well
A waves	atrial contraction waves
AWOL	absent without leave
AWP	average wholesale price
ax	axillary
A-Z test	Aschiem-Zondek test (diagnostic test for pregnancy)

b	twice *(bis)*
B	bacillus; bloody; both; buccal
B₁	thiamine HCl
B₂	riboflavin
B₆	pyridoxine HCl
B₉	folic acid
B₁₂	cyanocobalamin
Ba	barium
BA	backache; bile acid; blood alcohol; Bourns assist
BAC	blood alcohol content; bacterial artificial chromosome
BACOP	bleomycin, adriamycin, cyclophosphamide, oncovin (vincristine), prednisone
BAD	bipolar affective disorder
BaE	barium enema
BAE	bronchial artery embolization
BAEP	brain stem auditory evoked potential
BAL	blood alcohol level; bronchoalveolar lavage
BAN	British approved name
BAO	basal acid output
BAP	blood agar plate
baso	basophil
BAVP	balloon aortic valvuloplasty
BB	bed bath; bowel or bladder; breakthrough bleeding; blood bank; blow bottle
BBA	born before arrival
BBB	bundle branch block; blood-brain barrier
BBBB	bilateral bundle branch block
BBD	benign breast disease
BBM	banked breast milk
BBS	bilateral breath sounds
BBT	basal body temperature
BBVM	brush border vesicle membrane
BC	birth control; blood culture
BCA	balloon catheter angioplasty; basal cell atypia; brachiocephalic artery
BCAA	branched-chain amino acids
BCC	basal cell carcinoma
BCD	basal cell dysplasia
BCE	basal cell epithelioma
B cell	large lymphocyte
BCG	bacille bilié de Calmette-Guérin (vaccine)

BCL	basic cycle length
BCP	birth control pills
BCS	battered child syndrome; Budd-Chiari syndrome
BD	birth defect; brain dead; bronchial drainage
BDAE	Boston Diagnostic Aphasia Examination
BDI-SF	Beck's Depression Index—Short Form
BDR	background diabetic retinopathy
BE	barium enema; below elbow; bacterial endocarditis; base excess
BEAM	brain electrical activity mapping
BEC	bacterial endocarditis
BEE	basal energy expenditure
BEP	brainstem evoked potentials
BF	black female
BFP	biologic false positive
BFT	bentonite flocculation test
BG	blood glucose
BGC	basal ganglion calcification
BGM	blood glucose monitoring
BHI	biosynthetic human insulin
BHN	bridging hepatic necrosis
BHR	bronchial hyperresponsiveness
BHS	beta-hemolytic streptococci
BI	bladder irritation; bowel impaction; bioelectric impedance
BIB	brought in by
bid	twice daily *(bis in die)*
BIH	bilateral inguinal hernia; benign intracranial hypertension
bilat	bilateral
bilat SLC	bilateral short leg cast
bilat SXO	bilateral salpingo-oophorectomy
bili	bilirubin
bili-C	conjugated bilirubin
BIMA	bilateral internal mammary arteries
BIW	twice a week
BJ	bone and joint
BJE	bone and joint examination
BJM	bone, joint, and muscle
BJ protein	Bence-Jones protein
BK	below knee
BKA	below knee amputation

bkft	breakfast
bkg	background
BLE	both lower extremities
BLESS	bath, laxative, enema, shampoo, and shower
BLOBS	bladder obstruction
BLS	basic life support
BL unit	Bessey-Lowry unit
BM	basal metabolism; black male; bone marrow; bowel movement; breast milk
BMA	bone marrow aspirate
BMC	bone marrow cells
BMI	body mass index
BMJ	bone, muscle, joint; *British Medical Journal*
BMR	basal metabolic rate
BMT	bone marrow transplant; bilateral myringotomy tubes
BMTU	bone marrow transplant unit
BNDD	Bureau of Narcotics and Dangerous Drugs
BNO	bladder neck obstruction
BNR	bladder neck retraction
BO	body odor; bowel obstruction; behavioral objective
BOA	born on arrival; born out of asepsis
BOM	bilateral otitis media
BOO	bladder outlet obstruction
BOT	base of tongue
BP	bathroom privileges; blood pressure; boiling point; *British Pharmacopoeia*
BPC	*British Pharmaceutical Codex*
BPD	borderline personality disorder; bronchopulmonary dysplasia
BPF	bronchopleural fistula
BPG	bypass graft
BPH	benign prostatic hypertrophy/hyperplasia
BPM	breaths per minute; beats per minute
BPPV	benign paroxysmal positional vertigo
BPRS	Brief Psychiatric Rating Scale
BPS	Board of Pharmaceutical Specialities
BPSD	bronchopulmonary segmental drainage
BPV	benign paroxysmal vertigo
BR	bathroom; bed rest
BRAO	branch retinal artery occlusion
BRATT	bananas, rice, applesauce, tea, and toast (diet)
BRJ	brachial radialis jerk

BRM	biological response modifiers
BRP	bathroom privileges
BRR	blood-retinal barrier
BS	blood sugar; bowel sounds; breath sounds; bedside; before sleep
B&S	Bartholin and Skene (glands)
BSA	body surface area
BSB	body surface burned
BSC	bedside commode
BSE	breast self-examination; bovine spongiform encephalopathy
BSER	brainstem evoked responses
BSGA	beta streptococcus group A
BSOM	bilateral serous otitis media
BSPM	body surface potential mapping
BSS	balanced salt solution; black silk sutures; bismuth subsalicylate
BSU	Bartholin, Skene's, urethral (glands) (BUS)
BT	bladder tumor; brain tumor; breast tumor; blood transfusion; bedtime; bituberous
BTB	breakthrough bleeding
BTFS	breast tumor frozen section
BTL	bilateral tubal ligation
BTPS	body temperature pressure saturated
BTR	bladder tumor recheck
BTU	British thermal unit
BU	Bodansky unit
BUE	both upper extremities
BUN	blood urea nitrogen
BUR	backup rate (ventilator)
BUS	Bartholin, urethral, and Skene's (glands) (BSU)
BVL	bilateral vas ligation
BW	birth weight; body weight; body water
BWCS	bagged white cell study
BWFI	bacteriostatic water for injection
BWS	battered woman syndrome
Bx	biopsy
c	food *(cibus)* or meals *(cibos)*
C	carbohydrate; Celsius; hundred; cyanosis; clubbing
C_1	first cervical vertebra
C1 to C9	precursor molecules of the complement system

Ca	calcium
CA	cardiac arrest; carcinoma; carotid artery; chronological age; coronary artery
CAA	crystalline amino acids
CAB	coronary artery bypass
CABG	coronary artery bypass graft
CaBI	calcium bone index
CABS	coronary artery bypass surgery
CACI	computer-assisted continuous infusion
CAD	coronary artery disease
CAE	cellulose acetate electrophoresis
CAH	chronic active hepatitis; chronic aggressive hepatitis; congenital adrenal hyperplasia
CAL	calories; callus; chronic airflow limitation
CALD	chronic active liver disease
CALGB	Cancer and Leukemia Group B
CALLA	common acute lymphoblastic leukemia antigen
CAM	complementary and alternative medicine
cAMP	cyclic adenosine monophosphate
CAN	contrast associated nephropathy; cord around neck
CAO	chronic airway obstruction
CAP	community-acquired pneumonia
Ca/P	calcium-to-phosphorus ratio
CAPD	chronic/continuous ambulatory peritoneal dialysis
caps	capsule *(capsula)*
CAR	cardiac ambulation routine
carb	carbohydrate (C; CHO; COH)
CAS	carotid artery stenosis
CAT	computed axial tomography; children's apperception test; cataract
cath	catheter; catheterization
CAVB	complete atrioventricular block
CAVC	common atrioventricular canal
CAVH	continuous arteriovenous hemofiltration
CB	code blue; chronic bronchitis; cesarean birth; chair and bed
C&B	crown and bridge
CBA	chronic bronchitis and asthma; cost-benefit analysis
CBC	complete blood count
CBD	common bile duct; closed bladder drainage
CBF	cerebral blood flow; ciliary beat frequency
CBFV	cerebral blood flow velocity

CBG	capillary blood glucose; corticosteroid-binding globulin
CBI	continuous bladder irrigation
CBN	chronic benign neutropenia
CBR	complete bed rest; chronic bed rest; carotid bodies resected
CBS	chronic brain syndrome
CC	chief complaint; cubic centimeter; critical condition; creatinine clearance; cerebral concussion; clean catch (urine); cord compression
CCA	common carotid artery
CCAP	capsule cartilage articular preservation
CCB	calcium channel blocker
CC&C	colony count and culture
CCE	clubbing, cyanosis, and edema
CCF	compound comminuted fracture; crystal-induced chemostatic factor
CCG	Children's Cancer Group
CCGP	Commission for Certification in Geriatric Pharmacy
CCHD	cyanotic congenital heart disease
CCI	chronic coronary insufficiency
CCK	cholecystokinin
CCK-PZ	cholecystokinin-pancreozymin
CCL	cardiac catheterization lab
CCMSU	clean catch midstream urine
CCNS	cell cycle nonspecific
C-collar	cervical collar
CCPD	continuous cycling/cyclical peritoneal dialysis
CCR	continuous complete remission
CCRU	critical care recovery unit
CCS	cell cycle specific; Cooperative Care Suite
CCT	closed cerebral trauma
CCU	coronary care unit
CCX	complications
CD	cesarean delivery; chronic dialysis; continuous drainage; Crohn's disease
C&D	cystoscopy and dilatation
C/D	cup to disc ratio
CD4	antigenic marker on helper T cells
CD8	antigenic marker on suppressor T cells
CDA	congenital dyserythropoietic anemia
CDAI	Crohn's Disease Activity Index

CDB	cough, deep breathe
C&DB	cough and deep breath
CDC	Centers for Disease Control
CDE	Certified Diabetic Educator; common duct exploration
CDH	congenital dysplasia of the hip; chronic daily headache
CDLE	chronic discoid lupus erythematosus
CDS	chronic dieting syndrome
CDU	chemical dependency unit
CE	cardiac enlargement; contrast echocardiology; central episiotomy; continuing education
CEA	carcinoembryonic antigen; carotid endarterectomy; cost-effectiveness analysis
CECT	contrast enhancement computed tomography
CEI	continuous extravascular infusion
CEP	cardiac enzyme panel; congenital erythropoietic porphyria; countercurrent electrophoresis
ceph	cephalic
ceph floc	cephalic flocculation
CE&R	central episiotomy and repair
CERA	cortical evoked response audiometry
cerv	cervical
CES	cognitive environmental stimulation
CEU	continuing education units
CF	cystic fibrosis; complement fixation; cardiac failure; cancer-free; count fingers; contractile force
CFA	common femoral artery; complete Freund's adjuvant
CFIDS	chronic fatigue and immune dysfunction syndrome
CFM	close-fitting mask
CFP	cystic fibrosis protein
CFR	*Code of Federal Regulations* (United States)
CFS	cancer family syndrome; chronic fatigue syndrome
CFT	complement fixation test
CF test	complement fixation test
CFU	colony-forming units
CG	cholecystogram
CGB	chronic gastrointestinal bleeding
CGD	chronic granulomatous disease
CGI	Clinical Global Impression (scale)
CGL	chronic granulocytic leukemia
CGMP	Current Good Manufacturing Practices
CGN	chronic glomerulonephritis
cgs	centimeter-gram-second system of measurements

CGTT	cortisol glucose tolerance test
CH	child; chronic; chest; crown-heel; convalescent hospital; cluster headache
CHAI	continuous hepatic artery infusion
CHAMPUS	Civilian Health and Medical Program of the Uniformed Services
CHAMPVA	Civilian Health and Medical Program of the Veterans Administration
CHB	complete heart block
CHC	comprehensive health center
CHD	congenital heart disease; childhood diseases; coronary heart disease
CHE	chronic hepatic encephalopathy
CHF	congestive heart failure
CHFV	combined high frequency of ventilation
CHI	closed head injury
CHIP	Children's Health Insurance Program
CHO	carbohydrate (C; carb; COH)
chol	cholesterol
c hold	withhold
CHOP	cyclophosphamide, hydroxydaunomycin, oncovin (vincristine), and prednisone
CHPA	Consumer Healthcare Products Association
CHPB	Canadian Health Protection Branch (FDA equivalent)
chr	chronic
CHT	closed head trauma
CHU	closed head unit
Ci	Curie(s)
CI	cardiac index; cesium implant; complete iridectomy; confidence interval
CIA	chronic idiopathic anhidrosis
CIAED	collagen-induced autoimmune ear disease
CIB	cytomegalic inclusion bodies; crying-induced bronchospasm
CIBD	chronic inflammatory bowel disease
CIC	circulating immune complexes; coronary intensive care
CICE	combined intracapsular cataract extraction
CICU	cardiac intensive care unit
CID	cytomegalic inclusion disease
CIDS	continuous insulin delivery system; cellular immunodeficiency syndrome

CIE	counterimmunoelectrophoresis; crossed immunoelectrophoresis
CIN	chronic interstitial nephritis
CINE	chemotherapy-induced nausea and emesis
circ	circumcision; circumference; circulation
CIS	carcinoma in situ
CIU	chronic idiopathic urticaria
CJD	Creutzfeldt-Jakob disease
CK	check; creatinine kinase
CK-MB	creatine kinase isoenzyme with muscle and brain subunits (MB-CK)
cl	cloudy
Cl	chloride
CLA	community living arrangements
clav	clavicle
CLBBB	complete left bundle branch block
CLD	chronic lung disease
CLEAR	National Clearing House on Licensure Enforcement and Regulation
CLF	cholesterol-lecithin flocculation
CLH	chronic lobular hepatitis
CLIA	clinical laboratory improvement amendment
CLL	chronic lymphocytic leukemia
CLLE	columnar-lined lower esophagus
cl liq	clear liquid
CLO	cod liver oil; close
CL&P	cleft lip and palate
CL-VOID	clean voided specimen
CM	Caucasian male; costal margin; continuous murmur; contrast media; centimeter; cochlear microphonics; culture media; common migraine
CMA	certified medical assistant; cost-minimization analysis
CMBBT	cervical mucous basal body temperature
CMC	critical micelle concentration; carboxymethyl cellulose; chronic mucocutaneous candidosis
CME	continuing medical education; cystoid macular edema
CMF	cyclophosphamide, methotrexate, and fluorouracil
CMG	cystometrogram
CMHC	Community Mental Health Center
CMHN	Community Mental Health Nurse
CMI	cell-mediated immunity; Cornell Medical Index
CMJ	carpometacarpal joint

CMK	congenital multicystic kidney
CML	cell-mediated lympholysis; chronic myelogenous leukemia
CMM	cutaneous malignant melanoma
CMRNG	chromosomally resistant Neisseria gonorrhoeae
CMRO$_2$	cerebral metabolic rate for oxygen
CMS	Centers for Medicare and Medicaid Services (formerly HCFA); circulation motion sensation
CMSUA	clean midstream urinalysis
CMT	chiropractic manipulative treatment
CMV	cytomegalovirus; cool mist vaporizer; controlled mechanical ventilation
CN	cranial nerve
CNA	chart not available
CNH	central neurogenic hyperpnea
CNP	continuous negative pressure
CNS	central nervous system; clinical nurse specialist
Co	cobalt
CO	cardiac output; carbon monoxide
C/O	complains of; complaints; under care of
CO$_2$	carbon dioxide
CoA	coarctation of the aorta; coenzyme A
COA	certificate of authority
COAD	chronic obstructive airway disease; chronic obstructive arterial disease
COAG	chronic open angle glaucoma; coagulation
COBRA	Consolidated Omnibus Reconciliation Act
COC	combination oral contraceptive; certificate of coverage
COD	cause of death
COEPS	cortically originating extrapyramidal symptoms
COG	cognitive function tests; Central Oncology Group
COH	carbohydrate (C; carb; CHO)
CoHb	carboxyhemoglobin
COI	cost-of-illness analysis
COLD	chronic obstructive lung disease
COLD A	cold agglutinin titer
collyr	eyewash (collyrium)
col/ml	colonies per milliliter
comp	complications; compound
CON	certificate of need
conc	concentrated

cong	congenital
COP	cyclophosphamide, oncovin (vincristine), and prednisone
COPD	chronic obstructive pulmonary disease
COPE	chronic obstructive pulmonary emphysema
cor	coronary
CORF	comprehensive outpatient rehabilitation facility
COSTEP	Commissioned Officer Study Training and Externship Program
COT	content of thought
COU	cardiac observation unit
CP	cerebral palsy; cleft palate; creatine phosphokinase; chest pain; chronic pain; chondromalacia patella
C&P	cystoscopy and pyelography
CPA	costophrenic angle; cardiopulmonary arrest; cerebellar pontile angle
CPAF	chlorpropamide-alcohol flush
CPAP	continuous positive airway pressure
CPB	cardiopulmonary bypass
CPBA	competitive protein-binding assay
CPC	clinicopathological conference; cerebral palsy clinic
CPCR	cardiopulmonary-cerebral resuscitation
CPD	cephalopelvic disproportion; chronic peritoneal dialysis
CPDD	calcium pyrophosphate deposition disease
CPE	chronic pulmonary emphysema; cardiogenic pulmonary edema
CPGN	chronic progressive glomerulonephritis
CPH	chronic persistent hepatitis
CPhT	Certified Pharmacy Technician
CPI	Consumer Price Index
CPK	creatine phosphokinase
CPKD	childhood polycystic kidney disease
CPM	central pontine myelinolysis; continuous passive motion; continue present management; counts per minute
CPmax	peak serum concentration
CPmin	trough serum concentration
CPN	chronic pyelonephritis
CPP	cerebral perfusion pressure
CPPB	continuous positive pressure breathing
CPPV	continuous positive pressure ventilation

CPR	cardiopulmonary resuscitation
CPS	complex partial seizures
CPSC	Consumer Product Safety Commission
CPT	chest physiotherapy
CPT Codes	Current Procedural Terminology Codes
CPTH	chronic posttraumatic headache
CQI	continuous quality improvement
Cr	creatinine
CR	cardiorespiratory; controlled release; cardiac rehabilitation; colon resection; closed reduction; complete remission
CRA	central retinal artery; clinical research associate
CRBBB	complete right bundle branch block
CRC	colorectal cancer; child-resistant closure
CrCl	creatinine clearance
CRD	chronic renal disease
CREST	calcinosis, Raynaud's phenomenon, esophageal hypomotility, scleroderma, and telangiectasia
CRF	chronic renal failure; corticotropin-releasing factor
CRI	chronic renal insufficiency
cric	cricoidotomy
crit	hematocrit
CRO	clinical research organization
CRP	C-reactive protein
CRPF	choroquine-resistant *Plasmodium falciparum*
CRST	calcification, Raynaud's phenomenon, scleroderma, and telangiectasia
CRT	central reaction time; cadaver renal transplant
CRTZ	chemoreceptor trigger zone
CRUMBS	continuous remove, unobtrusive monitoring of biobehavioral systems
CRVO	central retinal vein occlusion
CS	coronary sclerosis; central supply; clinical stage; conjunctiva-sclera; consciousness; cat scratch; cycloserine
C&S	culture and sensitivity
CSBF	coronary sinus blood flow
CSC	cornea, sclera, conjunctiva
CS&CC	culture, sensitivity, and colony count
CSD	cat scratch disease; celiac sprue disease
CSE	cross section echocardiography
C sect	cesarean section

CSF	cerebrospinal fluid; colony-stimulating factor
CSH	carotid sinus hypersensitivity
CSICU	cardiac surgery intensive care unit
CSII	continuous subcutaneous insulin infusion
CSLU	chronic stasis leg ulcer
CSM	circulation, sensation, movement; cerebrospinal meningitis
CSOM	chronic serous otitis media
CSP	cellulose sodium phosphate
C spine	cervical spine
CSR	Cheyne-Stokes respiration; central supply room
CST	convulsive shock therapy; contraction stress test; cosyntropin stimulation test; certified surgical technologist
CSU	cardiac surveillance unit; cardiovascular surgery unit
CT	computed tomography; circulation time; coagulation time; clotting time; corneal thickness; cervical traction; Coomb's test; cardiothoracic; coated tablet
CTA	clear to auscultation
CTB	ceased to breathe
CTD	chest tube drainage; cumulative trauma disorder
CT&DB	cough, turn, and deep breathe
CTF	Colorado tick fever
CTL	cytotoxic T lymphocytes
CT/MPR	computed tomography with multiplanar reconstructions
cTNM	clinical-diagnostic staging of cancer (tumor, node, metastasis)
CTP	comprehensive treatment plan
CTS	carpal tunnel syndrome
CTSP	called to see patient
CTW	central terminal of Wilson
CTXN	contraction
CTZ	chemoreceptor trigger zone
CU	cause unknown
CUC	chronic ulcerative colitis
CUD	cause undetermined
CUG	cystourethrogram
CUS	chronic undifferentiated schizophrenia
CV	cardiovascular; cell volume; curriculum vita (vitae)
CVA	cerebrovascular accident; costovertebral angle
CVAT	costovertebral angle tenderness

CVC	central venous catheter
CVD	collagen vascular disease
CVI	cerebrovascular insufficiency; continuous venous infusion
CVID	common variable immune deficiency
CVO	central vein occlusion; conjugate diameter of pelvic inlet
CVP	central venous pressure
CVRI	coronary vascular resistance index
CVS	clean voided specimen; cardiovascular system; chorionic villus sampling
CVUG	cysto-void urethrogram
CW	crutch walking
C/W	consistent with
CWMS	color, warmth, movement, sensation
CWP	coal worker's pneumoconiosis
Cx	cervix; culture; cancel
CXR	chest X-ray
cysto	cystoscopy; cystogram
d	day *(dies)*; right *(dexter)*
D	diarrhea; divorced; distal; dead; diopter; cholecalciferol, vitamin D
D_1	first dorsal vertebra
D_2	second dorsal vertebra
D5LR	dextrose (5 percent) in lactated Ringer's solution
D5NS	5 percent dextrose in normal saline
D5W	5 percent dextrose in water
DA	direct admission
DAD	drug administration device
DAF	decay-accelerating factor
DAH	disordered action of the heart
DAI	diffuse axonal injury
DAL	drug analysis laboratory
DANA	drug-induced antinuclear antibodies
DAPT	draw-a-person test
DAT	direct agglutination test; diet as tolerated; dementia of the Alzheimer type
DAVE	average diameter
DAW	dispense as written
DAWN	Drug Abuse Warning Network
db	decibel (dB)

DB	date of birth
DBil	direct bilirubin
DBP	diastolic blood pressure
DBS	diminished breath sounds
DC	discontinue; discharge; decrease; diagonal conjugate; Doctor of Chiropractic
D&C	dilation and curettage
D/C	discontinue; discharge
DCH	delayed cutaneous hypersensitivity
DCI	duplicate coverage inquiry
DCO	diffusing capacity of carbon monoxide
DCR	delayed cutaneous reaction
DCSA	double contrast shoulder arthrography
DCT	direct (antiglobulin) Coombs test; deep chest therapy
DCTM	delay computer tomographic myelography
DD	differential diagnosis; down drain; dependent drainage; dry dressing; Duchenne's dystrophy
D&D	diarrhea and dehydration
DDD	degenerative disc disease; dense deposit (renal) disease
DDS	dialysis disequilibrium syndrome; Doctor of Dental Surgery
DDx	differential diagnosis
D&E	dilation and evacuation
DEA	Drug Enforcement Administration
decub	decubitus
DEF	decayed, extracted, or filled
degen	degenerative
DEHP	diethyl hexyl phthalate
del	delivery, delivered
DEP ST SEG	depressed ST segment
DER	disulfiram-ethanol reaction
derm	dermatology
DES	disequilibrium syndrome; diffuse esophageal spasm
DESI	Drug Efficacy Study Implementation
DEV	duck embryo vaccine; deviation
DEVR	dominant exudative vitreoretinopathy
dex	right
DEXA	dual energy X-ray absorpiometry
DF	decayed and filled
DFD	defined formula diets
DFE	distal femoral epiphysis

DFMC	daily fetal movement count
DFR	diabetic floor routine
DFU	dead fetus in uterus
dgeo	geometric diameter
DGI	disseminated gonococcal infection
DGM	ductal glandular mastectomy
DH	developmental history; diaphragmatic hernia; delayed hypersensitivity
DHF	dengue hemorrhagic fever
DHHS	Department of Health and Human Services
DHL	diffuse histiocytic lymphoma
DHS	duration of hospital stay
DI	diabetes insipidus (DIP); detrusor instability; drug information; drug interaction
DIA	Drug Information Association
diag	diagnosis
DIC	Drug Information Center; disseminated intravascular coagulation
diff	differential blood count
DIJOA	dominantly inherited juvenile optic atrophy
dil	dilute
DIL	drug-induced lupus erythematosus
DILD	diffuse infiltrative lung disease
dim	diminish
DIP	diabetes insipidus (DI); distal interphalangeal; desquamative interstitial pneumonia; drip infusion pyelogram
dis	dislocation
disch	discharge
DISH	diffuse idiopathic skeletal hyperostosis
dist	distilled
DIV	double inlet ventricle
DIVA	digital intravenous angiography
DJD	degenerative joint disease
DKA	diabetic ketoacidosis
dl	deciliter (dL; DL)
DL	danger list; direct laryngoscopy; diagnostic laparoscopy
DLE	discoid lupus erythematosus
DLIS	digitalis-like immunoreactive substance
DLMP	date of last menstrual period
DLNMP	date of last normal menstrual period

DM	diabetes mellitus; diastolic murmur; dermatomyositis; disease management
DMARD	disease-modifying antirheumatic drug
DMD	Duchenne's muscular dystrophy
DME	durable medical equipment
DMF	decayed, missing, or filled
DMFT	decayed, missing, and filled teeth
DMOOC	diabetes mellitus out of control
DMSO	dimethyl sulfoxide
DMT	dimethyltryptamine
DMX	diathermy, massage, and exercise
DN	down
DNA	deoxyribonucleic acid
DNI	do not intubate
DNKA	did not keep appointment
DNP	do not publish
DNR	do not resuscitate/report/refill
DNS	do not show; deviated nasal septum; dysplastic nevus syndrome
DO	right eye; Doctor of Osteopathy
DOA	dead on arrival; date of admission
DOA-DRA	dead on arrival, despite resuscitative attempts
DOB	date of birth
DOC	drug of choice; died of other causes
DOE	dyspnea on exertion
DOI	date of injury
DORV	double outlet right ventricle
DORx	date of treatment
DOT	Doppler ophthalmic test; died on table
DP	dorsalis pedis (pulse); diastolic pressure
DPC	discharge planning coordinator; delayed primary closure
DPDL	diffuse poorly differentiated lymphocytic lymphoma
DPM	disintegrations per minute; Doctor of Podiatric Medicine
DPN	diabetic peripheral neuropathy; diphosphopyridine nucleotide
DPT	diphtheria, pertussis, and tetanus (vaccine)
DPU	delayed pressure urticaria
DR	delivery room; diabetic retinopathy; doctor
DR&C	deep respiration and coughing
DRE	digital rectal exam

DREZ	dorsal root entry zone
DRG	diagnosis-related group
DRP	drug-related problem
DRR	drug regimen review
DRSG	dressing (dsg)
DS	discharge summary; Down's syndrome; double strength; disoriented; dextrose stick
DSA	digital subtraction angiography
DSAP	disseminated superficial actinic porokeratosis
DSC	differential scanning calorimetry
DSD	dry sterile dressing; discharge summary dictated
dsg	dressing (DRSG)
DSHEA	Dietary Supplement Health and Education Act of 1994
DSI	deep shock insulin
DSIAR	double-stapled ilenanal reservoir
DSM	disease state management
DSM-IV	*Diagnostic and Statistical Manual of Mental Disorders,* Fourth Edition
DSS	dengue shock syndrome
DST	dexamethasone suppression test; donor-specific transfusion
DT	diptheria-tetanus; diptheria-toxoid
DTA	differential thermal analysis
DTCA	direct-to-consumer advertising
dtd	give of such doses *(dentur tales doses)*
DTH	delayed-type hypersensitivity
DTP	drug therapy problem
DTR	deep tendon reflexes
DTs	delirium tremens
DTS	donor transfusion, specific
DTT	diphtheria tetanus toxoid
DTV	due to void
DTX	detoxification
DU	duodenal ulcer; duroxide uptake; diabetic urine; diagnosis undetermined
DUB	dysfunctional uterine bleeding
DUE	drug use evaluation
DUI	driving under the influence
DUR	drug utilization review
DVD	dissociated vertical deviation
DVIU	direct vision internal urethrotomy

DVR	double valve replacement
DVT	deep vein thrombosis
DW	distilled water; deionized water
DWDL	diffuse, well-differentiated lymphocytic lymphoma
Dx	diagnosis
Dz	disease; dozen
E	edema, enzyme
E^1	elimination reaction, monomolecular
E^2	elimination reaction, bimolecular
EAC	estimated acquisition cost; external auditory canal
EAHF	eczema, allergy, hay fever
EAM	external auditory meatus
EAR	early asthmatic response
EAST	external rotation, abduction stress test
EAT	ectopic atrial tachycardia
EB	epidermolysis bullosa
EBL	estimated blood loss
EBV	Epstein-Barr virus
EC	enteric coated; eyes closed; extracellular; Enzyme Commission (number)
ECBD	exploration of common bile duct
ECC	emergency cardiac care
ECCE	extracapsular cataract extraction
ECD	endocardial cushion defect
ECEMG	evoked compound electromyography
ECF	extracellular fluid; extended care facility; eosinophilic chemotactic factor
ECG	electrocardiogram (EKG)
echo	echocardiogram (ECHO)
ECHO	etoposide, cyclophosphamide, adriamycin (hydroxydaunomycin), and oncovin (vincristine)
ECL	extent of cerebral lesion; extracapillary lesions
ECM	erythema chronicum migrans
ECMO	extracorporeal membrane oxygenation
ECN	extended care nursery
EC No.	Enzyme Commission number
ECR	emergency chemical restraint
ECRL	extensor carpi radialis longus
ECT	electroconvulsive therapy; enhanced computer tomography; emission computed tomography
ECU	extensor carpi ulnaris

ECW	extracellular water
ED	emergency department; epidural
ED$_{50}$	median effective dose
EDC	estimated date of confinement; estimated date of conception; end diastolic counts
EDD	expected date of delivery
EDF	extension, derotation, flexion
EDM	early diastolic murmur
EDS	Ehlers-Danlos syndrome
EDTA	ethylenediaminetetraacetic acid; edetic acid (ethylenediamine tetracetic acid)
EDV	end-diastolic volume
EE	equine encephalitis; end to end
EEE	Eastern equine encephalomyelitis; edema, erythema, and exudate
EEG	electroencephalogram
EENT	eyes, ears, nose, throat
EES	erythromycin ethylsuccinate
EF	extended-field (radiotherapy); endurance factor; ejection fraction
EFAD	essential fatty acid deficiency
EFE	endocardial fibroelastosis
EFM	external fetal monitoring
EFW	estimated fetal weight
EGA	estimated gestational age
EGBUS	external genitalia, Bartholin, urethral, Skene's (glands)
EGD	esophagogastroduodenoscopy
EGF	epidermal growth factor
EGTA	esophageal gastric tube airway
EH	essential hypertension; enlarged heart; extramedullary hematopoiesis
EHB	elevate head of bed
EHF	epidemic hemorrhagic fever
E&I	endocrine and infertility
EIA	exercise-induced asthma; enzyme immunoassay
EIAB	extracranial-intracranial arterial bypass
EIB	exercise-induced bronchospasm
EID	electronic infusion device
EIF	eukaryotic initiation factor
EIS	endoscopic injection scleropathy
EJ	external jugular; elbow jerk

EKC	epidemic keratoconjunctivitis
EKG	electrocardiogram (ECG)
E-L	external lids
ELF	elective low forceps
ELH	endolymphatic hydrops
ELISA	enzyme-linked immunosorbent assay
elix	elixir
ELOP	estimated length of program
ELP	electrophoresis
EM	electron microscope; ejection murmur; erythema multiforme
EMB	endomyocardial biopsy
EMC	encephalomyocarditis; equilibrium moisture content
EMD	electromechanical dissociation
EMF	erythrocyte maturation factor; electromotive force
EMG	electromyography; essential monoclonal gammopathy
EMIC	emergency maternity and infant care
E-MICR	electron microscopy
EMIT	enzyme multiplied immunoassay technique
emp	as directed; in the manner prescribed *(ex modo praescripto)*
EMR	emergency mechanical restraint; empty, measure, and record; educable mentally retarded; electronic medical record
EMS	emergency medical services/systems
EMT	emergency medical technician
EMV	eye, motor, verbal
EMW	electromagnetic waves
EN	enteral nutrition
ENA	extractable nuclear antigen
endo	endotracheal
ENG	electronystagmography
ENL	erythema nodosum leprosum
ENP	extractable nucleoprotein
ENT	ears, nose, throat
EO	eyes open
EOA	examination, opinion, and advice; esophageal obturator airway
EOG	electro-oculogram
EOM	extraocular movement; extraocular muscles
EOMI	extraocular muscles intact

EORA	elderly onset rheumatoid arthritis
eos	eosinophil
EP	endogenous pyrogen; electrophysiologic
EPA	Environmental Protection Agency
EPB	extensor pollicis brevis
epis	episiotomy
epith	epithelial
EPL	extensor pollicis longus
EPM	electronic pacemaker
EPO	exclusive provider organization
EPP	erythropoietic protoporphyria
EPR	electrophrenic respiration; emergency physical restraint; electron paramagnetic resonance
EPS	electrophysiologic study; extrapyramidal syndrome/symptoms
EPT	early pregnancy test
EPTS	existed prior to service
ER	emergency room; estrogen receptor; external rotation
ERA	evoked response audiometry; estrogen receptor assay
ERCP	endoscopic retrograde cholangiopancreatography
ERFC	erythrocyte rosette-forming cells
ERG	electroretinogram
ERL	effective refractory length
ERP	estrogen receptor protein; endoscopic retrograde pancreatography
ERPF	effective renal plasma flow
ERPs	event-related potentials (of the brain)
ERT	estrogen replacement therapy
ERV	expiratory reserve volume
ESAP	evoked sensory (nerve) action potentiation
ESM	ejection systolic murmur
ESP	end systolic pressure
ESR	erythrocyte sedimentation rate; electron spin resonance
ESRD	end-stage renal disease
EST	electroshock therapy
ESU	electrostatic units
ESWL	extracorporeal shock wave lithotripsy
ET	endotracheal; esotropia; eustachian tube; ejection time; exercise treadmill
ETF	eustachian tubal function
ETO	estimated time of ovulation
EtOH	ethyl alcohol; ethanol

ETS	environmental tobacco smoke
ETT	endotracheal tube; exercise tolerance test
EU	excretory urography
EUA	examine under anesthesia
EUS	endoscopic ultrasonography
evac	evacuation
eval	evaluate
EWB	estrogen withdrawal bleeding
EWSCLs	extended-wear soft contact lenses
exam	examination
exp	exploration; experienced
exp lap	exploratory laparotomy
ext	extract *(extractum);* external
ext rot	external rotation
EX U	excretory urogram
F	Fahrenheit; female; flow; facial; firm; Faraday
F1	offspring from first generation
F2	offspring from second generation
FA	femoral artery
FAAP	family assessment adjustment pass
FAC	fractional area concentration
FACH	forceps to after-coming head
FACS	Fellow of the American College of Surgeons
FAD	Family Assessment Device; flavin adenine dinucleotide
FAHRB	Federation of Associations of Health Regulatory Boards
FAI	functional assessment inventory
fall	fallopian
fam	family
FANA	fluorescent antinuclear antibody
FAP	fibrillating action potential; familial amyloid polyneuropathy; familial adenomatous polyposis
FAPhA	Fellow of the American Pharmacists Association
FAS	fetal alcohol syndrome
FASHP	Fellow of the American Society of Health-System Pharmacists; Federal Association of Schools of Health Professionals
FAST	functional assessment staging test (of Alzheimer's disease); fluoro-allegro sorbent test; fetal acoustical stimulation test

FAT	fluorescent antibody test
FB	foreign body; finger breadth
FBG	fasting blood glucose
FBM	fetal breathing movements
FBN	fibronectin
FBP	fetal biophysical profile
FBS	fasting blood sugar; fetal bovine serum
FBU	fingers below umbilicus
FBW	fasting blood work
FC	Foley catheter; finger counting; fever, chills
F&C	foam and condom; flare and cells
F cath	Foley catheter
FCC	follicular center cells; familial colonic cancer; fracture compound comminuted
FCDB	fibrocystic disease of the breast
FCH	familial combined hyperlipedemia
FCMC	family-centered maternity care
FCMD	Fukuyama's congenital muscular dystrophy
FCMN	family-centered maternity nursing
FCR	flexor carpi radialis
FCRB	flexor carpi radialis brevis
FCSNVD	fever, chills, sweating, nausea, vomiting, diarrhea
FCU	flexor carpi ulnaris
FD	focal distance; familial dysautonomia
F&D	fixed and dilated
FDA	fronto-dextra anterior; Food and Drug Administration
FDC	Food, Drug, and Cosmetic (Act)
FDIU	fetal death in utero
FDLE	Federal Drug Law Examination
FDP	fibrin-degradation products; flexor digitorum profundus
FDS	flexor digitorum superficials; for duration of stay
Fe	iron
FEC	forced expiratory capacity
FEF	forced expiratory flow
FEHBP	Federal Employees Health Benefit Program
FEL	familial erythrophagocytic lymphohistiocytosis
fem	femoral
fem-pop	femoral popliteal (bypass)
FEN	fluid, electrolytes, nutrition
FE$_{na}$	fractional extraction of sodium

FEP	Federal Employee Plan; free erythrocyse protoporphyrin
FeSO$_4$	ferrous sulfate
FEV	forced expiratory volume
FEV$_1$	forced expiratory volume in one second
FF	filtration fraction; fundus firm; flat feet; fat free; force fluids
FFA	free fatty acid
F factor	fertility/sex factor
FFP	fresh frozen plasma
FFS	fee for service
FFT	fast-Fourier transforms
FGF	fibroblast growth factor
FH	family history
FHF	fulminant hepatic failure
FHH	familial hypocalciuric hypercalcemia
FHI	Fuchs heterochromic iridocyclitis
FHR	fetal heart rate
FHS	fetal heart sounds; fetal hydantoin syndrome
FHT	fetal heart tone
FICA	Federal Insurance Contributions Act
FiCO$_2$	fraction of inspired carbon dioxide
FIFO	first in, first out
FIM	functional independent measure
FiO$_2$	fraction of inspired oxygen
FIP	Federation Internationale Pharmaceutique (International Pharmaceutical Federation)
floc	flocculation
FLS	flashing lights and/or scotoma
FM	fetal movements; face mask
F&M	firm and midline (uterus)
FMC	fetal movement count
FMD	foot and mouth disease
FME	full-mouth extraction
FMF	forced midexpiratory flow; familial Mediterranean fever
FMG	foreign medical graduate; fine mesh gauze
FMH	family medical history; fibromuscular hyperplasia
FMN	flavin mononucleotide
FMP	fasting metabolic panel
FMS	fibromyalgia syndrome
FMX	full-mouth X-ray

FN	false negative; finger-to-nose (FTN)
FNAB	fine-needle aspiration biopsy
FNAC	fine-needle aspiration cytology
FNH	focal nodular hyperplasia; febrile nonhemolytic reaction
FNR	false negative rate
FNS	functional neuromuscular stimulation
FOB	foot of bed; fiberoptic bronchoscope; father of baby
FOBT	fecal occult blood test
FOC	father of child
FOD	free of disease
FOI	flight of ideas; freedom of information
FOOB	fell out of bed
FP	family planning; family practice; frozen plasma; flat plate; false positive; flavoprotein
FPAL	full-term, premature, abortion, living
FPB	flexor pollicis brevis
FPD	feto-pelvic disproportion; fixed partial denture
FPG	fasting plasma glucose
FPGEE	Foreign Pharmacy Graduate Equivalency Examination
FPIA	fluorescence-polarization immunoassay
FPL	flexor pollicis longus
FPNA	first-pass nuclear angiocardiography
FR	flow rate
F&R	flow and rhythm (pulse)
FRC	functional residual capacity
FRJM	full range of joint motion
FROM	full range of movement
FS	frozen section; flexible sigmoidoscopy
FSB	fetal scalp blood
FSBM	full-strength breast milk
FSE	fetal scalp electrode
FSG	focal segmental glomerulosclerosis
FSGS	focal and segmental glomerulosclerosis
FSH	follicle-stimulating hormone; facioscapulohumeral
FSHMD	facioscapulohumeral muscular dystrophy
FSHRF	follicle-stimulating hormone releasing factor
FSP	fibrin split products
FT	full term
FTA	fluorescent titer antibody; fluorescent treponemal antibody

FTC	Federal Trade Commission
FTD	failure to descend
FTI	free thyroxine index
FTLFC	full-term living female child
FTLMC	full-term living male child
FTN	finger-to-nose (FN); full-term nursery
FTND	full-term normal delivery
FTP	failure to progress
FTR	for the record
FTSG	full-thickness skin graft
FTT	failure to thrive
F&U	flanks and upper quadrants
F/U	follow-up; fundus at umbilicus
FUN	follow-up note
FUO	fever of undetermined origin
FUR	functional uterine bleeding
FVC	forced vital capacity
FVH	focal vascular headache
FVL	flow volume loop
FWB	full weight bearing
FWS	fetal warfarin syndrome
FWW	front wheel walker
Fx	fracture (Fxr); fractional urine; function (Fxn)
Fx-dis	fracture-dislocation
Fxn	function (Fx)
Fxr	fracture (Fx)
FY	fiscal year

g	gram (gm)
G	gauge; gallop
G 1-4	grades 1-4
G6PD	glucose-6-phosphate dehydrogenase
GA	gastric analysis; general appearance; general anesthesia; gestational age
GABA	gamma-aminobutyric acid
GABHS	group A beta hemolytic streptococci
GAD	generalized anxiety disorder
GAF	Global Assessment of Functioning (Scale)
GAO	General Accounting Office
GAS	general adaptation syndrome
GAT	group adjustment therapy
GB	gallbladder

GBM	glomerular basement membrane
GBP	gastric bypass
GBS	gallbladder series; Guillain-Barr syndrome; group B streptococci
GC	gonococci (gonorrhea); gas chromatography
G+C	gram-positive cocci
G–C	gram-negative cocci
GCA	giant cell arteritis
GCDFP	gross cystic disease fluid protein
GCIIS	glucose control insulin infusion system
GCS	Glasgow coma scale
GCT	giant cell tumor
GD	Graves disease
G&D	growth and development
GDF	gel diffusion precipitin
GDM	gestational diabetes mellitus
GDP	guanosine 5'-diphosphate
GE	gastroenteritis
GEP	general enrollment period; gastroenteropancreatic
GER	gastroesophageal reflux
GERD	gastroesophageal reflux disease (GRD)
GETA	general endotracheal anesthesia
GF	grandfather; gluten-free; gastric fistula
GFR	glomerular filtration rate
GFW	gram formula weight
GGE	generalized glandular enlargement
GH	growth hormone
GHD	growth hormone deficiency
GHQ	general health questionnaire
GI	gastrointestinal; granuloma inguinale
GIB	gastric ileal bypass
GIC	general immunocompetence
GIFT	gamete intrafallopian treatment
GIP	giant cell interstitial pneumonia; gastric inhibiting peptide; gastric inhibitory polypeptide
GIS	gastrointestinal series
GIT	gastrointestinal tract
GJ	gastrojejunostomy
GL	greatest length
GLA	gingivolinguoaxial
GLNH	giant lymph node hyperplasia
GLP	good laboratory practice(s)

GM	grandmother
GMC	general medicine clinic
GMP	good manufacturing practice(s)
GMT	geometric mean (antibody) titer
GN	glomerulonephritis; gram-negative
GnRH	gonadotropin-releasing hormone
GOT	glutamate oxaloacetate transaminase
GP	general practitioner; gutta percha
G/P	gravida/para
GPC	gram-positive cocci; giant papillary conjunctivitis
GPIA	Generic Pharmaceutical Industry Association
GPN	graduate practical nurse
GPO	group purchasing organization
GPPP	group practice prepayment plan
GPT	glutamate pyruvate transaminase
gr	grain
G+R	gram-positive rods
G–R	gram-negative rods
GRAS	generally regarded as safe
grav	gravid (pregnant)
GRD	gastroesophageal reflux disease (GERD)
GRN	granules
GSD	glycogen storage disease
GSE	grip strong and equal; gluten-sensitive enteropathy
GSI	genuine stress incontinence
GSP	general survey panel
GSPN	greater superficial petrosal neurectomy
GSR	galvanic skin resistance
GSW	gunshot wound
gt	drop *(gutta)*
GT	gastrotomy tube; gait training
GTF	glucose tolerance factor
GTN	gestational trophoblastic neoplasms
GTP	glutamyl transpeptidase; guanosine 5'-triphosphate
gtt	drops *(guttae)*
GTT	glucose tolerance test
GU	genitourinary
GUS	genitourinary sphincter; genitourinary system
GVF	good visual fields
GVHD	graft-versus-host disease
GWA	gunshot wound of the abdomen
GWT	gunshot wound of the throat

GXT	graded exercise testing
GYN	gynecology
H	hypodermic; hour; heroin; hydrogen; husband
H$_1$	histamine receptor subtype 1
H$_2$	histamine receptor subtype 2
H$_2$O	water
HA	headache; hyperalimentation; hypothalamic amenorrhea; hearing aid; hemolytic anemia; hospital admission; hepatitis, type A; hemagglutination assay
HAA	hepatitis-associated antigen
HAE	hereditary angioedema; hepatic artery embolization; hearing aid evaluation
HAI	hepatic arterial infusion
HAL	hyperalimentation
HAN	heroin-associated nephropathy
HANE	heredity angioneurotic edema
HAPS	hepatic arterial perfusion scintigraphy
HAQ	Health Assessment Questionnaire
HAS	hyperalimentation solution
HASHD	hypertensive arteriosclerotic heart disease
HAT	head, arms, and trunk
HAV	hepatitis A virus; hallux abducto valgus
Hb	hemoglobin
HB	hemoglobin; heart block; hepatitis, type B; hold breakfast; heartburn
HBA	hepatitis B antigen
HBBW	hold breakfast, blood work
HBD	has been drinking
HBF	hepatic blood flow
HBGM	home blood glucose monitoring
HBI	hemibody irradiation
HBO	hyperbaric oxygen
HBP	high blood pressure
HBS	Health Behavior Scale
HBsAg	hepatitis B surface antigen
HBV	hepatitis B virus; hepatitis B vaccine
HC	home care; head circumference; heel cord; house call; Hickman catheter
HCA	health care aide
HCC	hepatocellular carcinoma
HCFA	Health Care Financing Administration (now CMS)

HCG	human chorionic gonadotropin
HCL	hair cell leukemia
HCLs	hard contact lenses
HCM	health care maintenance; hypertropic cardiomyopathy
HCO$_3$	bicarbonate
HCP	hereditary coprophemia
HCT	hematocrit; histamine challenge test
HCV	hepatitis C virus
HCVD	hypertensive cardiovascular disease
HD	Hodgkin's disease; Huntington's disease; hearing distance; hemodialysis; hip disarticulation; high dose
HDC	high-dose chemotherapy
HDCV	human diploid cell vaccine
HDL	high-density lipoprotein
HDLW	hearing distance for watch ticking in left ear
HDMA	Health Distributors Manufacturers Association (formerly NWDA)
HDN	hemolytic disease of the newborn
HDPAA	heparin-dependent, platelet-associated antibody
HDRS	Hamilton Depression Rate Scale
HDRW	hearing distance for watch ticking in right ear
HDV	hepatitis D virus
H&E	hemorrhage and exudate; hematoxylin and eosin
HEDIS	Health Plan Employer Data and Information Set
HEENT	head, eyes, ears, nose, throat
HEK	human embryonic kidney
HEL	human embryonic lung
hemi	hemiplegia
HEMPAS	hereditary erythrocytic multinuclearity with positive acidified serum test
HEP	histamine equivalent prick; hepatic; heparin
HEPLOCK	heparin lock
HES	hypereosinophilic syndrome
HEV	hepatitis E virus
HF	heart failure
HFD	high forceps delivery
HFHL	high-frequency hearing loss
Hgb	hemoglobin
HGH	human growth hormone
HGPRT	hypoxanthine-guanine phosphoriboxyltranferase
HH	hiatal hernia; home health
H&H	hematocrit and hemoglobin

HHA	home health agency
HHC	home health care
HHD	hypertensive heart disease
HHFM	high-humidity face mask
HHH	high, hot, and a "hell of a lot" (order for an uncomfortable enema)
HHN	handheld nebulizer
HHNK	hyperglycemic hyperosmolar nonketotic (coma)
HHS	Health and Human Services (Department)
HHT	hereditary hemorrhagic telangiectasis
HHV-6	human herpes virus 6
HI	hemagglutination inhibition; head injury
HIA	hemagglutination inhibition antibody
HIB	health insurance benefits; hospital insurance benefits
HIBv	haemophilus influenzae type B vaccine
HICN	health insurance claim number
HID	headache, insomnia, depression
HIE	hypoxic-ischemic encephalopathy
HIF	higher integrative functions
HIL	hypoxic-ischemic lesion
HIM	health insurance manual
HIPAA	Health Insurance Portability and Accountability Act of 1996
HIR	health insurance regulations; head injury routine
HIS	Health Intention Scale
histo	histoplasmin skin test; histoplasmosis
HIT	heparin-induced thrombocytopenia; histamine inhalation test
HIV	human immunodeficiency virus
HIVD	herniated intervertebral disk
HJR	hepato-jugular reflex
H-K	hand to knee; heel to knee
HKAFO	hip-knee-ankle-foot orthosis
HKO	hip-knee orthosis
HL	heparin lock; harelip; hairline; hearing level; Hickman line
HLA	human leukocyte antigen
HLB	hydrophil-lipophil-balance
HLD	herniated lumbar disc
HLHS	hypoplastic left heart syndrome
HLV	hypoplastic left ventricle
HM	hand motion

HMD	hyaline membrane disease
HMG	human menopausal gonadotropin
HMI	healed myocardial infarction
HMO	health maintenance organization
HMP	hexose monophosphate; hot moist packs
HMR	histiocytic medullary reticulosis
HMX	heat massage exercise
HN	high nitrogen
H&N	head and neck
HNP	herniated nucleus pulposus
hnRNA	heterogeneous nuclear ribonucleic acid
HNV	has not voided
H/O	history of
HOB	head of bed
HOB UPSOB	head of bed up for shortness of breath
HOC	Health Officer Certificate
HOCM	hypertrophic obstructive cardiomyopathy
HOH	hard of hearing
HP	hemiplegia; hemipelvectomy; hot packs
H&P	history and physical
HPA	human papilloma virus (HPV); hypothalamic-pituitary-adrenal (axis)
HPF	high-power field
HPFH	hereditary persistence of fetal hemoglobin
HPG	human pituitary gonadotropin
HPI	history of present illness
HPL	human placental lactogen
HPLC	high-pressure (performance) liquid chromatography
HPM	hemiplegic migraine
HPN	home parenteral nutrition
HPO	hypertrophic pulmonary osteoarthropathy; hydrophilic ointment
HPT	hyperparathyroidism
HPV	human papilloma virus (HPA)
H&P	history and physical
HPZ	high-pressure zone
HR	heart rate; hour; hallux rigidus; hospital record; Harrington rod
HRA	histamine-releasing activity
HRIG	human rabies immune globulin
HRLA	human retrovirus-like agent
HRPC	Heat Responsive Pain Council

HRS	hepatorenal syndrome
HRT	hormone replacement therapy
hs	bedtime *(hora somni)*
HS	hereditary spherocytosis; heel spur; heel stick
H-S	heel to shin
HSA	human serum albumin; hypersomnia-sleep apnea; Health Systems Agency; health supports and appliances
HSBG	heelstick bloodgas
HSG	hysterosalpingogram
HSM	hepato-splenomegaly; holosystolic murmur
HSP	Henoch-Schonlein purpura
HSR	heated serum reagent
HSSE	high soap suds enema
HSV	herpes simplex virus
HT	hypertension; Hubbard tank; height; heart; hammertoe
ht aer	heated aerosol
HTC	hypertensive crisis
HTF	house tube feeding
HTL	human thymic leukemia
HTLV	human T-cell leukemia virus
HTLV III	human T-cell lymphotrophic virus type III
HTN	hypertension
HTP	House-Tree-Person test
HTR	hemolytic transfusion reaction
HTVD	hypertensive vascular disease
hum	humidifier (HUM)
HUS	hemolytic uremic syndrome
HV	hallux valgus; has voided
H&V	hemigastrectomy and vagotomy
HWB	hot water bottle
Hx	history; hospitalization
HXM	hexamethylmelamine
HZ	herpes zoster
HZO	herpes zoster ophthalmicus
I	independent; impression; incisal; one
IA	intra-amniotic
IAA	interrupted aortic arch
IABC	intra-aortic balloon counterpulsation
IABP	intra-aortic balloon pump
IAC	internal auditory canal

IAC-CPR	interposed abdominal compressions–cardiopulmonary resuscitation
IACP	intra-aortic counterpulsation
IADH	inappropriate antidiuretic hormone
IA DSA	intra-arterial digital subtraction arteriography
IAHA	immune adherence hemagglutination
IAI	intra-abdominal infection
IAM	internal auditory meatus
IAN	intern admission note
IAP	intermittent acute porphyria
IASD	interatrial septal defect
IAT	indirect antiglobulin test
IB	isolation bed
IBC	iron-binding capacity
IBD	inflammatory bowel disease
IBI	intermittent bladder irrigation
ibid	at the same place
IBNR	incurred but not reported
IBS	irritable bowel syndrome
IBW	ideal body weight
IC	irritable colon; intercostal; intracranial; individual counseling; inspiratory capacity
ICA	internal carotid artery; islet cell antibodies
ICBT	intercostobronchial trunk
ICC	Interstate Commerce Commission
ICCE	intracapsular cataract extraction
ICCU	intermediate coronary care unit
ICD	isocitrate dehydrogenase; instantaneous cardiac death
ICD-9-CM	*International Classification of Diseases,* Ninth Revision, *Clinical Modification*
ICF	intracellular fluid; intermediate care facility
ICF/MR	intermediate care facility for the mentally retarded
ICG	indocyanine green
ICH	intracranial hemorrhage
ICM	intracostal margin
ICN	intensive care nursery
ICP	intracranial pressure
ICPP	intubated continuous positive pressure
ICS	intercostal space
ICSH	interstitial cell-stimulating hormone
ICT	intensive conventional therapy; inflammation of connective tissue

ICU	intensive care unit
ICVH	ischemic cerebrovascular headache
ICW	intercellular water
ID	intradermal; initial dose, infectious disease; identification; identify
I&D	incision and drainage
IDDM	insulin-dependent diabetes mellitus
IDDS	implantable drug delivery system
IDE	Investigational Device Exemption
IDFC	immature dead female child
IDM	infant of a diabetic mother
IDMC	immature dead male child
IDV	intermittent demand ventilation
IEC	inpatient exercise center
IEF	isoelectric focusing
IEM	immune electron microscopy
IEP	individualized education program; immunoelectrophoresis; initial enrollment period
IF	intrinsic factor; immunofluorescence
IFA	indirect fluorescent antibody test
IFE	immunofixation electrophoresis
IFN	interferon
IG	Inspector General
IgA	immunoglobulin A
IgD	immunoglobulin D
IgE	immunoglobulin E
IGF	insulin-like growth factor
IgG	immunoglobulin G; immune gammaglobulin
IGIV	immune globulin intravenous
IgM	immunoglobulin M
IGR	intrauterine growth retardation
IGT	impaired glucose tolerance
IH	infectious hepatitis; inguinal hernia; indirect hemagglutination (IHA)
IHA	immune hemagglutination assay; indirect hemagglutination (IH)
IHC	immobilization hypercalcemia
IHD	ischemic heart disease; intrahepatic duct
IHH	idiopathic hypogonadotropic hypogonadism
IHs	iris hamartomas
IHS	Indian Health Service; Idiopathic Headache Score

IHSS	idiopathic hypertrophic subaortic stenosis; idiopathic hypertrophic supra-aortic stenosis
IHT	insulin hypoglycemia test
IICP	increased intracranial pressure
IICU	infant intensive care unit
IIT	intensive insulin therapy
IJ	internal jugular; ileojejunal
IL	intermediary letter; independent living
ILD	ischemic leg disease
ILFC	immature living female child
ILM	internal limiting membrane
ILMC	immature living male child
ILMI	inferolateral myocardial infarct
IM	intramuscular; infectious mononucleosis; information memorandum; intermetatarsal; internal medicine
IMA	inferior mesenteric artery; internal mammary artery
IMAG	internal mammary artery graft
IMB	intermenstrual bleeding
IMF	intermaxillary fixation
IMG	internal medicine group (practice)
IMH	indirect microhemagglutination (test)
IMI	inferior myocardial infarction
IMIG	intramuscular immunoglobulin
IMN	internal mammary (lymph) node
imp	impacted
INB	intermittent nebulized beta-agonists
inc	incomplete; incontinent
INC	inside-the-needle catheter
IND	investigational new drug
INDA	Investigational New Drug Application
INDM	infant of nondiabetic mother
inf	inferior; infusion; infant; infected
ing	inguinal
inj	injection; injury
INN	international nonproprietary name
ins	insurance
inst	instrumental (delivery)
int	internal
int-rot	internal rotation
inver	inversion
IO	intraocular pressure; inferior oblique; initial opening
I&O	intake and output

IOC	intraoperative cholangiogram
IOD	interorbital distance
IOF	intraocular fluid
IOFB	intraocular foreign body
IOH	idiopathic orthostatic hypotension
IOL	intraocular lens
ION	ischemic optic neuropathy
IOP	intraocular pressure
IORT	intraoperative radiation therapy
IOS	intraoperative sonography
IOV	initial office visit
IP	intraperitoneal; inpatient
IPA	invasive pulmonary aspergillosis; individual practice association
IPCD	infantile polycystic disease
IPD	immediate pigment darkening; intermittent peritoneal dialysis
IPFD	intrapartum fetal distress
IPG	impedance plethysmography
IPJ	interphalangeal joint
IPK	intractable plantar keratosis
IPMI	inferoposterior myocardial infarct
IPN	infantile periarteritis nodosa; intern progress note; independent practice network
IPP	inflatable penile prosthesis
IPPA	inspection, palpation, percussion, and auscultation
IPPB	intermittent positive pressure breathing
IPPV	intermittent positive pressure ventilation
IPR	independent professional review
IPV	inactivated polio vaccine
IQ	intelligence quotient
IR	internal rotation; infrared
IRBBB	incomplete right bundle branch block
IRMA	intraretinal microvascular abnormalities
IRR	intrarenal reflux
IRV	inspiratory reserve volume
IS	intercostal space; incentive spirometer; induced sputum
ISB	incentive spirometry breathing
ISC	irreversible sickle cells
ISG	immune serum globulin
ISH	isolated systolic hypertension

ISMA	infantile spinal muscular atrophy
ISO	internal standardization organization
ISS	Injury Severity Score
IST	insulin sensitivity test; insulin shock therapy
ISW	interstitial water
IT	intrathecal; inhalation therapy
ITE	insufficient therapeutic effect
ITP	idiopathic thrombocytopenic purpura; interim treatment plan
ITVAD	indwelling transcutaneous vascular access device
IU	international unit
IUB	International Union of Biochemistry
IUCD	intrauterine contraceptive device
IUD	intrauterine device; intrauterine death
IUFD	intrauterine fetal death
IUGR	intrauterine growth retardation
IUP	intrauterine pregnancy
IUPAC	International Union of Pure and Applied Chemistry
IUPD	intrauterine pregnancy delivered
IV	intravenous
IVC	intravenous cholangiogram; inferior vena cava; intraventricular catheter
IVD	intervertebral disk; intravenous drip
IVDA	intravenous drug abuse
IVF	in vitro fertilization; intravenous fluid
IVFE	intravenous fat emulsion
IVF-ET	in vitro fertilization, embryo transfer
IVGTT	intravenous glucose tolerance test
IVH	intravenous hyperalimentation; intraventricular hemorrhage
IVIG	intravenous immunoglobulin
IVLBW	infant of very low birth weight
IVP	intravenous pyelogram; intravenous push
IVPB	intravenous piggyback
IVR	idioventricular rhythm
IVS	intraventricular septum
IVSD	interventricular septal defect
IVSP	intravenous syringe pump
IVT	intravenous transfusion
IVU	intravenous urography
IWL	insensible water loss
IWMI	inferior wall myocardial infarct

J	joint
JAMA	*Journal of the American Medical Association*
JAMG	juvenile autoimmune myasthenia gravis
JC	junior clinician
JCAHO	Joint Commission on Accreditation of Healthcare Organizations
JDMS	juvenile dermatomyositis
JE	Japanese encephalitis
JF	joint fluid
JI	jejunoileal
JIB	jejunoileal bypass
JJ	jaw jerk
JODM	juvenile onset diabetes mellitus
JP	Jobst pump; Jackson-Pratt (drain)
JRA	juvenile rheumatoid arthritis
jt	joint
juv	juvenile
JVD	jugular venous distention
JVP	jugular venous pulse; jugular venous pressure
JVPT	jugular venous pulse tracing
K	potassium
K24H	potassium, urine 24 hour
KA	ketoacidosis
KAFO	knee-ankle-foot orthosis
KAO	knee-ankle orthosis
KAS	Katz Adjustment Scale
KCal	kilocalorie
KCl	potassium chloride
KCS	keratoconjunctivitis sicca
KD	Kawasaki's disease; knee disarticulation
KDA	known drug allergies
KDDM	kidney disease of diabetes mellitus
KF	kidney function
KFD	Kyasanur Forrest disease
kg	kilogram (kilo)
KI	karyopyknotic index; potassium iodide
KID	keratitis, ichthyosis, deafness
kilo	kilogram (kg)
KISS	saturated solution of potassium iodide
KJ	knee jerk
KK	knee kick

KLH	keyhole limpet hemocyanin (antibody)
KNO	keep needle open
KO	keep open
KP	keratoprecipitate
KS	ketosteroids; Kaposi's sarcoma
KTU	kidney transplant unit
KUB	kidney, ureter, bladder
KVO	keep vein open
KW	Keith Wagner (fundoscopic finding); Kimmelstiel-Wilson
K-wire	Kirschner wire

L	left; liter; lumbar; lingual; lymphocyte; fifty
L$_2$	second lumbar vertebra
LA	left atrium; local anesthesia; long acting; left arm; Latin American
L&A	light and accommodation
lab	laboratory
LAC	laceration; long arm cast
LAD	left anterior descending; left axis deviation
LAD-MIN	left axis deviation minimal
LAE	left atrial enlargement
LAF	lymphocyte-activating factor; laminar air flow; Latin American female
LAG	lymphangiogram; lymphangiosium
LAH	left atrial hypertrophy
LAL	left axillary line; limulus amebocyte lysate
LAN	lymphadenopathy
LAO	left anterior oblique
LAP	laparotomy; laparoscopy; left arterial pressure; leukocyte alkaline phosphatase; leucine amino peptidase
LAPMS	long arm posterior molded splint
LAR	late asthmatic response
L-ASP	L-asparaginase
LAT	left anterior thigh; lateral
L atm	liter-atmosphere
LATS	long-acting thyroid stimulator
LAV	lymphadenopathy-associated virus
LAVH	laparoscopic-assisted vaginal hysteroscopy
lb	pound
LB	low back; left buttock; large bowel; left breast

LBB	left breast biopsy
LBBB	left bundle branch block
LBCD	left border of cardiac dullness
LBD	left border dullness
LBF	*Lactobacillus bulgaricus* factor
LBM	lean body mass; loose bowel movement
LBO	large bowel obstruction
LBP	low back pain; low blood pressure
LBT	lupus band test
LBV	left brachial vein
LBW	low birth weight; lean body weight
LC	living children; low calorie
LCA	left coronary artery; Leber's congenital amaurosis
LCAT	lecithin cholesterol acyltransferase
LCCA	leukocytoclastic angitis; left common carotid artery
LCCS	low cervical cesarean section
LCD	liquor carbonis detergens (coal tar solution); localized collagen dystrophy
LCGU	local cerebral glucose utilization
LCLC	large cell lung carcinoma
LCM	left costal margin; lymphocytic choriomeningitis
LCR	late cutaneous reaction
LCS	low constant suction; low continuous suction
LCT	long-chain triglyceride; low cervical transverse; lymphocytotoxicity
LCV	low cervical vertical
LCX	left circumflex coronary artery
LD	lethal dose; loading dose; liver disease; labor and delivery
LDA	left dorsoanterior (position)
LDB	Legionnaires' disease bacterium
LDH	lactate dehydrogenase
LDL	low-density lipoprotein
LDP	left dorsoposterior position
LDV	laser Doppler velocimetry
LE	lupus erythematosus; lower extremities; left eye
LED	lupus erythematosus disseminatus
LEEP	loop electrocautery excision procedure
LEHPZ	lower esophageal high-pressure zone
L-ERX	leukoerythroblastic reaction
LES	lower esophageal sphincter; local excitatory state
LESP	lower esophageal sphincter pressure

LET	linear energy transfer
LF	low forceps; left foot
LFA	left fronto-anterior; low friction arthroplasty
LFC	living female child
LFD	low-fat diet; low-forceps delivery; lactose-free diet
LFP	left frontoposterior
LFS	liver function studies
LFT	liver function test; left frontotransverse; latex flocculation test
LG	lymph glands; large; left gluteus
LGA	large for gestational age
LGL	Lown-Ganong-Levine (syndrome)
LGV	lymphogranuloma venereum
LH	luteinizing hormone; left hyperphoria; left hand
LHL	left hemisphere lesions
LHP	left hemiparesis
LHR	leukocyte histamine release
LHRH	luteinizing hormone-releasing hormone
LHT	left hypertropia
LI	lactose intolerance
LIB	left in bottle
LIC	left iliac crest; left internal carotid
LICA	left internal carotid artery
LIF	left iliac fossa; liver inhibitory factor
lig	ligament
LIH	left inguinal hernia
LIMA	left internal mammary artery (graft)
LIP	lymphocytic interstitial pneumonia
liq	liquid
LIQ	lower inner quadrant
LIS	low intermittent suction
LISS	low ionic strength saline
LK	left kidney
LKS	liver/kidney/spleen
LL	large lymphocyte; lumbar length; lymphoblastic lymphoma; left leg; lower lip
LLB	long leg brace
LLC	long leg case
LLE	left lower extremity
LLETZ	large loop excision of transformation zone (of cervix)
LL-GXT	low-level graded exercise test
LLL	left lower lobe; left lower lid

LLO	Legionella-like organism
LLPDD	late luteal phase dysphoric disorder
LLQ	left lower quadrant
LLS	lazy leukocyte syndrome
LLSB	left lower sternal border
LLT	left lateral thigh
LMA	left mento-anterior; liver membrane autoantibody
LMB	Laurence-Moon-Biedl (syndrome)
LMC	living male child
LMCA	left main coronary artery
LMD	low molecular weight dextran (LMWD)
LMEE	left middle ear exploration
L/min	liters per minute
LML	left medial lateral/lobe
LMM	lentigo maligna melanoma
LMP	last menstrual period; left mentoposterior
LMT	left mentotransverse
LMWD	low molecular weight dextran (LMD)
LN	lymph nodes
LND	lymph node dissection
LNMP	last normal menstrual period
LO	lateral oblique
LOA	left occiput anterior; leave of absence
LOC	loss of consciousness; level of consciousness; level of care; laxative of choice; local
LOD	line of duty; loss on drying
LOM	limitation of motion; left otitis media
LOP	left occiput posterior; leave on pass
LOQ	lower outer quadrant
LORS	Level of Rehabilitation Scale
LOS	length of stay
LOT	left occiput transverse
LOV	loss of vision
loz	lozenge
LP	lumbar puncture; light perception
LPC	laser photocoagulation
LPD	luteal phase defect
LPF	low power field
LPH	left posterior hemiblock
LPN	licensed practical nurse
LPO	left posterior oblique; light perception only
lpp	lipoprotein

LR	light reflex; labor room; left-right
L>R	left greater than right
L-R	left to right
LRD	living renal donor
LRND	left radical neck dissection
LRQ	lower right quadrant
L/S	lecithin-sphingomyelin ratio
L-S	lumbo-sacral
LSA	left sacrum anterior; lipid-bound sialic acid; lymphosarcoma
LSB	left sternal border
LS BPS	laparoscopic bilateral partial salpingectomy
LSE	local side effects
LSF	low saturated fat
LSKM	liver-spleen-kidney-megaly
LSM	late systolic murmur
LSO	left salpingo-oophorectomy
LSP	left sacrum posterior; liver-specific (membrane)
LSS	liver-spleen scan
LST	left sacrum transverse
LSTL	laparoscopic tubal ligation
LT	light; left; left thigh; lumbar traction; Levin tube; leukotrienes
LTB	laparoscopic tubal banding; laryngotracheobronchitis
LTC	long-term care; left to count; lean tissue compartment
LTCF	long-term care facility
LTCS	low transverse cesarean section
LTGA	left transposition of great artery
LTL	laparoscopic tubal ligation
LTT	lymphocyte transformation test
L&U	lower and upper
LUE	left upper extremity
LUL	left upper lobe
LUQ	left upper quadrant
LUSB	left upper sternal border
LV	left ventricle
LVA	left ventricular aneurysm
LVAD	left ventricular assist device
LVE	left ventricular enlargement
LVEDP	left ventricular end diastolic pressure
LVEDV	left ventricular end diastolic volume
LVEF	left ventricular ejection fraction

LVF	left ventricular failure
LVFP	left ventricular filling pressure
LVH	left ventricular hypertrophy
LVL	left vastus lateralis
LVMM	left ventricular muscle mass
LVP	left ventricular pressure; large volume parenteral
LVPW	left ventricular posterior wall
LVSWI	left ventricular stroke work index
LVV	left ventricular volume
L&W	living and well
LWCT	Lee-White clotting time
LYG	lymphomatoid granulomatosis
lymphs	lymphocytes
lytes	electrolytes
m	meter
M	murmur; medial; myopia; monocytes; male; molar; thousand; minum; mix
m²	square meters (body surface)
M₁	first mitral sound
MA	mental age; medical assistance; milliamps; menstrual age
M/A	mood and/or affect
MAA	Medical Assistance for the Aged; macroaggregates of albumin
MAb	monoclonal antibody
MABP	mean arterial blood pressure
MAC	maximum allowable concentration; midarm circumference; minimum alveolar concentration; mycobacterium avium complex, maximum allowable cost
MAE	moves all extremities
MAEEW	moves all extremities equally well
MAFAs	movement-associated fetal (heart rate) accelerations
MAHA	microangiopathic hemolytic anemia
MAI	mycobacterium avium-intracellular
MAL	midaxillary line
MALT	mucosa-associated lymphoid tissue
MAMC	mid-arm muscle circumference
mammo	mammography
mand	mandibular
MAOI	monoamine oxidase inhibitor (MOI)

MAP	mean arterial pressure
MAPC	maximum allowable prevailing charge
MAS	meconium aspiration syndrome; mobile arm support
MAT	multifocal atrial tachycardia
max	maximal; maxillary; maximum
MBC	maximum breathing capacity; minimal bactericidal concentration
MB-CK	creatinine kinase isoenzyme with muscle and brain subunits (CK-MB)
MBD	minimal brain damage; minimal brain dysfunction
MBI	methylene blue installation
MBM	mother's breast milk
MC	mixed cellularity; metatarso-cuneiform; moisture content; methyl cellulose
MCA	middle cerebral aneurysm; middle cerebral artery; motorcycle accident
MCCU	midstream clean-catch urine
MCD	minimal change disease
mcg	microgram
MCGN	minimal change glomerular nephritis
MCH	mean corpuscular hemoglobin; muscle contraction headache
MCHC	mean corpuscular hemoglobin concentration
MCHS	Maternal and Child Health Services
MCL	midclavicular line; midcostal line
MCLNS	mucocutaneous lymph node syndrome
MCO	managed care organization
MCP	metacarpophalangeal (joint)
MCS	microculture and sensitivity
MCSA	minimal cross-sectional area
MCT	medium chain triglyceride; mean circulation time
MCTD	mixed connective tissue disease
MCV	mean corpuscular volume
MD	medical doctor; mental deficiency; muscular dystrophy; manic depression
MDA	manual dilation of the anus; micrometastases detection assay
MDC	medial dorsal cutaneous (nerve); major diagnostic category
MDD	manic-depressive disorder; major depressive disorder
MDF	myocardial depressant factor
MDI	metered dose inhaler

MDM	mid-diastolic murmur; minor determinant mix
MDR	minimum daily requirement
MDS	maternal deprivation syndrome; minimum data set
MDTP	multidisciplinary treatment plan
ME	macula edema; medical examiner; middle ear
MEA-1	multiple endocrine adenomutosis type 1
mec	meconium
MEC	minimum effective concentration
med	medial; medical; medication; medicine; medium
MED	median erythrocyte diameter; minimum erythema dose
MEDAC	multiple endocrine deficiency autoimmune candidiasis
MEE	middle ear effusion
MEF	maximum expired flow (rate)
MEFV	maximum expiratory flow volume
MEN (II)	multiple endocrine neoplasia (type II)
MEOS	microsomal ethanol oxidizing system
mEq	milliequivalent
M/E	myeloid-to-erythroid ratio
meta	metamyelocytes
METS	metabolic equivalents (multiples of resting oxygen uptake); metastases
MF	myocardial fibrosis; mycosis fungoides
M&F	mother and father; male and female
MFA	mid-forceps delivery
MFAT	multifocal atrial tachycardia
MFEM	maximal forced expiratory maneuver
MFH	malignant fibrous histiocytoma
MFR	mid-forceps rotation
mg	milligram
MG	myasthenia gravis
MGF	maternal grandfather
MGM	maternal grandmother
MGN	membranous glomerulonephritis
MgO	magnesium oxide
MgSO$_4$	magnesium sulfate
MGUS	monoclonal gammopathies of undetermined significance
M-GXT	multistage graded exercise test
MH	marital history; menstrual history; mental health; malignant hyperthermia
MHA	microangiopathic hemolytic anemia

MHB	maximum hospital benefit
MHC	major histocompatibility complex; mental health center
MH/MR	mental health and mental retardation
MI	myocardial infarction; mitral insufficiency; mental institution
MIA	medically indigent adult
MIC	minimum inhibitory concentration; maternal and infant care
MICN	mobile intensive care nurse
MICU	medical intensive care unit
MID	multi-infarct dementia
MIF	migration inhibitory factor
MIH	migraine with interparoxysmal headache
min	minimum; minute; minor
MIO	minimum identifiable odor
MIRP	myocardial infarction rehabilitation program
MKAB	may keep at bedside
mL	milliliter
ML	midline; middle lobe
MLC	mixed lymphocyte culture; minimal lethal concentration
MLD	metachromatic leukodystrophy; minimal lethal dose
MLF	median longitudinal fasciculus
MLNS	mucocutaneous lymph node syndrome
MLR	mixed lymphocyte reaction; medical loss ratio
mm	millimeter
mM	millimole (mmol)
MM	mucous membrane; multiple myeloma
M&M	morbidity and mortality
MMA	monocyte monolayer assay
MMECT	multiple monitor electroconvulsive therapy
MMEFR	maximal mid-expiratory flow rate
MMF	mean maximum flow
mmHg	millimeters of mercury
MMIS	Medicaid Management Information System
MMK	Marshall-Marchetti-Krantz (cystourethropexy)
MMOA	maxillary mandibular odontectomy alveolectomy
mmol	millimole (mM)
MMPI	Minnesota Multiphasic Personality Inventory
MMR	measles, mumps, rubella; midline malignant reticulosis

MMS	Mini-Mental State (examination)
MMT	manual muscle test
Mn	manganese
MN	midnight
M&N	morning and night
MNC	mononuclear leukocytes
MNG	multinodular goiter
MNR	marrow neutrophil reserve
MN SSEPs	median nerve somatosensory evoked potentials
MNTB	medial nucleus of the trapezoid body
MO	month; medial oblique; mineral oil
MOA	mechanism of action
mod	moderate
MOD	medical officer of the day
MODY	maturity onset diabetes of youth
MOF	multiple organ failure
MOI	monoamine oxidase inhibitor (MAOI)
MOM	milk of magnesia
mono	monocyte; infectious mononucleosis
mOsm	milliosmole
MP	metacarpal phalangeal (joint)
MPBB	maximum permissible body burden
MPGN	membranoproliferative glomerulonephritis
MPJ	metacarpophalangeal joint
MPJE	Multistate Pharmacy Jurisprudence Examination
MPL	maximum permissible level
MPPPA	Medical Prudent Pharmaceutical Purchasing Act
MPR	multifetal pregnancy reduction
MPS	mucopolysaccharidosis
MQ	memory quotient
MR	mental retardation; may repeat; magnetic resonance; mitral regurgitation
MR × 1	may repeat times one
MRA	medical record administrator; magnetic resonance angiography
MRD	Medical Records Department
MRG	murmurs, rubs, and gallops
MRI	magnetic resonance imaging
mRNA	messenger ribonucleic acid
MRS	magnetic resonance spectroscopy
MRSA	methicillin-resistant *Staphylococcus aureus*

MS	multiple sclerosis; mitral stenosis; mental status; musculoskeletal; minimal support
M&S	microculture and sensitivity
MSAF	meconium-stained amniotic fluid
MSAFP	maternal serum alpha fetoprotein
MSE	Mental Status Examination
MSK	medullary sponge kidney
MSL	midsternal line; medical science liasion
MSR	muscle stretch reflexes
MSS	minor surgery suite; muscular subaortic stenosis; Marital Satisfaction Scale
MST	mean survival time
MSTA	mumps skin test antigen
MSU	midstream urine
MSUD	maple syrup urine disease
MSW	multiple stab wounds
MT	music therapy; medical technologist
MTAL	medullary thick ascending limb
MTC	minimum toxic concentration
MTD	Monro Tidal drainage
MTI	malignant teratoma interminate
MTM	modified Thayer-Martin (medium)
MTP	metatarsal phalangeal
MTU	malignant teratoma undifferentiated
MU	million units
MUDPIES	methanol, uremia, diabetes, paraldehyde, iron, ethanol or ethylene glycol, salicylates (possible causes of metabolic acidosis)
MUGA	multiple gated acquisition
MULEPAK	methanol, uremia, lactic acidosis, ethylene glycol, paraldehyde, aspirin, diabetic ketoacidosis (possible causes of metabolic acidosis)
MVA	motor vehicle accident; malignant ventricular arrhythmias
MVB	mixed venous blood
MVC	maximal voluntary contraction
MVO_2	myocardial oxygen consumption
MVP	mitral valve prolapse
MVR	mitral valve replacement; mitral valve regurgitation
MVS	mitral valve stenosis
MVV	maximum voluntary ventilation; mixed vespid venom
MWS	Mickey-Wilson syndrome

My	myopia
myelo	myelocyte
N	normal; negative
NA	nursing assistant; nurse anesthetist; not applicable
NAA	neutron activation analysis
NABP	National Association of Boards of Pharmacy
NABPF	National Association of Boards of Pharmacy Foundation
NABS	normoactive bowel sounds
NACDS	National Association of Chain Drug Stores
NaCl	sodium chloride
NAD	no acute distress; no apparent distress; no appreciable disease; normal axis deviation; nothing abnormal detected; nicotinamide adenine dinucleotide
NADH	nicotinamide adenine dinucleotide (reduced form)
NADP	nicotinamide adenine dinucleotide phosphate
NADPH	nicotinamide adenine dinucleotide phosphate (reduced form)
NaF	sodium fluoride
NAG	narrow angle glaucoma
NaHCO$_3$	sodium bicarbonate
NANB	non-A, non-B (hepatitis)
NANC	nonadrenergic, noncholinergic
NAPLEX	North American Pharmacist Licensure Examination
NARD	National Association of Retail Druggists (now NCPA)
NAS	no added salt; neonatal abstinence syndrome
NAS/NRC	National Academy of Science/National Research Council
NAT	no action taken
NB	newborn; note well *(nota bene);* needle biopsy
NBM	normal bowel movement
NBN	newborn nursery
NBS	normal bowel sound; no bacteria seen; National Bureau of Standards
NBT	nitroblue tetrazolium (reduction test)
NBTE	nonbacterial thrombotic endocarditis
NC	neurologic check; no complaints; not completed; nasal cannula
NCA	neurocirculatory asthenia
NC/AT	normal cephalic atraumatic

NCB	no code blue
NCD	normal childhood diseases; not considered disabling
NCF	neutrophilic chemotactic factor
NCI	National Cancer Institute
NCJ	needle catheter jejunostomy
NCL	neuronal ceroid lipofuscinosis
NCM	nailfold capillary microscopy
NCNC	normochromic, normocytic
NCPA	National Community Pharmacists Association (formerly NARD)
NCPDP	National Council for Prescription Drug Programs
NCPIE	National Council on Patient Information and Education
NCPR	no cardiopulmonary resuscitation
NCQA	National Committee for Quality Assurance
NCS	no concentrated sweets; nerve conduction studies
NCSPAE	National Council of State Pharmaceutical Association Executives
NCTC	national collection of type cultures
NCV	nerve conduction velocity
ND	normal delivery; normal development; not done; not diagnosed; nasal deformity
NDA	New Drug Application
NDAC	Nonprescription Drugs Advisory Committee
NDC	National Drug Code
NDD	no dialysis days
NDMA	Nonprescription Drug Manufacturers Association
NDT	neurodevelopmental treatment
NDV	Newcastle disease virus
NE	norepinephrine; not elevated; not examined
NEC	necrotizing enterocolitis
NED	no evidence of disease
neg	negative
NEMD	nonspecific esophageal motility disorder
NERD	nonerosive reflux disease
NET	naso-endotracheal tube
neuro	neurology; neurological
neut	neutrophil
NF	not found; neurofibromatosis; *National Formulary*
NFL	nerve fiber layer
NFTD	normal full-term delivery
NFTT	nonorganic failure to thrive

NFW	nursed fairly well
NG	nasogastric; nanogram
NGF	nerve growth factor
NGR	nasogastric replacement
NGT	nasogastric tube
NGU	nongonococcal urethritis
NH	nursing home
NHBA	National Heartburn Alliance
NHD	normal hair distribution
NHL	non-Hodgkin's lymphoma; nodular histiocytic lymphoma
NHP	nursing home placement
NICC	neonatal intensive care center
NICU	neurosurgical intensive care unit; neonatal intensive care unit
NIDD	non-insulin-dependent diabetes
NIDDM	non-insulin-dependent diabetes mellitus
NIF	negative inspiratory force
NIH	National Institutes of Health
NIMH	National Institute of Mental Health
NINVS	noninvasive neurovascular studies
NIOSH	National Institute for Occupational Safety and Health
NISPC	National Institute for Standards in Pharmacist Credentialing
NJ	nasojejunal
NK	natural killer (cells)
NKA	no known allergies
NKDA	no known drug allergies
NKHS	nonketotic hyperosmolar syndrome
NKMA	no known medication allergies
NL	normal; normal limits
NLD	necrobiosis lipoidica diabeticorum; nasolacrimal duct
NLF	nasolabial fold
NLP	nodular liquefying panniculitis; no light perception
NLT	not later than; not less than
NM	nodular melanoma
NMD	normal muscle development
NMI	no middle initial
NMR	nuclear magnetic resonance
NMS	neuroleptic malignant syndrome
NMT	no more than
NN	neonatal; nursing notes

NND	neonatal death
NNE	neonatal necrotizing enterocolitis
NNO	no new orders
NNU	net nitrogen utilization
no	number *(numero)*
noc	night
noct	at night *(nocte)*
NOD	notify of death
NOMI	nonocclusive mesenteric infarction
NOOB	not out of bed
NOS	not otherwise specified
NOSIE	Nurse Observation Scale for Inpatient Evaluation
NP	neuropsychiatric; nasopharyngeal; newly presented; no pain; not pregnant; not present; nursed poorly; nasal prongs; nurse practitioner
NPA	near point of accommodation
NPC	near point convergences; nodal premature contractions; nonpatient contact; National Pharmaceutical Council
NPDL	nodular poorly differentiated lymphocytic
NPDR	nonproliferative diabetic retinopathy
NPH	normal pressure hydrocephalus; no previous history; neutral protamine Hagedorn (insulin)
NPhA	National Pharmaceutical Association
NPO	nothing by mouth *(per os)*
NPR	noncardiogenic pulmonary reaction
NPT	normal pressure and temperature; nocturnal penile tumescence
NR	nonreactive
NRBS	nonrebreathing system
NRC	normal retinal correspondence
NREM	nonrapid eye movement
NREMS	nonrapid eye movement sleep
NRT	neuromuscular reeducation techniques
NS	nephrotic syndrome; nuclear sclerosis; not seen; not significant; nylon suture; normal saline solution; nasal spray
NSA	normal serum albumin; no significant abnormality
NSAID	nonsteroidal anti-inflammatory drug
NSC	no significant change; not service connected
NSCLC	non-small-cell lung cancer
NSD	normal spontaneous delivery; nominal standard dose

NSDA	non-steroid-dependent asthmatic
NSE	neuron-specific enolase
NSF	National Science Foundation
NSFTD	normal spontaneous full-term delivery
NSG	nursing
NSILA	nonsuppressible insulin-like activity
NSN	nephrotoxic serum nephritis
NSPVT	nonsustained polymorphic ventricular tachycardia
NSR	normal sinus rhythm; not seen regularly; nonspecific reaction; nasoseptal repair
NSS	normal saline solution (0.9 percent sodium chloride)
NSSTT	nonspecific ST and T (waves)
NST	nutritional support team; nonstress test; not sooner than
NSU	nonspecific urethritis
NSV	nonspecific vaginitis
NSVD	normal spontaneous vaginal delivery
NT	not tested; nasotracheal; not tender
N&T	nose and throat
NTC	neurotrauma center
NTD	neural tube defects
NTE	not to exceed
NTF	normal throat flora
NTG	nontreatment group
NTMB	nontuberculous mycobacteria
NTMI	nontransmural myocardial infarction
NTP	normal temperature and pressure
NTS	nasotracheal suction; nucleus tractus solitarii
NTT	nasotracheal tube
NUD	nonulcer dyspepsia
nullip	nullipara
NV	neurovascular; nausea and vomiting
N&V	nausea and vomiting
NVD	nausea, vomiting, and diarrhea; neck vein distention; no venereal disease; neurovesicle dysfunction; nonvalvular disease; neovascularization of the disc
NVE	neovascularization elsewhere
NVG	neovascular glaucoma
NVS	neurological vital signs
NWB	non-weight bearing
NWDA	National Wholesale Druggists Association (formerly HDMA)

NYD	not yet diagnosed
O	objective (finding); eye *(oculus);* oral; open
O₂	oxygen
O × 3	oriented to time, place, and person
OA	oral alimentation; occiput anterior; osteoarthritis
O&A	observation and assessment
OAA	Old Age Assistance
OAF	osteoclast activating factor
OASDI	Old Age, Survivors, and Disability Insurance
OASI	Old Age and Survivors Insurance
OAW	once a week
OB	obstetrics; occult blood
OB-GYN	obstetrics and gynecology
OBRA '90	Omnibus Budget Reconcilliation Act of 1990
OBS	organic brain syndrome
OC	oral contraceptive; obstetrical conjugate; oral care; on call; office call
OCA	oculocutaneous albinism
OCCC	open chest cardiac compression
OCCM	open chest cardiac massage
OCD	obsessive-compulsive disorder
OCG	oral cholecystogram
OCP	ova, cysts, parasites
OCT	oxytocin challenge test; optical coherence tomography; ornithine carbamyl transferase
OCU	observation care unit
od	right eye *(oculus dexter)*
OD	overdose; optical density; on duty; Doctor of Optometry
OER	oxygen enhancement ratios
OFC	occipital-frontal circumference
OG	orogastric (feeding)
OGTT	oral glucose tolerance test
OH	occupational history; open heart; outpatient hospital
OHD	organic heart disease
OHG	oral hypoglycemic
OHP	oxygen under hyperbaric pressure
OHRR	open heart recovery room
OHS	open heart surgery
OI	osteogenesis imperfecta
OIF	oil-immersion field

OIG	Office of Inspector General
OJ	orange juice
OKAN	optokinetic after nystagmus
OKN	optokinetic nystagmus
ol	left eye *(oculus laevus)*
OLA	occiput left anterior
OM	otitis media
OME	Office of the Medical Examiner; otitis media with effusion
OMI	old myocardial infarct
OMR	operative mortality rate
OMSC	otitis media secretory/suppurative chronic
ON	overnight
ONC	over-the-needle catheter
OOB	out of bed
OOBBRP	out of bed with bathroom privileges
OOC	out of control
OOP	out on pass; out of pelvis
OOR	out of room
OOS	out of stock
OOT	out of town
OP	outpatient; operation; occiput posterior; open
O&P	ova and parasites
OPB	outpatient basis
OPC	outpatient clinic
OPCA	olivopontocerebellar atrophy
OPD	outpatient department
OPG	ocular plethysmography
OPM	occult primary malignancy
OPPG	oculopneumoplethysmography
OPS	operations
OPT	outpatient physical therapy
OPV	oral polio vaccine
OR	operating room; oil retention
ORIF	open reduction internal fixation
ORL	otorhinolaryngology
os	left eye *(oculus sinister)*
OS	opening snap
O/S	out-of-stock
OSA	obstructive sleep apnea
OSD	overside drainage
OSHA	Occupational Safety and Health Administration

OSM S	osmolarity serum
OSM U	osmolarity urine
OSN	off-service note
oss	osseous
OT	old tuberculin; occupational therapy; occupational therapist
OTC	over-the-counter
OTD	out the door
oto	otology
OTR	Occupational Therapist, Registered
OTS	orotracheal suction
OTT	orotracheal tube
ou	both eyes *(oculus uterque)*
OV	office visit; ovum; ovary
OW	out of wedlock
oz	ounce

p	plan; protein; pint; pulse; peripheral; para-
P_2	pulmonic second sound
PA	pernicious anemia; physician assistant; professional association; proprietary association; professional associates; physician associates; posterior-anterior; pulmonary artery; presents again; psychiatric aide
P&A	percussion and auscultation
PAB	premature atrial beat
PABA	*p*-aminobenzoic acid
PAC	premature atrial contraction
PACO	pivot ambulating crutchless orthosis
$PaCO_2$	arterial carbon dioxide tension
PACU	postanesthesia care unit
PADP	pulmonary artery diastolic pressure
PAF	paroxysmal atrial fibrillation; platelet activating factors
PAGE	polyacrylamide gel electrophoresis
PAH	para-aminohippurate
PAIVS	pulmonary atresia with intact ventricle septum
PA line	pulmonary artery line
PALN	para-aortic lymph node
PAN	periodic alternating nystagmus; polyarteritis nodosa
PAO_2	arterial oxygen tension
POAG	primary open-angle glaucoma
PAOP	pulmonary artery occlusion pressure

PAP	pulmonary artery pressure; prostatic acid phosphatase
PA/PS	pulmonary atresia/pulmonary stenosis
Pap smear	Papanicolaou smear
PAR	postanesthetic recovery; platelet aggregate ratio
para	paraplegic
PARA	number of pregnancies producing viable offspring
PARU	postanesthetic recovery unit
PAS	periodic acid-Schiff (reagent); peripheral anterior synechia; pulmonary artery stenosis
Pas Ex	passive exercise
PAT	paroxysmal atrial tachycardia; preadmission testing; percent acceleration time
path	pathology
PAWP	pulmonary artery wedge pressure
Pb	lead
PB	powder board; paraffin bath
PBA	percutaneous bladder aspiration
PBC	point of basal convergence; primary biliary cirrhosis
PBD	percutaneous biliary drainage
PBI	protein-bound iodine
PBL	peripheral blood lymphocyte
PBM	pharmacy benefits manager
PBMC	peripheral blood mononuclear cell (PBMNC)
PBMNC	peripheral blood mononuclear cell (PBMC)
PBO	placebo
PBP	provider-based physician
pc	after meals *(post cibos);* after food *(post cibus)*
PC	packed cells; professional corporation; platelet concentrate; pharmaceutical care
PCA	patient care assistant/aide; patient-controlled analgesia; posterior cerebral artery; procoagulation activity; passive cutaneous anaphylaxis
PCCF	Patient Care Claim Form
PCCM	primary care case management
PCCU	postcoronary care unit
PCG	phonocardiogram
PCH	paroxysmal cold hemoglobinuria
PCI	prophylactic cranial irradiation; percutaneous coronary intervention
PCIOL	posterior chamber intraocular lens
PCL	posterior chamber lens; posterior cruciate ligament
PCM	protein-calorie malnutrition

PCO	polycystic ovary
PCO$_2$	carbon dioxide pressure/tension
P~CO$_2$	partial pressure of carbon dioxide
PCOD	polycystic ovarian disease
PCP	*Pneumonocystis carinii* pneumonia; pulmonary capillary pressure; phencyclidine; primary care physician
PCR	protein catabolic/caloric rate; polymerase chain reaction
PCT	porphyria cutanea
PCTA	percutaneous transluminal angioplasty
PCU	progressive care unit
PCV	packed cell volume
PCWP	pulmonary capillary wedge pressure
PD	peritoneal dialysis; postural drainage; Parkinson's disease; percutaneous drain
P/D	packs per day (cigarettes) (PPD)
PDA	patent ductus arteriosus
PDE	paroxysmal dyspnea on exertion; pulsed Doppler echocardiography
PDFC	premature dead female child
PDGF	platelet-derived growth factor
PDGXT	predischarge graded exercise test
PDL	poorly differentiated lymphocyte
PDMC	premature dead male child
PDR	proliferative diabetic reinopathy; *Physician's Desk Reference*
PDS	pain dysfunction syndrome
PDT	photodynamic therapy
PDU	pulsed Doppler ultrasonography
PE	physical examination; physical exercise; pulmonary embolism; pleural effusion
PEcho	prostatic echogram
peds	pediatrics
PEEP	positive end expiratory pressure
PEFR	peak expiratory flow rate
PEG	pneumoencephalogram; percutaneous endoscopic gastrostomy; polyethylene glycol
PEN	parenteral and enteral nutrition
PENS	percutaneous epidural nerve stimulator
PEP	protein electrophoresis; preejection period
perf	perforation

PERL	pupils equal, reactive to light
PERRLA	pupils, equal, round, reactive to light and accommodation
PES	preexcitation syndrome
PET	positron-emission tomography; preeclamptic toxemia; pressure-equalizing tubes
PF	power factor
PFC	persistent fetal circulation
PFR	peak flow rate; parotid flow rate
PFT	pulmonary function test
PFU	plaque-forming unit
pg	picogram
PG	pregnant
PGA	pteroylglutamic acid
PGF	parenteral grandfather
PGH	pituitary growth hormone
PGL	persistent generalized lymphadenopathy
PGM	paternal grandmother
PgR	progesterone receptor
PGU	postgonococcal urethritis
pH	negative log of hydrogen ion concentration
PH	past history; poor health; public health
pHA	arterial blood hydrogen tension
PHA	phytohemagglutin; passive hemagglutination
Pharm	pharmacy
PharmD	doctor of pharmacy
PhC	pharmaceutical chemist
PHC	primary hepatocellular carcinoma
PhD	doctor of philosophy
PhG	graduate in pharmacy
PHH	posthemorrhagic hydrocephalus
PhI	*Pharmacopoeia Internationalis*
PHN	public health nurse; postherpetic neuralgia
PHP	prepaid health plan
PHPT	primary hyperparathyroidism
PHPV	persistent hyperplastic primary vitreous
PhRMA	Pharmaceutical Research and Manufacturers of America (formerly PMA)
PHS	Public Health Service (United States) (USPHS)
phx	pharynx
PI	present illness; pulmonary infarction; peripheral iridectomy; package insert; principal investigator

PICA	posterior inferior communicating artery; posterior inferior cerebellar artery
PICU	pediatric intensive care unit
PID	pelvic inflammatory disease; prolapsed intervertebral disc
PIE	pulmonary infiltration with eosinophilia; pulmonary interstitial emphysema
PIFR	peak inspiratory flow rate
PIH	pregnancy-induced hypertension
PIP	proximal interphalangeal joint; postinspiratory pressure
PISA	phase invariant signature algorithm
PITR	plasma iron turnover rate
PIV	peripheral intravenous
PIVD	protruded intervertebral disc
PJB	premature junctional beat
PJC	premature junctional contraction
PJS	Peutz-Jeghers syndrome
PK	penetrating keratoplasty
PKD	polycystic kidney disease
PKU	phenylketonuria
PL	plantar; place; perception of light
PLAP	placental alkaline phosphatase
PLFC	premature living female child
PLH	paroxysmal localized hyperhidrosis
PLL	prolymphocytic leukemia
PLMC	premature living male child
PLN	pelvic lymph node; popliteal lymph node
PLS	primary lateral sclerosis
PLTs	platelets
PM	postmortem; evening *(post meridiem);* pretibial myxedema
PMA	Prinzmetal's angina; premenstrual asthma; Pharmaceutical Manufacturers Association (now PhRMA)
PMB	postmenopausal bleeding; polymorphonuclear basophils
PMC	pseudomembranous colitis
PMD	private medical doctor
PME	postmenopausal estrogen
PMF	progressive massive fibrosis
PMH	past medical history

PMI	point of maximal impulse; patient medication instructions
PML	progressive multifocal leukoencephalopathy
PMN	polymorphonuclear neutrophil
PMP	pain management program; previous menstrual period
PMPM	per member per month
PMPY	per member per year
PMR	polymyalgia rheumatica; polymorphic reticulosis; proton magnetic resonance
PM&R	physical medicine and rehabilitation
PMS	premenstrual syndrome
PMT	premenstrual tension
PMTS	premenstrual tension syndrome
PMV	prolapse of mitral valve
PMW	pacemaker wires
PN	parenteral nutrition; progress note; percussion note
PNAS	prudent no added salt
PNB	premature nodal beat
PNC	premature nodal contraction; peripheral nerve conduction
PND	paroxysmal nocturnal dyspnea; postnasal drip
PNF	proprioceptive neuromuscular fasciculation (reaction)
PNH	paroxysmal nocturnal hemoglobinuria
PNI	prognostic nutrition index; peripheral nerve injury
PNMG	persistent neonatal myasthenia gravis
PNP	Pediatric Nurse Practitioner; progressive nuclear palsy
PNS	peripheral nervous system; partial nonprogressing stroke
PNT	percutaneous nephrostomy tube
PNU	protein nitrogen units
PNV	prenatal vitamins
PNX	pneumothorax
po	by mouth (*per os*)
PO	phone order
PO₂	partial pressure of oxygen
POA	pancreatic oncofetal antigen
POAG	primary open-angle glaucoma
POC	product of conception; postoperative care
POD 1	postoperative day one

POEMS	polyneuropathy, organomegaly, endocrinopathy, monoclonal (M)-protein, skin changes (with plasma cell dyscrasia)
poik	poikilocytosis
POL	premature onset of labor
poly	polymorphonucleocytes
POMR	problem-oriented medical record
poplit	popliteal
POPR	problem-oriented patient record
PORT	postoperative respiratory therapy
POS	parosteal osteosarcoma; point of service
POSM	patient-operated selector mechanism
POST	postmortem examination (autopsy)
post-op	after surgery (postoperative)
PP	postpartum; postprandial; paradoxical pulse; pinprick; patient profile; protoporphyria; proximal phalanx
PPA	prudent purchaser agreement
PPAC	pharmacy practice activity classification
ppb	parts per billion
PPBG	postprandial blood glucose
PPBS	postprandial blood sugar
PPC	progressive patient care
PPD	packs per day (P/D); postpartum day; posterior polymorphous dystrophy; purified protein derivative
P&PD	percussion and postural drainage
PPD-B	purified protein derivative—Battey
PPD-S	purified protein derivative—standard
PPF	plasma protein fraction
PPG	photoplethysmography
PPH	postpartum hemorrhage
PPHN	persistent pulmonary hypertension of the newborn
PPI	patient package insert; protein pump inhibitor
PPL	pars planus lensectomy
PPLO	pleuro-pneumonia-like organism
ppm	parts per million
PPN	peripheral parenteral nutrition
PPNG	penicillinase-producing *Neisseria gonorrhoeae*
PPO	preferred provider organization
PPP	preferred pharmacy program; postpartum psychosis
PPPBL	peripheral pulses palpable both legs
PPPG	postprandial plasma glucose
PPROM	prolonged premature rupture of membranes

PPS	postpartum sterilization; pneumococcal polysaccharide (vaccine); prospective payment system
PPS codes	professional pharmacy service codes
PPTL	postpartum tubal ligation
PR	per rectum; pulse rate; profile
P&R	pulse and respiration; pelvic and rectal
PRA	plasma renin angiotensin; plasma renin activity
PRAT	platelet radioactive antiglobulin test
PRBC	packed red blood cells
PRC	packed red cells
PRCA	pure red cell aplasia
PRE	progressive/passive resistive exercise
pre-op	before surgery (preoperative)
prep	prepare (for surgery)
PRG	phleborrheogram
PRIMP	primipara (first pregnancy)
prn	as needed *(pro re nata)*
pro	protein
PRO	peer/professional review organization
prob	probable
procto	proctology; proctoscopic
prog	prognosis; prognathism
PROM	passive range of motion; premature rupture of membranes
prov	provisional
PRP	panretinal photocoagulation; polyribose ribital phosphate
PRRB	Provider Reimbursement Review Board
PRRE	pupils round, regular, equal
PRSs	positive rolandic spikes
PRTH-C	prothrombin time control
PRV	polycythemia rubra vera
PRW	polymerized ragweed
PS	pulmonary stenosis; paradoxic sleep; pathologic stage; plastic surgery; serum from pregnant women; performance status
P&S	paracentesis and suction; pain and suffering
PS I	healthy patient with localized pathological process
PS II	patient with mild to moderate systemic disease
PS III	patient with severe systemic disease limiting activity, but not incapacitating

PS IV	patient with incapacitating systemic disease
PS V	moribund patient not expected to live
PSA	prostate-specific antigen; psoriatic arthritis
PSAO	pharmacy services administrative organization
PSC	posterior subcapsular cataract; primary sclerosing cholangitis
PSE	portal systemic encephalopathy
PSF	posterior spinal fusion
PSG	polysomnography
PSGN	poststreptococcal glomerulonephritis
PSH	postspinal headache
psi	pounds per square inch
PSM	presystolic murmur
PSP	pancreatic spasmolytic peptide; progressive supranuclear palsy
PSRBOW	premature spontaneous rupture of bag of waters
PSRO	professional standards review organization
PSS	progressive systemic sclerosis; physiologic saline solution
PSVT	paroxysmal supraventricular tachycardia
PSW	psychiatric social worker
PT	physical therapy; patient; prothrombin time; physical therapist
P&T	pharmacy and therapeutics (committee)
PTA	prior to admission; plasma thromboplastin antecedent; pretreatment anxiety; puretone average; physical therapy assistant; percutaneous transluminal angioplasty
PTB	patellar tendon bearing
PTBD-EF	percutaneous transhepatic biliary drainage–enteric feeding
PTC	plasma thromboplastin components; percutaneous transhepatic cholangiography
PTCA	percutaneous transluminal coronary angioplasty
PTCB	Pharmacy Technician Certification Board
PTD	period to discharge; permanent and total disability
PTE	proximal tibial epiphysis; pulmonary thromboembolism; pretibial edema
PTF	plasma thromboplastin factor
PTH	posttransfusion hepatitis; parathyroid hormone
PTL	preterm labor
PTMDF	pupils, tension, media, disc, fundus

PTPM	posttraumatic progressive myelopathy
PTPN	peripheral (vein) total parenteral nutrition
PTS	prior to surgery
PTSD	post-traumatic stress disorder
PTT	partial thromboplastin time
PTx	parathyroidectomy
PTX	pneumothorax
PU	peptic ulcer; pregnancy urine
PUBS	percutaneous umbilical blood sampling
PUD	peptic ulcer disease
PUFA	polyunsaturated fatty acids
pul	pulmonary
PUN	plasma urea nitrogen
PUO	pyrexia of undetermined origin
PUPPP	pruritic urticariat papules and plaques of pregnancy
PUVA	psoralen-ultraviolet A (light)
PV	polycythemia vera; polio vaccine; portal vein; pulmonary vein; per vagina
P&V	pyloroplasty and vagotomy
PVB	premature ventricular beat
PVC	premature ventricular contraction; pulmonary venous congestion; polyvinyl chloride
PVD	peripheral vascular disease; posterior vitreous detachment
PVE	premature ventricular extrasystole; perivenous encephalomyelitis
PVO	peripheral vascular occlusion; pulmonary venous occlusion
PVOD	pulmonary vascular obstructive disease
PVP	peripheral venous pressure
PVR	peripheral vascular resistance; postvoiding residual; proliferative vitreoretinopathy; pulse-volume recording
PVS	peritoneovenous shunt; pulmonic valve stenosis; percussion, vibration, and suction
PVT	paroxysmal ventricular tachycardia; private
PWB	partial weight bearing
PWLV	posterior wall of left ventricle
PWP	pulmonary wedge pressure
PWV	polistes wasp venom
Px	physical exam; prognosis; pneumothorax; practice
PXE	pseudoxanthoma elasticum

PY	pack years
q	every, each *(quodque);* quantity
q4h	every four hours
QA	quality assurance
qAM	every morning
QCA	quantitative coronary angiography
qd	every day
QEEG	quantitative electroencephalogram
qhs	every night
qid	four times daily *(quarter in die)*
qns	quantity not sufficient
QRRB	Qualified Railroad Retirement Beneficiary
qs	sufficient quantity *(quantum sufficiat);* every shift
QSAR	quantitative structure-activity relationship
qwk	once a week
r	correlation coefficient
R	respiration; right; rectum; regular; rate
R (AW)	airway resistance
RA	rheumatoid arthritis; right atrium; right auricle; right arm; room air
RABG	room air blood gas
RAC	right atrial catheter
RAD	right axis deviation; radical
RAE	right atrial enlargement
RAEB	refractory anemia, erythroblastic
RAI	radioactive iodine
RAIU	radioactive iodine uptake
RALT	routine admission laboratory tests
RAM	rapid alternating movements
RAN	resident admission notes
RAO	right anterior oblique
RAP	right atrial pressure; resident assessment protocol
RAPD	relative afferent pupillary defect
RAS	renal artery stenosis
RAST	radioallergosorbent test
RAT	right anterior thigh
RAU	recurrent aphthous stomatitis
RB	retrobulbar; right buttock
R&B	right and below
RBA	right brachial artery

RBB	right breast biopsy
RBBB	right bundle branch block
RBC	red blood cells
RBCD	right border cardiac dullness
RBD	right border of dullness
RBE	relative biological equivalent/effectiveness
RBF	renal blood flow
RBOW	rupture bag of water
RBP	retinol-binding protein
RBRVS	resource-based relative value scale
RBV	right brachial vein
RCA	right coronary artery; radionuclide cerebral angiogram; regional citrate anticoagulation
RCC	renal cell carcinoma
RCD	relative cardiac dullness
RCM	right costal margin; radiographic contrast media
RCR	replication-competent retrovirus
RCS	reticulum cell sarcoma
RCT	root canal therapy; randomized clinical trial
RCV	red cell volume
RD	registered dietitian; renal disease; retinal detachment; respiratory disease
R&D	research and development
RDA	recommended daily allowance
RDH	registered dental hygienist
RDI	respiratory distress index
RDPE	reticular degeneration of pigment epithelium
RDS	respiratory distress syndrome
RDT	regular dialysis/hemodialysis treatment
RDVT	recurrent deep vein thrombosis
RDW	red cell size distribution width
RE	reticuloendothelial; rectal examination; regional enteritis; right eye; concerning
REE	resting energy expenditure
REF	renal erythropoietic factor; referred
rehab	rehabilitation
rel	religion
REM	rapid eye movement; roentgen equivalent in man
REMS	rapid eye movement sleep
rep	repeat; report; repair
repol	repolarization

RER	renal excretion rate; rough-surfaced endoplasmic reticulum
RES	reticuloendothelial system; resident; rehabilitation evaluation system
resc	resuscitation
resp	respiratory; respiration
retic	reticulocyte
rev	revolutions; review; reverse
RF	rheumatoid factor; renal failure; rheumatic fever
RFA	right frontoanterior; right femoral artery
RFL	right frontolateral
RFP	right frontoposterior
RFT	right frontotransverse
RF test	rheumatoid factor test
RG	right gluteal
RGM	right gluteus medius
Rh	Rhesus factor (in blood)
RH	right hyperphoria; right hand; room humidifier
RHB	raise head of bed
RHC	respiration has ceased; rural health clinic
RHD	rheumatic heart disease; relative hepatic dullness
RHE	recombinant human erythropoietin (R-HuEPO)
RHF	right heart failure
RHL	right hemisphere lesions
RHT	right hypertropia
R-HuEPO	recombinant human erythropoietin (RHE)
RIA	radioimmunoassay
RIC	right iliac crest; right internal carotid (artery)
RICE	rest and immobilization, ice, compression, elevation
RICS	right intercostal space
RICU	respiratory intensive care unit
RID	radial immunodiffusion
RIF	rigid internal fixation; right iliac fossa
RIG	rabies immune globulin
RIH	right inguinal hernia
RIMA	right internal mammary anastomosis
RIND	reversible ischemic neurologic defect
RIP	radioimmunoprecipitin (test); rapid infusion pump
RISA	radioiodinated serum albumin
RIST	radioimmunosorbent test
RK	radial keratotomy
RL	right leg; right lung; right lateral

RLE	right lower extremity
RLF	retrolental fibroplasia
RLL	right lower lobe
RLQ	right lower quadrant
RLR	right lateral rectus
RLT	right lateral thigh
RM	repetitions maximum; room; radical mastectomy; respiratory movement
R&M	routine and microscopic
RMA	right menoanterior
RMCA	right main coronary artery
RMCL	right midclavicular line
RMD	rapid movement disorder
RME	right medilateral episiotomy
RMEE	right middle ear exploration
RMI	repetitive motion injuries
RML	right middle lobe
RMP	right mentoposterior
RMR	right medial rectus; resting metabolic rate
RMSF	Rocky Mountain spotted fever
RMT	right mentotransverse; registered music therapist
RN	registered nurse
RNA	radionuclide angiography; ribonucleic acid
RND	radial neck dissection
RNEF	resting/radionuclide ejection fraction
RO	rule out (R/O); routine order
ROA	right occiput anterior
ROI	return on investment
ROM	range of motion
ROP	right occiput posterior; retinopathy of prematurity
ROS	review of systems
ROSC	restoration of spontaneous circulation
ROT	right occipital transverse; remedial occupational therapy
RP	retinitis pigmentosa; retrograde pyelogram; Raynaud's phenomenon
RPA	right pulmonary artery; radial photon absorptiometry; registered physician assistant/associate
RPCF	Reiter protein complement fixation
RPD	removable partial denture
RPE	retinal pigment epithelium; rating of perceived exertion

RPF	renal plasma flow; relaxed pelvic floor
RPGN	rapidly progressive glomerulonephritis
RPh	registered pharmacist
RPH	retroperitoneal hemorrhage
RPICCE	round pupil intracapsular cataract extraction
rpm	revolutions per minute
RPM	renal parenchymal malacoplakia
RPN	renal papillary necrosis
RPO	right posterior oblique
RPP	rate-pressure product
RPT	registered physical therapist
RQ	respiratory quotient
RR	recovery room; respiratory rate; regular respirations
R&R	rate and rhythm
RRE	round, regular, and equal (pupils)
RREF	resting radionuclide ejection fraction
rRNA	ribosomal ribonucleic acid
RRND	right radical neck dissection
RRR	regular rhythm and rate
RRRN	round, regular, react normally
RS	Reiter's syndrome; Reye's syndrome; rhythm strip; right side
RSA	right sacrum anterior; right subclavian artery
RSDS	reflex-sympathetic dystrophy syndrome
RSI	repetitive stress injury
R-SICU	respiratory-surgical intensive care unit
RSO	right salpingo-oophorectomy; radiation safety officer
RSP	right sacroposterior
RSR	regular sinus rhythm; relative survival rate
RSV	respiratory syncytial virus
RSW	right-sided weakness
R/t	related to
RT	right; radiation therapy; recreational therapy; renal transplant; running total; respiratory therapist; radiologic technician
RT3U	resin tri-iodothyronine uptake
RTA	renal tubular acidosis
RTC	return to clinic; round the clock
RTECS	Registry of Toxic Effects of Chemical Substances
RTL	reactive to light
rTNM	retreatment staging of cancer (tumor, node, metastasis)
RTO	return to office

rtPA	recombinant tissue-type plasminogen
RTRR	return to recovery room
RTS	real-time scan
RTx	radiation therapy
RU	rehabilitation unit
RUA	routine urine analysis
RUE	right upper extremity
RUG	retrograde urethrogram
RUL	right upper lobe
rupt	ruptured
RUQ	right upper quadrant
RURTI	recurrent upper respiratory tract infection
RUSB	right upper sternal border
RV	right ventricle; residual volume; rectovaginal; rubella vaccine
RVD	relative vertebral density
RVE	right ventricular enlargement
RVET	right ventricular ejection time
RVG	radionuclide ventriculography
RVH	right ventricular hypertrophy; renovascular hypertension
RVL	right vastus lateralis
RVO	retinal vein occlusion; relaxed vaginal outlet
RVOT	right ventricular outflow tract
RVP	red veterinary petrolatum
RVR	rapid ventricular response
RVSWI	right ventricular stroke work index
RV/TLC	residual volume to total lung capacity
Rx	therapy; drug; medication; treatment; take; prescription
RXN	reaction
S	subjective (finding); serum; suction; sacral; single; sister; without
S$_1$	first heart sound; first sacral vertebrae
S$_2$	second heart sound
SA	sinoatrial; sustained action; surface area
S&A	sugar and acetone
SAARD	slow-acting antirheumatic drugs
SAB	subarachnoid block/bleed
SAC	short arm cast
SACH	solid ankle cushion heel

SAD	sugar and acetone determination; seasonal affective disorder
SAE	signal-averaged electrocardiogram
SAF	self-articulating femoral
SAFE	stationary attachment and flexible endoskeletal (prosthesis)
Sag D	sagittal diameter
SAH	subarachnoid hemorrhage; systemic arterial hypertension
SAL12	sequential analysis of 12 chemistry constituents
SAM	systolic anterior motion; self-administered medication
SAN	sinoatrial node (S-A node)
S-A node	sinoatrial node (SAN)
SAPD	self-administration of psychotropic drugs
SAPHO	synovitis, acne, pustulosis, hyperostosis, osteitis
SAR	structure-activity relationship
SAS	sleep apnea syndrome
SAT	subacute thyroiditis; saturation
SAVD	spontaneous assisted vaginal delivery
SB	stillbirth; stillborn; spina bifida; sternal border; Sengstaken-Blakemore (tube); sinus bradycardia; small bowel
SBE	subacute bacterial endocarditis
SBFT	small bowel follow-through
SBGM	self blood glucose monitoring
SB-LM	Stanford Binet Intelligence Test—Form LM
SBO	small bowel obstruction
SBP	systolic blood pressure; spontaneous bacterial peritonitis
SBR	strict bed rest
SBT	serum bacterial titers
SC	subcutaneous; subclavian; sternoclavicular; sickle-cell
SCA	subcutaneous abdominal (block)
SCB	strictly confined to bed
SCBC	small cell bronchogenic carcinoma
SCC	squamous cell carcinoma; sickle cell crisis
SCCA	semiclosed circle absorber
SCD	sudden cardiac death; sickle cell disease; subacute combined degeneration; service connected disability; spinal cord disease
SCE	sister chromatic exchange

SCI	spinal cord injury
SCID	severe combined immunodeficiency disease/disorders
SCIV	subclavian intravenous
SCLC	small-cell lung cancer
SCLE	subcutaneous lupus erythematosis
SCLs	soft contact lenses
SCM	sternocleidomastoid; spondylitic caudal myelopathy
SCP	sodium cellulose phosphate
SCR	spondylitic caudal radiculopathy
SC/SP	supracondylar/suprapatellar prosthesis
SCT	sickle-cell trait; sugar-coated tablet; sentence completion test
SCUT	schizophrenia chronic undifferentiated type
SCV	subcutaneous vaginal (block)
SD	senile dementia; scleroderma; spontaneous delivery; sterile dressing; surgical drain
S&D	stomach and duodenum
SDA	steroid-dependent asthmatic
SDAT	senile dementia of Alzheimer's type
SDH	subdural hematoma
SDL	serum digoxin level
SDS	same-day surgery; sodium dodecyl sulfate
SDT	speech detection threshold
SE	side effect
sec	secondary
sed	sedimentation
sed rt	sedimentation rate
SEER	Surveillance, Epidemiology, and End Results (Program)
seg	segment; segmented neutrophil
SEM	systolic ejection murmur; scanning electron microscopy; standard error of mean
SEMI	subendocardial myocardial infarction
sens	sensorium
SEP	systolic ejection period; somatosensory evoked potential; separate
SER-IV	supination external rotation, type 4
SERs	somatosensory-evoked responses
SES	socioeconomic status
SF	scarlet fever; sugar free; salt free; symptom free; spinal fluid
SFA	superficial femoral artery; saturated fatty acids

SFC	spinal fluid count
SFEMG	single-fiber electromyography
SFP	spinal fluid pressure
SFPT	standard fixation preference test
SG	specific gravity; serum glucose; Swan-Ganz
SGA	small for gestational age
SGD	straight gravity drainage
SGE	significant glandular enlargement
SGOT	serum glutamic oxaloacetic transaminase
SGPT	serum glutamic pyruvic transaminase
SH	serum hepatitis; social history; shower; shoulder
S&H	speech and hearing
S/H	suicidal/homicidal (ideation)
SHA	super heater aerosol
SHb	sickle hemoglobin
SHEENT	skin, head, eyes, ears, nose, throat
SI	sacroiliac
S&I	suction and irrigation
SIADH	syndrome of inappropriate antidiuretic hormone secretion
SIB	self-injurious behavior
sibs	siblings
SICT	selective intracoronary thrombolysis
SICU	surgical intensive care unit
SIDS	sudden infant death syndrome
SIJ	sacroiliac joint
SIMV	synchronized intermittent mandatory ventilation
SIRS	systemic inflammatory response syndrome
SISI	short increment sensitivity index
SIT	sperm immobilization test; Slossen Intelligence Test
SIW	self-inflicted wound
SJS	Stevens-Johnson syndrome
SL	sublingual; slight
SLB	short leg brace
SLC	short leg cast
SLE	systemic lupus erythematosus; slit lamp examination
SLGXT	symptom limited graded exercise test
SLK	superior limbic keratoconjunctivitis
SLR	straight leg raising
SLRC	straight leg raising cast
SLS	sedation level score
SLWC	short leg walking cast

SM	systolic murmur; small
SMA	sequential multiple analyzer; simultaneous multichannel autoanalyzer; superior mesenteric artery; spinal muscular atrophy
SMC	special mouth care; somatomedin-C
SMD	senile macular degeneration
SMI	small volume infusion; sustained maximal inspiration; supplementary medical insurance
SMM	*State Medicaid Manual*
SMON	subacute myelopticoneuropathy
SMP	self-management program
SMR	submucosal resection; standardized mortality ratio; skeletal muscle relaxant
SMSA	standard metropolitan statistical area
SMVT	sustained monomorphic ventricular tachycardia
SNAP	sensory nerve action potential
SNCV	sensory nerve conduction velocity
SND	sinus node dysfunction
SNE	subacute necrotizing encephalomyelopathy
SNF	skilled nursing facility
SNGFR	single nephron glomerular filtration rate
SNT	Suppan nail technique
S-O	salpingo-oophorectomy
SO$_4$	sulfate
SOA	swelling of ankles; supraorbital artery
SOAA	signed out against advice
SOAP	subjective, objective, assessment, and plan
SOB	shortness of breath
S&OC	signed and on chart (permission)
SOD	superoxide dismutase
SOFAS	Social and Occupational Functioning Assessment Scale
sol	solution *(solutio)*
SOM	serous otitis media
SOMI	sterno-occipital mandibular immobilizer
sono	sonogram
SONP	solid organs not palpable
SOP	standard operating procedure
SP	suprapubic; sequential pulse; sacrum to pubis; speech pathologist; status post
S/P	status post
SPA	stimulation-produced analgesia

SPAG	small-particle aerosol generator
SPBI	serum protein bound iodine
SPBT	suprapubic bladder tap
SPE	serum protein electrolytes
spec	specimen
SPECT	single photon emission computer tomography
SPEP	serum protein electrophoresis
SPF	sun protection factor
sp fl	spinal fluid
sp gr	specific gravity
SPK	superficial punctate keratitis
SPMA	spinal progressive muscle atrophy
SPMSQ	Short Portable Mental Status Questionnaire
SPN	solitary pulmonary nodule
SPP	suprapubic prostatectomy
SPROM	spontaneous premature rupture of membrane
SPS	sodium polyethanol sulfanate
SPT	skin prick test
sp tap	spinal tap
SPU	short procedure unit
SPVR	systemic peripheral vascular resistance
SQ	subcutaneous
Sq CCa	squamous cell carcinoma
SR	sedimentation rate; sustained release; side rails; system review; sinus rhythm; sensitivity requirement
SRBC	sickle/sheep red blood cells
SRBOW	spontaneous rupture of bag of waters
SRC	scleroderma renal crisis
Sr Cr	serum creatinine
SRF	somatotropin-releasing factor
SRF-A	slow-releasing factor of anaphylaxis
SRIF	somatotropin-release-inhibiting factor
SRMD	stress-related mucosal damage
SR/NE	sinus rhythm, no ectopy
SRNS	steroid-responsive nephrotic syndrome
SROM	spontaneous rupture of membrane
SRP	signal recognition protein
SRS-A	slow-reacting substance of anaphylaxis
SRT	speech reception threshold; sedimentation rate test
SRU	side rails up
SS	salt substitute; Social Security; social services; slip sent; symmetrical strength; saturated solution

S&S	signs and symptoms
SSA	Social Security Administration
SSD	Social Security Disability; source to skin distance
SSDI	Social Security Disability Income
SSE	saline solution enema; soapsuds enema; systemic side effects
SSEP	somatosensory evoked potential
SSI	Supplemental Security Income
SSKI	saturated solution of potassium iodide
SSM	superficial spreading melanoma
SSN	Social Security number
SSPE	subacute sclerosing panencephalitis
SSRI	selective serotonin reuptake inhibitor
SSS	sick sinus syndrome; sterile saline soak
SSSS	staphylococcal scalded skin syndrome
ST	speech therapist; sinus tachycardia; split thickness
STA	superficial temporal artery
staph	*Staphylococcus aureus*
stat	immediately *(statim)*
STB	stillborn
STBY	standby
STD	sexually transmitted disease; skin test dose
STD TF	standard tube feeding
STET	submaximal treadmill exercise test
STF	special tube feeding
STG	short-term goals
STH	soft tissue hemorrhage; somatotrophic hormone
STIIPCH	systematic, totally integrated, individualized, patient-centered health care
STJ	subtalar joint
STM	short-term memory
sTNM	surgical-evaluative staging of cancer (tumor, node, metastasis)
STNR	symmetrical tonic neck reflex
STORCH	syphilis, toxoplasmosis, other agents, rubella, cytomegalovirus, and herpes
STP	standard temperature and pressure
STPD	standard temperature and pressure, dry
STR	short tandem repeat
strep	streptococcus; streptomycin
STS	serologic test for syphilis
STSG	split thickness skin graft

STU	shock trauma unit
SU	sensory urgency; Somogyi units
S&U	supine and upright
SUB	Skene's, urethral, and Bartholin (glands)
subq	subcutaneous
SUD	sudden unexpected death
SUID	sudden unexplained infant death
SUND	sudden unexpected nocturnal death
SUP	syndrome supinator; superior
suppos	suppository *(suppositoria)*
sur	surgery; surgical
SV	single ventricle; stock volume; sigmoid volvulus
SVC	superior vena cava
SVCO	superior vena cava obstruction
SVD	spontaneous vaginal delivery
SVE	sterile vaginal examination
SVPB	supraventricular premature beat
SVR	supraventricular rhythm; systemic vascular resistance
SVRI	systemic vascular resistance index
SVT	supraventricular tachycardia
SWD	short-wave diathermy
SWFI	sterile water for injection
SWI	sterile water for injection
SWS	slow-wave sleep; Sturge-Weber syndrome
SWT	stab wound of the throat
Sx	symptom; signs; surgery
Sz	seizure; suction; schizophrenic
T	temperature (TPR)
T(A)	axillary temperature
T(O)	oral temperature
T(R)	rectal temperature
T ½	half-life
T_1	tricuspid first sound; first thoracic vertebra
T_3	tri-iodothyronine
T_3RU	tri-iodothyroxine resin uptake
T_3UR	tri-iodothyronine uptake ratio
T_4	thyroxine
T_7	free thyroxine factor
TA	therapeutic abortion; temperature axillary; tricuspid atresia, tonometry applanation
T&A	tonsillectomy and adenoidectomy

TAA	total ankle arthroplasty; thoracic aortic aneurysm; tumor-associated antigen (antibodies); transverse aortic arch
tab	tablet *(tabella)*
TAB	therapeutic abortion; triple antibiotic
TAD	transverse abdominal diameter
TAE	transcatheter arterial embolization
TAF	tissue angiogenesis factor
TAH	total abdominal hysterectomy; total artificial heart
TAL	tendon Achilles lengthening
TANF	Temporary Assistance for Needy Families
TANI	total axial lymph node irradiation
TAO	thromboangitis obliterans
TAPVC	total anomalous pulmonary venous connection
TAPVD	total anomalous pulmonary venous drainage
TAPVR	total anamalous pulmonary venous return
TAR	thrombocytopenia with absent radius
TARA	total articular replacement arthroplasty
TAS	therapeutics activities specialist
TAT	tetanus antitoxin; till all taken; Thematic Apperception Test; turnaround time
TB	tuberculosis
TBA	to be admitted; to be absorbed
TBB	transbronchial biopsy
TBE	tick-borne encephalitis
TBG	thyroxine-binding globulin
TBI	total body irradiation
T bili	total bilirubin
tbl	tablespoon or tablespoonful (15 mL) (tbs; tbsp)
TBM	tubule basement membrane
TBNA	treated but not admitted
TBPA	thyroxine-binding prealbumin
TBR	total bed rest
tbs	tablespoon or tablespoonful (15 mL) (tbl; tbs)
TBSA	total burn surface area
tbsp	tablespoon or tablespoonful (15 mL) (tbl; tbs)
TBV	total blood volume; transluminal balloon valvuloplasty
TBW	total body water
TC	throat culture; total cholesterol; true conjugate; transcobalamin
T&C	type and crossmatch; turn and cough
T/C	to consider

TCA	tricyclic antidepressant; tricarboxylic acid cycle; tricuspid atresia; terminal cancer
TCABG	triple coronary artery bypass graft
TCBS agar	thiosulfate-citrate-bile salt-sucrose agar
TCCB	transitional cell carcinoma of bladder
TCDB	turn, cough, and deep breathe
T cell	small lymphocyte
TCH	turn, cough, hyperventilate
TCID 5O	median tissue culture doses
TCM	transcutaneous monitor; tissue culture media
TCMH	tumor-direct cell-mediated hypersensitivity
TCT	thrombin clotting time
TCVA	thromboembolic cerebral vascular accident
TD	tardive dyskinesia (TDK); travelers diarrhea; treatment discontinued; tetanus-diphtheria (toxoid)
TDD	thoracic duct drainage
TDE	total daily energy (requirement)
TDF	tumor dose fractionation
TDK	tardive dyskinesia (TD)
TDM	therapeutic drug monitoring
TdP	Torsades de Pointes
TDT	tentative discharge tomorrow
TE	tracheoesophageal; trace elements; thromboembolism
T&E	trial and error
TEA	total elbow arthroplasty; thromboendarterectomy
TEC	total eosinophil count
TED	tool for evaluation of documentation
TEE	transesophageal echocardiography
TEF	tracheoesophageal fistula
TEFRA	Tax Equity and Fiscal Responsibility Act of 1982
TEG	thromboelastogram
tele	telemetry
TEM	transmission electron microscopy
TEN	toxic epidermal necrolysis
TENS	transcutaneous electrical nerve stimulation
tert	tertiary
TES	treatment emergent symptoms; trace element solution
TET	treadmill exercise test
TF	tetralogy of Fallot (TOF); tactile fremitus; tube feeding; to follow
TFB	trifascicular block
TFT	thyroid function test

TG	triglycerides
TGA	transient global amnesia; transposition of the great arteries
TGF	tissue/transforming growth factor
TGFA	triglyceride fatty acid
TGS	tincture of green soap
TGT	thromboplastin generation test
TH	total hysterectomy; thyroid hormone
THA	total hip arthroplasty; transient hemispheric attack
THC	transhepatic cholangiogram; tetrahydrocannibinol
th-cult	throat culture
THE	transhepatic embolization
Ther Ex	therapeutic exercise
THI	transient hypogammaglobulinemia of infancy
THR	total hip replacement
TIA	transient ischemic attack
tib	tibia
TIBC	total iron-binding capacity
tid	three times a day *(ter in die)*
TIE	transient ischemia episode
TIG	tetanus immune globulin
TIN	tubulointerstitial nephritis
tinct	tincture *(tinctura)*
TJ	triceps jerk
TJN	twin jet nebulizer
TKA	total knee arthroplasty
TKNO	to keep needle open
TKO	to keep open
TKP	thermokeratoplasty
TKR	total knee replacement
TL	tubal ligation; team leader; trial leave
TLC	triple lumen catheter; thin layer chromatography; total lung capacity; total lymphocyte count; tender loving care
TLI	total lymphoid irradiation
TLS	tumor lysis syndrome
TLV	total lung volume
TM	tympanic membrane; travecular meshwork
TMA	transmetatarsal amputation
TMB	transient monocular blindness
TMC	transmural colitis
TMET	treadmill exercise test

TMI	threatened myocardial infarction
TMJ	temporomandibular joint
TMP	thallium myocardial perfusion
TMS	trace metal solution
TMTC	too many to count
Tn	intraocular tension, normal
TNF	tumor necrosis factor
TNI	total nodal irradiation
TNM	tumor/nodes/metastasis (classification)
TNTC	too numerous to count
TO	telephone order
TOA	tubo-ovarian abscess; time of arrival
TOF	tetralogy of Fallot (TF)
TOGV	transposition of the great vessels
TOL	trial of labor
tomo	tomography
TOP	termination of pregnancy
TOPV	trivalent oral polio vaccine
TORCH	toxoplasmosis, other (syphilis, hepatitis, Zoster), rubella, cytomegalovirus, and herpes simplex
TORP	total ossicular replacement prosthesis
TOS	thoracic outlet syndrome
tox	toxicology
TP	total protein
TPA	tissue plasminogen activator; tissue polypeptide antigen; total parenteral alimentation, third-party administrator
TPC	total patient care
TPD	tropical pancreatic diabetes
TPE	total protective environment
TPH	thromboembolic pulmonary hypertension
TPL	third-party liability
TPM	temporary pacemaker
TPN	total parenteral nutrition
TP&P	time, place, and person
TPP&E	time, person, place, and event
TPPN	total peripheral parenteral nutrition
TPPP	third-party prescription program
TPR	temperature, pulse, and respiration; temperature (T); total peripheral resistance
TPT	time to peak tension; total parenteral therapeutics
TPVR	total peripheral vascular resistance
TQM	total quality management

tr	trace; tremor; treatment; tincture
TRA	to run at
trach	tracheal; tracheostomy
Trans D	transverse diameter
TRC	tanned red cells
TRD	traction retinal detachment
TRH	thyrotropin-releasing hormone
trig	triglycerides
tRNA	transfer ribonucleic acid
TRNG	tetracycline resistant *Neisseria gonorrhea*
TRP	tubular reabsorption of phosphate, tamper-resistant packaging
TRT	thermoradiotherapy
TS	test solution; Tourette's syndrome
T&S	type and screen
TSA	total shoulder arthroplasty
TSBB	transtracheal selective bronchial brushing
TSD	Tay-Sachs disease; target to skin distance
T set	tracheotomy set
TSF	triceps skin fold
TSH	thyroid-stimulating hormone
tsp	teaspoon (5 mL)
TSP	total serum protein
T spine	thoracic spine
TSR	total shoulder replacement
TSS	toxic shock syndrome
TT	thrombin time; thymol turbidity; twitch tension; transtracheal; tilt table
TT$_3$	total serum tri-iodothyronine
TT$_4$	total thyroxine
T&T	touch and tone
TTA	total toe arthroplasty
TTN	transient tachypnea of the newborn (TTNB)
TTNB	transient tachypnea of the newborn (TTN)
TTP	thrombotic thrombocytopenic purpura
TTS	through the skin
TTVP	temporary transvenous pacemaker
TTY-TDD	teletypewriter for the deaf
TU	tuberculin units
TUN	total urinary nitrogen
TUR	transurethral resection
turb	turbidity

TURBN	transurethral resection bladder tumor
TURP	transurethral resection of prostate
TURV	transurethral resection valves
TV	tidal volume; trial visit
TVC	triple voiding cystogram; true vocal cord
TVH	total vaginal hysterectomy
TVP	transvenous pacemaker
TW	test weight
TWD	total white and differential count
TWE	tapwater enema
TWETC	tapwater enema till clear
TWWD	tapwater wet dressing
Tx	treatment; therapy; traction; transfuse; transplant
TxA2	thromboxane A2
U	units; urine
UA	uric acid; urinalysis; unauthorized absence; uncertain about
UAC	umbilical artery catheter
UAE	urinary albumin excretion
UAL	umbilical artery line
UAO	upper airway obstruction
UAT	up as tolerated
UAVC	univentricular atrioventricular connection
UB	uniform bill; uniform billing
UBF	unknown black female
UBI	ultraviolet blood irradiation
UBM	unknown black male
UC	urine culture; urethral catheter; uterine contraction; ulcerative colitis
U&C	urethral and cervical; usual and customary
UCC	Uniform Commercial Code
UCD	usual childhood diseases
UCG	urinary chorionic gonadotropins
UCHD	usual childhood diseases
UCI	urethral catheter in
UCO	urethral catheter out
UCR	usual, customary, and reasonable
UC	urine culture
UD	urethral discharge; unit dose
UDC	usual diseases of childhood
UDP	uridine 5'-diphosphate

UE	upper extremity
UES	upper esophageal sphincter
UFO	unflagged order
UFM	uroflowmetry
UG	urogenital
UGH	uveitis, glaucoma, hyphema
UGI	upper gastrointestinal (series)
UHBI	upper hemibody irradiation
UHDDS	Uniform Hospital Discharge Data Set
UIQ	upper inner quadrant
UK	urokinase; unknown (unk)
U/L	upper and lower
ULN	upper limits of normal
ULQ	upper left quadrant
UN	urinary nitrogen
UNA	urinary nitrogen appearance
ung	ointment *(unguentum)*
unk	unknown (UK)
UO	urine output
UOQ	upper outer quadrant
U/P	urine-to-plasma ratio
UPC	universal product code
UPEP	urine protein electrophoresis
UPJ	ureteropelvic junction
UPP	urethral pressure profile (studies)
UPT	urine pregnancy test
UR	utilization review
URAC	Utilization Review Accreditation Commission
URC	utilization review committee
URI	upper respiratory infection
urol	urology
US	ultrasound; ultrasonography
USAEC	United States Atomic Energy Commission
USAN	United States Adopted Names (Council)
USB	upper sternal border
USC	United States Code (a drug code)
USD	United States Dispensatory
USFDA	United States Food and Drug Administration
USG	ultrasonography
USI	urinary stress incontinence
USN	ultrasonic nebulizer
USP	*United States Pharmacopeia*

USPC	United States Pharmacopeial Convention
USP DI	*United States Pharmacopeial Dispensing Information*
USPHS	United States Public Health Service (PHS)
USP-NF	*United States Pharmacopeia–National Formulary*
USRDS	United States Renal Data System
UTD	up to date
ut dict	as directed *(ut dictum)*
UTF	usual throat flora
UTI	urinary tract infection
UTO	upper tibial osteotomy
UTP	uridine triphosphate
UTS	ultrasound
UUN	urine urea nitrogen
UV	ultraviolet
UVA	ultraviolet A (light); ureterovesical angle
UVB	ultraviolet B (light)
UVC	umbilical vein catheter; ultraviolet C (light)
UVJ	ureterovesical junction
UVL	ultraviolet light
UVR	ultraviolet rays
UWF	unknown white female
UWM	unknown white male
V	vomiting; vein; vagina; five
VA	Veterans Administration; visual acuity; vacuum aspiration
VAC	ventriculoarterial connections
VAD	vascular/venous access device; vincristine, adriamycin, dexamthasone
vag	vagina
vag hyst	vaginal hysterectomy
VAH	Veterans Administration Hospital
VAMC	Veterans Administration Medical Center
var	variant
VAS	vascular; visual analogue scale
VASC	Visual-Auditory Screen Test for Children
vas rad	vascular radiology
VB	VanBuren (catheter)
VBAC	vaginal birth after cesarean
VBI	vertebrobasilar insufficiency
VBS	vertebral-basilar system

VC	vital capacity; vena cava; vocal cords; color vision; vomiting center
VCG	vectorcardiography
VCT	venous clotting time
VCU	voiding cystourethrogram
VCUG	vesicoureterogram; voiding cystourethrogram
VD	venereal disease; volume of distribution; voided
VDA	visual discriminatory acuity; venous digital angiogram
VDG	venereal disease—gonorrhea
VDH	valvular disease of the heart
VDRR	vitamin D–resistant rickets
VDS	venereal disease—syphilis
VE	vaginal examination; vertex; volume of expired gas
VEB	ventricular ectopic beat
VEE	Venezuelan equine encephalitis
vent	ventricular; ventral; ventilator
VEP	visual evoked potential
VER	visual evoked response; ventricular escape rhythm
VF	ventricular fibrillation; vision field; vocal fremitus
V fib	ventricular fibrillation
VFP	vitreous fluorophotometry
VG	vein graft; ventricular gallop; very good
VH	vaginal hysterectomy; viral hepatitis; vitreous hemorrhage; Veterans Hospital
VI	volume index
vib	vibration
VID	videodensitometry
VIG	vaccinia immune globulin
VIP	voluntary interruption of pregnancy; vasoactive intestinal peptide
VIPPS	Verified Internet Pharmacy Practice Site (program)
V-Q	Ventilation-Perfusion (Scan)
VISC	vitreous infusion suction cutter
VIT	vitamin; vital; venom immunotherapy
vit cap	vital capacity
viz	namely
VKC	vernal keratoconjunctivitis
VLBW	very low birth weight
VLDL	very low density lipoprotein
VLH	ventrolateral nucleus of the hypothalamus
VMA	vanillylmandelic acid
VMH	ventromedial hypothalamus

VO	verbal order
VOCTOR	void on call to operating room
VOD	vision right eye *(oculus dexter);* venocclusive disease
vol	voluntary
VOR	vestibular ocular reflex
VOS	vision left eye *(oculus sinister)*
VOU	vision both eyes *(oculus uterque)*
VP	venous pressure; variegate porphyria; ventriculoperitoneal; ventricular-peritoneal
V&P	ventilation and perfusion; vagotomy and pyloroplasty
VPB	ventricular premature beat
VPC	ventricular premature contraction
VPD	ventricular premature depolarization
VPL	ventroposterolateral
VR	ventricular rhythm; verbal reprimand
VRA	visual reinforcement audiometry
vs	versus (VS)
VS	vital signs; versus (vs)
VSR	venous stasis retinopathy
VSS	vital signs stable
VT	ventricular tachycardia (V tach); tidal volume
V tach	ventricular tachycardia (VT)
VTE	venous thromboembolism
VTX	vertex
v/v	volume-to-volume ratio
VV	varicose veins
V&V	vulva and vagina
VVC	vulvovaginal candidiasis
VVFR	vesicovaginal fistula repair
VVOR	visual-vestibulo-ocular reflex
VW	vessel wall
VWM	ventricular wall motion
VZ	varicella zoster
VZIG	varicella zoster immune globulin
VZV	varicella zoster virus
w	white; with; widowed
WA	while awake; when awake
WAC	wholesale acquisition cost
WAIS	Wechsler Adult Intelligence Scale
WAIS-R	Wechsler Adult Intelligence Scale—Revised
WAP	wandering atrial pacemaker

WAS	Wiskott-Aldrich syndrome
WASS	Wasserman test
WB	whole blood; weight bearing
WBAT	weight bearing as tolerated
WBC	white blood cell count
WBH	whole-body hyperthermia
WBN	wellborn nursery
WC	wheelchair; white count; whooping cough; workers' compensation
W/D	warm and dry; withdrawal
W-D	wet to dry
WDHA	watery diarrhea, hypokalemia, and achlorhydria
WDL	well-differentiated lymphocytes
WDLL	well-differentiated lymphocytic lymphoma
WDWN-BF	well-developed, well-nourished black female
WDWN-BM	well-developed, well-nourished black male
WDWN-WF	well-developed, well-nourished white female
WDWN-WM	well-developed, well-nourished white male
WE	weekend
WEE	western equine encephalitis
WEP	weekend pass
WF	white female
WFI	water for injection
WFL	within functional limits
WFR	wheel-and-flare reaction
WHO	World Health Organization
WHV	woodchuck hepatitis virus
WHVP	wedged hepatic venous pressure
WIC	Women, Infants, and Children (Program)
wid	widow; widower
WISC	Wechsler Intelligence Scale for Children
WKS	Wernicke-Korsakoff syndrome
WLS	wet lung syndrome
WLT	waterload test
WM	white male
WMA	wall motion abnormality
WN	well-nourished
WND	wound
WNL	within normal limits
WO	written order; week(s) old
W/O	without
WP	whirlpool

WPFM	Wright peak flow meter
WPPSI	Wechsler Preschool Primary Scale of Intelligence
WPW	Wolff-Parkinson-White (syndrome)
WR	Wasserman reaction; wrist
wt	weight
W/U	workup
w/v	weight-to-volume ratio
w/w	weight-to-weight ratio
WWAC	walk with aid of cane
X	cross-match; start of anesthesia; except; times; ten; break
X × 3	orientation as to person, place, and time
X&D	examination and diagnosis
XL	extended release
XM	cross-match (X-mat)
X-mat	cross-match (XM)
XMM	xeromammography
XRT	X-ray therapy; radiotherapy
XS-LIM	exceeds limits (of procedure)
XT	exotropia
XX	normal female sex chromosome type
XY	normal male sex chromosome type
YACP	young adult chronic patient
YAG	yttrium aluminum garnert (laser)
YF	yellow fever
YJV	yellow jacket venom
YLC	youngest living child
YO	year(s) old
YSC	yolk sac carcinoma
ZEEP	zero end-expiratory pressure
ZES	Zollinger-Ellison syndrome
Z-ESR	zeta erythrocyte sedimentation rate
ZIFT	zygote intrafallopian transfer
ZIG	zoster serum immune globulin
ZIP	zoster immune plasma
ZMC	zygomatic
ZnO	zinc oxide

Latin/Greek Terminology

Abbreviation	Latin/Greek Words	English Definition
a	*ante*	before
aa, a	*ana (Greek)*	of each
ad	*ad*	to, up to
add	*adde*	add
ad hib	*ad hibendus*	to be administered
ad lib	*ad libitum*	at pleasure
admov	*admove*	apply
ad sat	*ad saturatum*	to saturation
aeq	*aequales*	equal
agit	*agita*	shake, stir
agit ante sum	*agita ante sumendum*	shake before taking
alb	*albus*	white
alt	*alter*	the other
alt hor	*alyernis horis*	every other hour
AM	*ante meridiem*	before noon
ampul	*ampulla*	ampoule, ampule, ampul
aq	*aqua*	water
bull	*aqua bulliens*	boiling water
cal	*aqua calida*	warm water
aq dest	*aqua destillata*	distilled water
ferv	*aqua fervens*	hot water
font	*aqua fontis*	spring water
frig	*aqua frigida*	cold water
aq pur	*aqua pura*	pure water
aur, a	*auris*	ear
aut	*aut*	or
b	*bis*	twice
bene	*bene*	well
bib	*bibe*	drink
bid	*bis in die*	twice daily
bin	*bis in noctus*	twice at night
bis	*bis*	twice

Abbreviation	Latin/Greek Words	English Definition
bol	*bolus*	large pill
brevis	*brevis*	short
bull	*bulliat*	let (it) boil
caps	*capsula*	capsule
cerat	*ceratum*	wax ointment
chart	*charta*	paper, powder paper
cint	*contra*	against
coch mag	*cochleare magnum*	tablespoonful
coch med	*cochleare medium*	dessertspoonful
coch parv	*cochleare parvum*	teaspoonful
collut	*collutorium*	mouthwash
collyr	*collyrium*	eyewash
commisce	*commisce*	mix together
comp	*compositus*	compounded of
cong	*congius*	gallon
contus	*contusus*	bruised
cotula	*cotula*	measure
cuj lib	*cujus libet*	of any you please
d	*da*	give
d	*dexter*	right
d	*dies*	day
de d in d	*de die in dieum*	from day to day
dec	*decanta*	pour off
dent tal dos	*dentur tales doses*	give of such doses
det	*detur*	let it be given
dieb alt	*diebus alternis*	every other day
dieb tert	*diebus tertiis*	every third day
dil	*dilue, dilutus*	dilute, diluted
dim	*dimidus*	one-half
disp	*dispensa*	dispense
div	*divide*	divide
div in par aeq	*dividatur in partes aequales*	let it be divided into equal parts
dos, d	*dosis*	dose
dtd	*dentur tales doses*	give of such doses
dulc	*dulcis*	sweet
dur	*durus*	hard
dur dolor	*durante dolore*	while pain lasts

Abbreviation	Latin/Greek Words	English Definition
emp	*ex modo praescripto*	as directed
emp	*emplastrum*	plaster
emuls	*emulsio*	emulsion
epistom	*epistomium*	stopper
ex	*ex*	out of
ext	*extende; extractum*	spread; extract
ferv	*fervens*	boiling
filt	*filtra*	filter
fl	*fluidus*	fluid
fort	*fortis*	strong
frig	*frigidus*	cold
ft	*fiat*	let it be made
garg	*gargarisma*	gargle
gm	*gramma*	gram
gr	*granum*	grain
grad	*gradatim*	by degrees
gran	*granulatus*	granulated
gt, gtt	*gutta, guttae*	drop, drops
guttat	*guttae guttatim*	by drops
haust	*haustus*	draught
hor decub	*hora decubitus*	bedtime
hor 1 spat	*horae unius spatio*	one hour's time
hs	*hora somni*	bedtime
ic	*inter cibos*	between meals
idem	*idem*	the same
inf	*infusum*	let it infuse
int	*intime*	thoroughly
juxt	*juxta*	near
la	*lege artis*	according to the art
laev	*laevus*	left
lb	*libra*	pound
lev	*levis*	light
lin	*linimentum*	liniment
liq	*liquor*	solution

Abbreviation	Latin/Greek Words	English Definition
lot	*lotio*	lotion
m	*mane*	in the morning
m	*mitte*	send
M	*misce*	mix
mac	*macera*	macerate
man prim	*mane primo*	first thing in the morning
mas	*massa*	mass
m dict	*more dicto*	as directed
med	*medicamentum*	medicine
m et n	*mane et nocte*	morning and night
mist	*mistura*	mixture
mitt	*mitte*	send
mod	*modicus*	moderate sized
mod praesc	*modo praescripto*	in the manner written
moll	*mollis*	soft
mor dict	*more dicto*	in the manner directed
mor sol	*more solito*	as accustomed
nebul	*nebula*	spray
no	*numero*	number
noct	*nocte*	at night
noct maneq	*nocte maneque*	night and morning
non rep	*non repetatur*	do not repeat
nunc	*nunc*	now
O	*Octarius*	pint
od	*oculus dexter*	right eye
ol	*oculus laevus*	left eye
om mane vel noc	*omni mane vel nocte*	every morning or night
omn bid	*omnibus bidendis*	every two days
omn bih	*omni bihoris*	every second hour
omn hor	*omni hora*	every hour
om 1/4 h	*omni quadrantae horae*	every 15 minutes
os	*oculus sinister*	left eye
ou	*oculus uterque*	both eyes
part aeq	*partes aequales*	equal parts
part vic	*partitus vicibus*	individual doses
parv	*parvus*	small

Abbreviation	Latin/Greek Words	English Definition
pc	*post cibus; post cibos*	after food; after meals
pil	*pilula*	pill
PM	*post meridiem*	after noon
po	*per os*	by mouth
ppa	*phiala prius agitate*	bottle being first shaken
prn	*pro re nata*	as needed
pro rat aet	*pro ratione aetatis*	according to patient's age
pulv	*pulvis*	powder
q, qq	*quodque*	each, every
qid	*quarter in die*	four times a day
qq hor	*quaque hora*	every hour
qs	*quantum sufficiat*	sufficient quantity
quot op cit	*quoties opus sit*	as often as necessary
qv	*quantum voleris*	as much as you wish
red in pulv	*redactus in pulverem*	reduced to powder
rept	*repetatur*	to be repeated
rub	*ruber*	red
S, Sig	*signa, signetur*	write
sa	*secundum artem*	according to art
sic	*siccus*	dried
sig	*signa; signetur*	write; let it be labeled
sing	*singulorum*	of each
sol	*solutio*	solution
solv	*solve*	dissolve
sos	*si opus sit*	if there is need
ss	*semi, semisse*	half
stat	*statim*	immediately
subind	*subinde*	frequently
suc	*succus*	juice
sum	*sume*	take
sum tal	*summat talem*	take one such
suppos	*suppositoria*	suppository
syr	*syrupus*	syrup
tab	*tabella*	tablet
tid	*ter in die*	three times a day
tinct	*tinctura*	tincture

Abbreviation	Latin/Greek Words	English Definition
tnt	*tritura*	triturate or grind
ult praes	*ultimus praescriptus*	the last ordered
ung	*unguentum*	ointment
ut dict	*ut dictum*	as directed

Weights and Measures

APOTHECARY SYSTEM

Weight units (Basic unit is the grain.)

Name of unit	Symbol	Equivalent weights			
grain	gr				
scruple	Э	20 gr			
drachm	Ʒ	60 gr	3 Э		
ounce	℥	480 gr	24 Э	8 Ʒ	
pound	℔	5,760 gr	288 Э	96 Ʒ	12 ℥

Volume units (Basic unit is the minim.)

Name of unit	Symbol	Equivalent volumes				
minim	♏					
fluid drachm	fl Ʒ	60 ♏				
fluid ounce	fl ℥	480 ♏	8 fl Ʒ			
pint	pt or 0	7,680 ♏	128 fl Ʒ	16 fl ℥		
quart	qt	15,360 ♏	256 fl Ʒ	32 fl ℥	2 pt	
gallon	gal or C	61,440 ♏	1,024 fl Ʒ	128 fl ℥	8 pt	4 qt

AVOIRDUPOIS SYSTEM

Weight units (Basic unit is the grain.)

Name of unit	Symbol	Equivalent weights	
grain	gr		
ounce	oz	437.5 gr	
pound	lb	7,000 gr	16 oz

IMPERIAL MEASURE (BRITISH)

Volume units (Basic unit is the minim.)

Name of unit	Symbol	Volume equivalents			
minim	♏				
fluid dram	fldr	60 ♏			
fluid ounce	floz	480 ♏	8 fldr		
pint	0 (pt)	9,600 ♏	160 fldr	20 floz	
gallon	cong	76,800 ♏	1,280 fldr	160 floz	8 pt

METRIC SYSTEM

Length units (Basic unit is the meter.)

Name of unit	Symbol	Length equivalent (meters)
nanometer	nm	0.000,000,001
micrometer	μm	0.000,001
millimeter	mm	0.001
centimeter	cm	0.01
decimeter	dm	0.10
meter	m	1.0
decameter	Dm or dam	10.0
hectometer	Hm or hm	100.0
kilometer	km	1000.0

Weight units (Basic unit is the gram.)

Name of unit	Symbol	Weight equivalents (grams)
nanogram	ng	0.000,000,001
microgram	μm or mcg	0.000,001
milligram	mg	0.001
centigram	cg	0.01

decigram	dg	0.1
gram	gm or g	1.0
decagram	dg or dag	10.0
hectogram	Hg or hg	100.0
kilogram	Kg or kg	1000.0

Volume units (Basic unit is the liter.)

Name of unit	Symbol	Volume equivalents (liters)
microliter	μl	0.000,001
milliliter	ml	0.001
centiliter	cl	0.01
deciliter	dl	0.1
liter	l	1.0
decaliter	dal	10.0
hectoliter	hl	100.0
kiloliter	kl	1000.0

CONVERSION EQUIVALENTS

Weight measure	Weight equivalents	
1 milligram	0.015432	grain
1 gram	15.432	grains
1 gram	0.25720	apothecary drachm
1 gram	0.03527	avoirdupois ounce
1 gram	0.03215	apothecary ounce
1 kilogram	35.274	avoirdupois ounces
1 kilogram	32.151	apothecary ounces
1 kilogram	2.2046	avoirdupois pounds
1 grain	64.7989	milligrams
1 grain	0.0647989	gram
1 apothecary drachm	3.88	grams

1 avoirdupois ounce	28.3495	grams
1 apothecary ounce	31.1035	grams
1 avoirdupois pound	453.5924	grams
1 apothecary pound	373.25038	grams

Liquid measure	Volume equivalents	
1 U.S. gallon	0.8326394	British gallon
1 British gallon	1.201	U.S. gallons
1 milliliter	16.23	minims
1 milliliter	0.2705	fluid drachm
1 milliliter	0.0338146	fluid ounces
1 liter	33.8148	fluid ounces
1 liter	2.1134	pints
1 liter	1.0567	quarts

Liquid measure	Volume equivalents	
1 liter	0.2642	gallon
1 fluid drachm	3.697	milliliters
1 fluid ounce	29.573	milliliters
1 pint	473.168	milliliters
1 quart	946.332	milliliters
1 gallon	3.785	liters
1 liter	1.0567	quarts

Length measure	Volume equivalents	
1 inch	2.54	centimeters
1 foot	30.48	centimeters
1 yard	91.44	centimeters
1 yard	0.9144	meter
1 centimeter	0.3937	inch
1 centimeter	0.03281	foot
1 meter	1.0936	yards

U.S. Schools and Associations

ACCREDITED SCHOOLS AND COLLEGES OF PHARMACY

Alabama

Auburn University Harrison School of Pharmacy
217 Pharmacy Building
Auburn, AL 36849-5501
334-844-8350
334-844-8353 (fax)
pharmacy.auburn.edu

Samford University McWhorter School of Pharmacy
800 Lakeshore Drive
Birmingham, AL 35229
205-726-2820
205-726-2759 (fax)
www.samford.edu/schools/pharmacy.html

Arkansas

University of Arkansas for Medical Sciences College of Pharmacy
4301 West Markham, Slot 522
Little Rock, AR 72205-7122
501-686-5557
501-686-8315 (fax)
www.uams.edu/cop

Arizona

Midwestern University College of Pharmacy—Glendale
19555 North Fifty-Ninth Avenue
Glendale, AZ 85308
623-572-3500
623-572-3510 (fax)
www.midwestern.edu/cpg

The University of Arizona College of Pharmacy
1703 East Mabel Street
P.O. Box 210207
Tucson, AZ 85721
520-626-1427
520-626-4063 (fax)
www.pharmacy.arizona.edu/

California

Loma Linda University School of Pharmacy
West Hall
Loma Linda, CA 92350
909-558-1300
909-558-4849 (fax)
www.llu.edu/llu/sps/index.html

University of California at San Diego School of Pharmacy
    and Pharmaceutical Sciences
9500 Gelman Drive
San Diego, CA 92093-0657
858-822-4900
858-822-5591 (fax)
www.pharmacy.ucsd.edu

University of California at San Francisco School of Pharmacy
513 Parnassus Avenue
San Francisco, CA 94143-0446
415-476-2733
415-476-0688 (fax)
pharmacy.ucsf.edu/

University of the Pacific Thomas J. Long School of Pharmacy
    and Health Sciences
3601 Pacific Avenue
Stockton, CA 95211
209-946-2561
209-946-2410 (fax)
www.uop.edu/

University of Southern California School of Pharmacy
1985 Zonal Avenue
Los Angeles, CA 90089
323-442-1369
323-442-1681 (fax)
pharmacy.usc.edu

Western University of Health Sciences School of Pharmacy
College Plaza
309 East Second Street
Pomona, CA 91766-1889
909-469-5500
909-469-5539 (fax)
www.westernu.edu

Colorado

University of Colorado Health Sciences Center School of Pharmacy
4200 East Ninth Avenue
Denver, CO 80262-0238
303-315-5055
303-315-6281 (fax)
www.uchsc.edu/sop/

Connecticut

The University of Connecticut School of Pharmacy
372 Fairfield Road, Unit 2092
Storrs, CT 06269-2092
860-486-2129
860-486-1553 (fax)
pharmacy.uconn.edu

District of Columbia

Howard University College of Pharmacy, Nursing and AHS
2300 Fourth Street, NW
Washington, DC 20059
202-806-6530
202-806-4636 (fax)
www.cpnahs.howard.edu/pharmacy/index.htm

Florida

Florida Agricultural and Mechanical University College of Pharmacy and Pharmaceutical Sciences
201 Dyson Pharmacy Building
P.O. Box 367
Tallahassee, FL 32307
850-599-3593
850-599-3347 (fax)
www.pharmacy.famu.edu

Nova Southeastern University College of Pharmacy
3200 South University Drive
Fort Lauderdale, FL 33328
954-262-1300
954-262-2278 (fax)
pharmacy.nova.edu

Palm Beach Atlantic College School of Pharmacy
901 South Flager Drive
West Palm Beach, FL 33416
561-803-2000
561-803-2437 (fax)
www.pbac.edu

University of Florida College of Pharmacy
1600 SW Archer Road, M-454
P.O. Box 100484 JHMHC
Gainesville, FL 32610-0484
352-392-9713
352-392-3480 (fax)
www.cop.ufl.edu/

Georgia

Mercer University Southern School of Pharmacy
3001 Mercer University Drive
Atlanta, GA 30341-4155
678-547-6304
678-547-6315 (fax)
www.mercer.edu/pharmacy

South University School of Pharmacy
709 Mall Boulevard
Savannah, GA 31406
912-201-8123
912-201-8154 (fax)
www.southcollege.edu/campus/SchoolsIndex.asp?id=1

University of Georgia College of Pharmacy
D.W. Brooks Drive
Athens, GA 30602
706-542-1911
706-542-5269 (fax)
www.rx.uga.edu

Iowa

Drake University College of Pharmacy and Health Sciences
2507 University Avenue
Des Moines, IA 50311
515-271-2172
515-271-4171 (fax)
pharmacy.drake.edu

The University of Iowa College of Pharmacy
115 South Grand Avenue
118 Pharmacy Building
Iowa City, IA 52242
319-335-8794
319-335-9418 (fax)
www.uiowa.edu/pharmacy/

Idaho

Idaho State University College of Pharmacy
970 South Fifth Avenue
Campus Box 8288
Pocatello, ID 83209
208-282-2175
208-282-4482 (fax)
pharmacy.isu.edu

Illinois

Midwestern University Chicago College of Pharmacy
555 Thirty-First Street
Downers Grove, IL 60515-1235
630-971-6417
630-971-6097 (fax)
www.midwestern.edu/pages/ccp.html

Southern Illinois University at Edwardsville School of Pharmacy
Campus Box 2000
Edwardsville, IL 62026-200
618-650-5150
618-650-5152 (fax)
www.siue.edu/PHARMACY

University of Illinois at Chicago College of Pharmacy
833 South Wood Street, Suite 145
Chicago, IL 60612
312-996-7240
312-996-3272 (fax)
www.uic.edu/pharmacy

Indiana

Butler University College of Pharmacy and Health Sciences
4600 Sunset Avenue
Indianapolis, IN 46208
317-940-9322
317-940-6172 (fax)
www.butler.edu/www/cophs

Purdue University School of Pharmacy and Pharmacal Sciences
1330 Heine Pharmacy Building
West Lafayette, IN 47907-1330
765-494-1368
765-494-7880 (fax)
www.pharmacy.purdue.edu

Kansas

University of Kansas School of Pharmacy
1251 Wescoe Hall Drive
2056 Malot Hall
Lawrence, KS 66045-2500
785-864-3591
785-864-5265 (fax)
www.pharm.ukans.edu/dean/index.htm

Kentucky

University of Kentucky College of Pharmacy
Rose Street—Pharmacy Building
Lexington, KY 40536-0082
859-323-7601
859-257-2128 (fax)
www.mc.uky.edu/Pharmacy/

Louisiana

The University of Louisiana at Monroe College of Pharmacy
700 University Avenue
Monroe, LA 71209-0470
318-342-1600
318-342-1606 (fax)
www.Rxweb.ulm.edu/pharmacy

Xavier University of Louisiana College of Pharmacy
1 Drexel Drive
New Orleans, LA 70125
504-483-7500
504-485-7930 (fax)
www.xula.edu

Massachusetts

Massachusetts College of Pharmacy and Health Sciences School
   of Pharmacy—Boston
179 Longwood Avenue
Boston, MA 02115
617-732-2825
617-732-2244 (fax)
www.mcp.edu

Massachusetts College of Pharmacy and Health Sciences School
  of Pharmacy—Worcester
19 Foster Street
Worcester, MA 01608
508-890-8855
508-890-8515 (fax)
www.mcp.edu

Northeastern University School of Pharmacy, Bouve College
  of Health Sciences
206 Mugar Hall
Boston, MA 02115
617-373-3380
617-373-7655 (fax)
www.neu.edu/bouve/pharma.html

Maryland

University of Maryland School of Pharmacy
20 North Pine Street
Baltimore, MD 21201-1180
410-706-7651
410-706-4012 (fax)
www.pharmacy.umaryland.edu

Michigan

Ferris State University College of Pharmacy
220 Ferris Drive
Big Rapids, MI 49307-2740
231-591-2254
231-591-3829 (fax)
www.pharmacy.ferris.edu

The University of Michigan College of Pharmacy
428 Church Street
Ann Arbor, MI 48109-1065
734-764-7312
734-763-2022 (fax)
www.umich.edu/~pharmacy/

Wayne State University
Eugene Applebaum College of Pharmacy and Health Sciences
259 Mack Avenue
Detroit, MI 48201
313-577-1574
313-577-5589 (fax)
www.cphs.wayne.edu/

Minnesota

University of Minnesota College of Pharmacy
308 Harvard Street SE
5-130 Weaver-Densford Hall
Minneapolis, MN 55455-0343
612-624-1900
612-624-2974 (fax)
www.pharmacy.umn.edu

University of Minnesota—Duluth College of Pharmacy
Room 386 Kirby Plaza
Duluth, MN 55812-2496
218-726-6000
218-726-6500 (fax)
www.pharmacy.umn.edu/duluth

Missouri

University of Missouri—Kansas City School of Pharmacy
5005 Rockhill Road
Kansas City, MO 64110-2499
816-235-1609
816-235-5190 (fax)
www.umkc.edu/pharmacy

St. Louis College of Pharmacy
4588 Parkview Place
St. Louis, MO 63110
314-367-8700
314-367-2784 (fax)
www.stlcop.edu

Mississippi

The University of Mississippi School of Pharmacy
Thad Cochran Research Center
P.O. Box 1848
University, MS 38655-9814
662-915-7265
662-915-5704 (fax)
www.olemiss.edu/depts/pharm_school/

Montana

University of Montana School of Pharmacy and Allied Health Sciences
32 Campus Drive #1512
Missoula, MT 59812-1075
406-243-4621
406-243-4209 (fax)
www.umt.edu/pharmacy

Nebraska

University of Nebraska College of Pharmacy
986000 Nebraska Medical Center
Omaha, NE 68198-6000
402-559-4333
402-559-5060 (fax)
www.unmc.edu/pharmacy/college.html

Creighton University School of Pharmacy and Health Professions
2500 California Plaza
Omaha, NE 68178
402-280-2950
402-280-5738 (fax)
pharmacy.creighton.edu

Nevada

Nevada College of Pharmacy
5740 South Eastern Avenue, Suite 240
Las Vegas, NV 89119
702-990-4433
702-990-4435 (fax)
www.nvcp.edu

New Jersey

Rutgers, The State University of New Jersey
Ernest Mario College of Pharmacy
160 Frelinghuysen Road
Piscataway, NJ 08854
732-445-2675
732-445-5767 (fax)
www.rutgers.edu/aboutru/colleges/collphar.htm

New Mexico

University of New Mexico College of Pharmacy
2502 Marble Northeast
Albuquerque, NM 87131
505-272-2461
505-272-6749 (fax)
hsc.unm.edu/pharmacy/

New York

Long Island University
Arnold and Marie Schwartz College of Pharmacy and Health Sciences
75 DeKalb Avenue
Brooklyn, NY 11201
718-488-1234
718-488-0628 (fax)
www.liu.edu/cwis/pharmacy/pharmacy/html

St. John's University College of Pharmacy and Allied Health
    Professions
800 Utopia Parkway
Jamaica, NY 11439
718-990-1415
718-990-1871 (fax)
www.stjohns.edu

Union University Albany College of Pharmacy
106 New Scotland
Albany, NY 12208
518-445-7200
518-445-7202 (fax)
www.acp.edu

University of Buffalo School of Pharmacy and Pharmaceutical Sciences
C126 Cooke-Hall
Box 601200
Buffalo, NY 14260-1200
716-645-2823
716-645-3688 (fax)
www.pharmacy.buffalo.edu

North Carolina

Campbell University School of Pharmacy
101 Main Street
P.O. Box 1090
Buies Creek, NC 27506
910-893-1685
910-893-1697 (fax)
www.campbell.edu/pharmacy/index.html

University of North Carolina School of Pharmacy
7360 Beard Hall
Chapel Hill, NC 27599-7360
919-966-1121
919-966-6919 (fax)
www.pharmacy.unc.edu

Wingate University School of Pharmacy
P.O. Box 3087
Wingate, NC 28174-0159
704-233-8331
704-233-8332 (fax)
www.pharmacy.wingate.edu/faculty/home.asp

North Dakota

North Dakota State University College of Pharmacy
123 Sudro Hall
Fargo, ND 58105
701-231-6469
701-231-7606 (fax)
www.ndsu.nodak.edu/pharmacy/

Ohio

Ohio Northern University College of Pharmacy
525 South Main
Ada, OH 45810
419-772-2275
419-772-2720 (fax)
www.onu.edu/pharmacy

University of Cincinnati College of Pharmacy
3223 Eden Avenue
P.O. Box 670004
Cincinnati, OH 45267
513-558-3784
513-558-4372 (fax)
pharmacy.uc.edu

The Ohio State University College of Pharmacy
500 West Twelfth Avenue
217 Parks Hall
Columbus, OH 43210-1291
614-292-2266
614-292-2588 (fax)
www.pharmacy.ohio-state.edu

The University of Toledo College of Pharmacy
2801 West Bancroft Street
Toledo, OH 43606
419-530-1904
419-530-1994 (fax)
www.utoledo.edu/pharmacy

Oklahoma

Southwestern Oklahoma State University School of Pharmacy
100 Campus Drive
Weatherford, OK 73096
580-774-3105
580-774-7020 (fax)
www.swosu.edu/depts/pharmacy/index.htm

University of Oklahoma College of Pharmacy
1110 North Stonewall Avenue
P.O. Box 26901
Oklahoma City, OK 73190-5040
405-271-6484
405-271-3830 (fax)
www.oupharmacy.com

Oregon

Oregon State University College of Pharmacy
203 Pharmacy Building
Corvallis, OR 97331
541-737-3424
541-737-3999 (fax)
pharmacy.oregonstate.edu

Pennsylvania

Duquesne University Mylan School of Pharmacy
306 Bayer Learning Center
Pittsburgh, PA 15282
412-396-6380
412-396-1810 (fax)
www.duq.edu/pharmacy/

Lake Erie College of Osteopathic Medicine
LECOM School of Pharmacy
1858 West Grandview Boulevard
Erie, PA 16509
814-866-6641
814-866-8450 (fax)
www/lecom.edu/pharmacy

Temple University of the Commonwealth of Higher Education
School of Pharmacy
3307 North Broad Street
Philadelphia, PA 19140
215-707-4990
215-707-3678 (fax)
www.temple.edu/pharmacy

University of Pittsburgh School of Pharmacy
1104 Salk Hall
Pittsburgh, PA 15261
412-648-8579
412-648-1086 (fax)
www.pharmacy.pitt.edu

University of the Sciences in Philadelphia
Philadelphia College of Pharmacy
600 South Forty-Third Street
Philadelphia, PA 19104
215-596-8870
215-596-8977 (fax)
www.usip.edu/academics/pharmacy.html

Wilkes University Nesbitt School of Pharmacy
Stark Learning Center
P.O. Box 111
Wilkes-Barre, PA 18766
570-408-4280
570-408-7828 (fax)
pharmacy.wilkes.edu

Rhode Island

University of Rhode Island College of Pharmacy
41 Lower College Road
Kingston, RI 02881-0809
401-874-2614
401-874-5014 (fax)
www.uri.edu/pharm/

South Carolina

Medical University of South Carolina College of Pharmacy
280 Calhoun Street
Charleston, SC 29425-2301
843-792-3115
843-792-9081 (fax)
www.musc.edu/pharmacy/

University of South Carolina School of Pharmacy
700 Sumter Street
Columbia, SC 29208
803-777-4151
803-777-2775 (fax)
www.pharm.sc.edu

South Dakota

South Dakota State University College of Pharmacy
Pharmacy Building
Brookings, SD 57007-0099
605-688-6197
605-688-6232 (fax)
www3.sdstate.edu/academics/collegeofpharmacy/

Tennessee

University of Tennessee College of Pharmacy
874 Monroe Avenue, Suite 226
Memphis, TN 38163
901-448-6036
901-448-7053 (fax)
www.utmem.edu/pharm/pharm.html

Texas

Texas Southern University College of Pharmacy and Health Sciences
3100 Cleburne
Houston, TX 77004
713-313-7164
713-313-1091 (fax)
www.tsu.edu/pharmacy/index.htm

Texas Tech University School of Pharmacy
1300 South Coulter Street
Amarillo, TX 79106
806-354-5463
806-354-4017 (fax)
ismo.ama.ttuhsc.edu

University of Houston College of Pharmacy
141 Science and Research 2 Building
Houston, TX 77204
713-743-1300
713-743-1259 (fax)
www.uh.edu/pharmacy

University of Texas at Austin College of Pharmacy
2409 University Avenue
Austin, TX 78712-1074
512-471-3718
512-471-8783 (fax)
www.utexas.edu/pharmacy

Utah

University of Utah College of Pharmacy
201 Skaggs Hall
Salt Lake City, UT 84112
801-581-6731
801-581-3716 (fax)
www.pharmacy.utah.edu/

Virginia

Hampton University School of Pharmacy
Kittrell Hall
Hampton, VA 23668
757-727-5071
757-727-5840 (fax)
www.hampton.edu/pharm/index.htm

Shenandoah University
Bernard J. Dunn School of Pharmacy
1460 University Drive
Winchester, VA 22601
540-665-1282
540-665-1283 (fax)
pharmacy.su.edu

Virginia Commonwealth University School of Pharmacy
410 North Twelfth Street
MCV Campus-Box 581
Richmond, VA 23298-0581
804-828-3006
804-827-0002 (fax)
views.vcu.edu/pharmacy

Washington

University of Washington School of Pharmacy
Health Science Building
Seattle, WA 98195
206-543-2030
206-685-9297 (fax)
depts.washington.edu/pha/

Washington State University College of Pharmacy
105 Wegner Hall
Pullman, WA 99164-6501
509-335-5901
509-335-0162 (fax)
www.pharmacy.wsu.edu

West Virginia

West Virginia University School of Pharmacy
Health Science Center
1136 HSN
Morgantown, WV 26506
304-293-5101
304-293-5483 (fax)
www.hsc.wvu.edu/sop

Wisconsin

University of Wisconsin—Madison School of Pharmacy
777 Highland Avenue
Madison, WI 53705
608-262-1416
608-262-3397 (fax)
www.pharmacy.wisc.edu/

Wyoming

University of Wyoming School of Pharmacy
P.O. Box 3375
Laramie, WY 82071
307-766-6120
307-766-2953 (fax)
www.uwyo.edu/pharmacy/

NATIONAL PHARMACY ASSOCIATIONS

Academy of Managed Care Pharmacy (AMCP)
100 North Pitt Street, Suite 400
Alexandria, VA 22314
703-683-8416
703-683-8417 (fax)
www.amcp.org/

American Association of Colleges of Pharmacy (AACP)
1426 Prince Street
Alexandria, VA 22314-2841
703-739-2330
703-836-8982 (fax)
www.aacp.org

American Association of Pharmaceutical Scientists (AAPS)
2107 Wilson Blvd, Suite 700
Arlington, VA 22201-3046
703-243-2800
703-243-9650 (fax)
www.aaps.org

American College of Apothecaries (ACA)
P.O. Box 341266
Memphis, TN 38184
901-383-8119
901-383-8882 (fax)
www.acainfo.org

American College of Clinical Pharmacy (ACCP)
3101 Broadway, Suite 650
Kansas City, MO 64111
816-531-2177
816-531-4990 (fax)
www.accp.com

American Council of Pharmaceutical Education (ACPE)
20 North Clark Street
Chicago, IL 60602-5109
312-664-3575
312-664-4652 (fax)
www.acpe-accredit.org

American Foundation for Pharmaceutical Education (AFPE)
1 Church Street, Suite 202
Rockville, MD 20850
301-738-2160
301-738-2161 (fax)
www.afpenet.org

American Institute for the History of Pharmacy (AIHP)
777 Highland Avenue
Madison, WI 53705-2222
608-262-5378
608-262-3397 (fax)
www.aihp.org

Association of Natural Medicine Pharmacists (ANMP)
P.O. Box 150727
San Rafael, CA 94915-0727
415-868-1909
415-868-1996 (fax)
www.anmp.org

American Pharmacists Association (APhA)
2215 Constitution Avenue, NW
Washington, DC 20037-2985
202-628-4410
202-783-2351 (fax)
www.aphanet.org

American Society of Automation in Pharmacy (ASAP)
492 Norristown Road, Suite 160
Blue Bell, PA 19422
610-825-7783
610-825-7641 (fax)
www.asapnet.org

American Society of Consultant Pharmacists (ASCP)
1321 Duke Street
Alexandria, VA 22314-3563
703-739-1300
703-739-1321 (fax)
www.ascp.com

American Society of Health-System Pharmacists (ASHP)
7272 Wisconsin Avenue
Bethesda, MD 20814
301-657-3000
301-664-8877 (fax)
www.ashp.org

American Society for Pharmacy Law (ASPL)
1224 Centre West, Suite 400B
Springfield, IL 62704
217-391-0219
217-793-0041 (fax)
www.aspl.org

Board of Pharmaceutical Specialties (BPS)
2215 Constitution Avenue, NW
Washington, DC 20037-2985
202-429-7591
202-429-6304 (fax)
www.bpsweb.org

National Association of Boards of Pharmacy (NABP)
700 Busse Highway
Park Ridge, IL 60068-2402
847-698-6227
847-698-0124 (fax)
www.nabp.net

National Association of Chain Drug Stores (NACDS)
P.O. Box 1417-D49
Alexandria, VA 22313-1480
703-549-3001
703-836-4869 (fax)
www.nacds.org

National Community Pharmacists Association (NCPA)
205 Daingerfield Road
Alexandria, VA 22314
703-683-8200
703-683-3619 (fax)
www.ncpanet.org

National Council on Patient Information and Education (NCPIE)
4915 Saint Elmo Avenue, Suite 505
Bethesda, MD 20814-6082
301-656-8565
301-656-4464 (fax)
www.talkaboutrx.org

National Pharmaceutical Association (NPhA)
107 Kilmayne Drive, Suite C
Cary, NC 27511
800-944-6742
919-469-5870 (fax)
www.npha.net

Pharmaceutical Care Management Association (PCMA)
2300 Ninth Street, Suite 210
Arlington, VA 22204
703-920-8480
703-920-8491 (fax)
www.pcmanet.org

United States Pharmacopoeial Convention, Inc. (USPC)
12601 Twinbrook Parkway
Rockville, MD 20852
301-881-0666
301-816-8299 (fax)
www.usp.org

U.S. Public Health Service (USPHS)
5600 Fishers Lane, Room 9A-05
Rockville, MD 20857
301-443-4010
301-443-3847 (fax)
www.usphs.gov

STATE PHARMACY ASSOCIATIONS

Alabama Pharmacy Association
1211 Carmichael Way
Montgomery, AL 36106-3672
334-271-5422
334-271-5423 (fax)
www.aparx.org

Alaska Pharmaceutical Association
4107 Laurel Street, #101
Anchorage, AK 99508
907-563-8880
907-563-7880 (fax)
www.alaskapharmacy.org

Arizona Pharmacy Association
1845 East Southern Avenue
Tempe, AZ 85282-5831
480-838-3385
480-838-3557 (fax)
www.azpharmacy.org

Arkansas Pharmacists Association
417 South Victory
Little Rock, AR 72201
501-372-5250
501-372-0546 (fax)
www.arpharmacists.org

California Pharmacists Association
1112 I Street, Suite 300
Sacramento, CA 95814
916-444-7811
916-444-7929 (fax)
www.cpha.com

Colorado Pharmacists Society
6825 East Tennessee Avenue, Suite 440
Denver, CO 80224
303-756-3069
303-756-3649 (fax)
www.copharm.org

Connecticut Pharmacists Association
35 Cold Spring Road, Suite 121
Rocky Hill, CT 06067
860-563-4619
860-257-8241 (fax)
www.ctpharmacists.org

Delaware Pharmacists Society
27 North Main Street
P.O. Box 454
Smyrna, DE 19977-0454
302-659-3088
302-659-3089 (fax)
www.depharmacy.org/Index.htm

Florida Pharmacy Association
610 North Adams Street
Tallahassee, FL 32301
850-222-2400
850-561-6758 (fax)
www.pharmview.com

Georgia Pharmacy Association
50 Lenox Pointe NE
Atlanta, GA 30324
404-231-5074
404-237-8435 (fax)
www.gpha.org

Hawaii Pharmacists Association
P.O. Box 22472
Honolulu, HI 96823-2472
808-432-5536
808-432-5535 (fax)

Idaho State Pharmacy Association
P.O. Box 140117
Boise, ID 83714-0117
208-424-1107
208-424-3131 (fax)
www.idahopharmacy.org

Illinois Pharmacists Association
204 West Cook
Springfield, IL 62704-2526
217-522-7300
217-522-7349 (fax)
www.ipha.org

Indiana Pharmacists Alliance
729 North Pennsylvania Street
Indianapolis, IN 46204-1171
317-634-4968
317-632-1219 (fax)
www.indianapharmacists.org

Iowa Pharmacy Association
8515 Douglas Avenue, Suite 16
Des Moines, IA 50322
515-270-0713
515-270-2979 (fax)
www.iarx.org

Kansas Pharmacists Association
1020 SW Fairlawn Road
Topeka, KS 66604
785-228-2327
785-228-9147 (fax)
www.kansaspharmacy.org

Kentucky Pharmacists Association
1228 U.S. 127 South
Frankfort, KY 40601-4330
502-227-2303
502-227-2258 (fax)
www.kphanet.org

Louisiana Pharmacists Association
525 Florida Street, Suite 300
Baton Rouge, LA 70801
225-408-5900
225-408-8270 (fax)
www.louisianapharmacists.com

Maine Pharmacy Association
725 Main Street
South Portland, ME 04106
800-639-1609
207-989-6743 (fax)
www.mparx.com

Maryland Pharmacists Association
650 West Lombard Street
Baltimore, MD 21201-1572
410-727-0746
410-727-2253 (fax)
www.erols.com/mpha

Massachusetts Pharmacists Association
681 Main Street, Suite 3-32
Waltham, MA 02451-0621
781-736-0101
781-736-0080 (fax)
www.masspharmacists.org

Michigan Pharmacists Association
815 North Washington Avenue
Lansing, MI 48906-5198
517-484-1466
517-484-4893 (fax)
www.michiganpharmacists.org

Minnesota Pharmacists Association
1935 West County Road B2
Roseville, MN 55113-2722
651-697-1771
651-697-1776 (fax)
www.mpha.org

Mississippi Pharmacists Association
341 Edgewood Terrace Drive
Jackson, MS 39206-6299
601-981-0416
601-981-0451 (fax)
www.mspharm.org

Missouri Pharmacy Association
211 East Capitol
Jefferson City, MO 65101
573-636-7522
573-636-7485 (fax)
www.morx.com

Montana Pharmacy Association
34 West Sixth Street 2E
Helena, MT 59601
406-449-3843
406-443-1592 (fax)
www.rxmt.com

Nebraska Pharmacists Association
6221 South Fifty-Eighth Street, Suite A
Lincoln, NE 68516-3687
402-420-1500
402-420-1406 (fax)
www.npharm.org

Nevada Pharmacy Alliance
5740 South Eastern, Suite 24 C
Las Vegas, NV 89119
702-259-3449
702-259-3521 (fax)
www.nvphall.org

New Hampshire Pharmacists Association
2 Eagle Square, Suite 400
Concord, NH 03301-4956
603-229-0292
603-224-7769 (fax)
www.nphanet.org

New Jersey Pharmacists Association
760 Alexander Road, CN1
Princeton, NJ 08543
609-275-4246
609-275-4066 (fax)
www.njpharma.org

New Mexico Pharmaceutical Association
4800 Zuni Southeast
Albuquerque, NM 87108
505-265-8729
505-255-8476 (fax)
www.nm-pharmacy.com

New York, Pharmacists Society of the State of
210 Washington Avenue Extension
Albany, NY 12203
518-869-6595
518-464-0618 (fax)
www.pssny.org

North Carolina Association of Pharmacists
109 Church Street
Chapel Hill, NC 27516
919-967-2237
919-968-9430 (fax)
www.ncpharmacists.org

North Dakota Pharmaceutical Association
1906 East Broadway Avenue
Bismarck, ND 58501-4700
701-258-4968
701-258-9312 (fax)
www.nodakpharmacy.com

Ohio Pharmacists Association
6037 Franz Road, Suite 106
Dublin, OH 43017
614-798-0037
614-798-0978 (fax)
www.ohiopharmacists.org

Oklahoma Pharmacists Association
45 NE Fifty-Second Street
P.O. Box 18731
Oklahoma City, OK 73154
405-528-3338
405-528-1417 (fax)
www.opha.com

Oregon State Pharmacists Association
29702-B SW Town Center Loop West
Wilsonville, OR 97070
503-582-9055
503-582-9046 (fax)
www.oregonpharmacists.com

Pennsylvania Pharmacists Association
508 North Third Street
Harrisburg, PA 17101-1199
717-234-6151
717-236-1618 (fax)
www.papharmacists.com

Puerto Rico, Colegio de Farmeceuticos de
P.O. Box 360206
San Juan, PR 00936-0206
787-753-7157
787-759-9793 (fax)
www.cfpr.org

Rhode Island Pharmacists Association
1643 Warwick Avenue
Warwick, RI 02889
401-737-2600
401-737-0959 (fax)
www.ripharm.com

South Carolina Pharmacy Association
1350 Browning Road
Columbia, SC 29210
803-354-9977
803-354-9207 (fax)
www.scrx.org

South Dakota Pharmacists Association
215 West Sioux Avenue
P.O. Box 518
Pierre, SD 57501
605-224-2338
605-224-1280 (fax)
www.sdpha.org

Tennessee Pharmacists Association
226 Capitol Boulevard, Suite 810
Nashville, TN 37219-1893
615-256-3023
615-255-3528 (fax)
www.tnpharm.org

Texas Pharmacy Association
P.O. Box 14709
Austin, TX 78761-4709
512-836-8350
512-836-0308 (fax)
www.txpharmacy.com

Utah Pharmaceutical Association
1850 South Columbia Lane
Orem, UT 84097
801-762-0452
801-762-0454 (fax)
www.upha.com

Vermont Pharmacists Association
P.O. Box 90
Woodstock, VT 05091
802-483-2646
802-483-6315 (fax)
www.vtpharmacists.org

Virginia Pharmacists Association
5501 Patterson Avenue, Suite 200
Richmond, VA 23226
804-285-4145
804-285-4227 (fax)
www.vapharmacy.org

Washington DC Pharmaceutical Association
908 Caddington Avenue
Silver Spring, MD 20901-1109
301-593-3292
301-593-7215 (fax)

Washington State Pharmacists Association
1501 Taylor Avenue SW
Renton, WA 98055-3139
425-228-7171
425-277-3897 (fax)
www.wsparx.org

West Virginia Pharmacists Association
2003 Quarrier Street
Charleston, WV 25311-2212
304-344-5302
304-344-5316 (fax)

Wisconsin, Pharmacy Society of
701 Heartland Trail
Madison, WI 53717
608-827-9200
608-827-9292 (fax)
www.pswi.org

Wyoming Pharmacists Association
1022 Ponderosa Court
Powell, WY 82435
307-754-4663
307-754-4145 (fax)
www.wpha.net

STATE BOARDS OF PHARMACY

Alabama Board of Pharmacy
1 Perimeter Park South, Suite 425 South
Birmingham, AL 35243
205-967-0130
205-967-1009 (fax)
www.albop.com

Alaska Board of Pharmacy
333 Willoughby Avenue
P.O. Box 110806
Juneau, AK 99811
907-465-2589
907-465-2974 (fax)
www.dced.state.ak.us/occ/ppha.htm

Arizona State Board of Pharmacy
4425 West Olive Avenue, Suite 140
Glendale, AZ 85302
623-463-2727
623-934-0583 (fax)
www.pharmacy.state.az.us

Arkansas State Board of Pharmacy
101 East Capitol, Suite 218
Little Rock, AR 72201
501-682-0190
501-682-0195 (fax)
www.state.ar.us/asbp

California Board of Pharmacy
400 R Street, Suite 4070
Sacramento, CA 95814
916-445-5014
916-327-6308 (fax)
www.pharmacy.ca.gov/

Colorado State Board of Pharmacy
1560 Broadway, Suite 1310
Denver, CO 80202-5146
303-894-7750
303-894-7764 (fax)
www.dora.state.co.us/pharmacy

Connecticut Commission of Pharmacy
165 Capitol Avenue
State Office Building, Room 147
Hartford, CT 06106
860-713-6070
860-713-7242 (fax)
www.ctdrugcontrol.com/rxcommision.htm

Delaware State Board of Pharmacy
P.O. Box 637
Dover, DE 19901
302-739-4798
302-739-3071 (fax)
www.professionallicensing.state.de.us

District of Columbia Board of Pharmacy
825 North Capitol Street NE, Room 2224
Washington, DC 20002
202-442-9200
202-442-9431 (fax)

Florida Board of Pharmacy
4052 Bald Cypress Way, Bin #C04
Tallahassee, FL 32399-3254
850-245-4292
850-413-6982 (fax)
www.doh.state.fl.us/mqa

Georgia State Board of Pharmacy
237 Coliseum Drive
Macon, GA 31217-3858
478-207-1686
438-207-1699 (fax)
www.sos.state.ga.us/plb/pharmacy/

Hawaii State Board of Pharmacy
P.O. Box 3469
Honolulu, HI 96801
808-586-2694
808-586-2689 (fax)
www.state.hi.us/dcca/pvl/

Idaho Board of Pharmacy
3380 American Terrace, Suite 320
P.O. Box 83720
Boise, ID 83720-0067
208-334-2356
208-334-3536 (fax)
www.state.id.us/bop

Illinois Department of Professional Regulation
320 West Washington Street, Third Floor
Springfield, IL 62786
217-785-0800
217-782-7645 (fax)
www.dpr.state.il.us

Indiana Board of Pharmacy
402 West Washington Street, Room 041
Indianapolis, IN 46204-2739
317-232-2960
317-233-4236 (fax)
www.in.gov/hpb/boards/isbp/

Iowa Board of Pharmacy Examiners
400 SW Eighth Street, Suite F
Des Moines, IA 50309-4688
515-281-5944
515-281-4609 (fax)
www.state.ia.us/ibpe

Kansas State Board of Pharmacy
900 Jackson, Room 513
Topeka, KS 66612
785-296-4056
785-296-8420 (fax)
www.accesskansas.org/pharmacy

Kentucky Board of Pharmacy
23 Millcreek Parkway
Frankfort, KY 40601-9230
502-573-1580
502-573-1582 (fax)
www.state.ky.us/boards/pharmacy

Louisiana Board of Pharmacy
5615 Corporate Boulevard, Suite 8E
Baton Rouge, LA 70808-2537
225-925-6496
225-925-6499 (fax)
www.labp.com

Maine Board of Pharmacy
35 State House Station
Augusta, ME 04333
207-624-8603
207-624-8637 (fax)
www.maineprofessionalreg.org

Maryland Board of Pharmacy
4201 Patterson Avenue
Baltimore, MD 21215-2299
410-764-4755
410-358-6207 (fax)
www.dhmh.state.md.us/pharmacyboard/

Massachusetts Board of Registration in Pharmacy
239 Causeway Street
Boston, MA 02113
617-727-9953
617-727-2197 (fax)
www.state.ma.us/reg/boards/ph

Michigan Board of Pharmacy
611 West Ottawa, First Floor
P.O. Box 30670
Lansing, MI 48909-8170
517-373-9102
517-373-2179 (fax)
www.michigan.gov/cis/0,1607,7-154-10568_17671_17688-42779
   --,00.html

Minnesota Board of Pharmacy
2829 University Avenue SE, Suite 530
Minneapolis, MN 55414-3251
612-617-2201
612-617-2212 (fax)
www.phcybrd.state.mn.us

Mississippi Board of Pharmacy
P.O. Box 24507
Jackson, MS 39225-4507
601-354-6750
601-354-6071 (fax)
www.mbp.state.ms.us

Missouri Board of Pharmacy
3605 Missouri Boulevard
P.O. Box 625
Jefferson City, MO 65102
573-751-0091
573-526-3464 (fax)
www.ecodev.state.mo.us/pr/pharmacy

Montana Board of Pharmacy
111 North Jackson
P.O. Box 200513
Helena, MT 59620-0513
406-841-2356
406-841-2343 (fax)
http://discoveringmontana.com/dli/bsd/license/bsd_boards/pha_board/
    board_page.htm

Nebraska Board of Examiners in Pharmacy
301 Centennial Mall South
P.O. Box 94986
Lincoln, NE 68509
402-471-2115
402-471-0555 (fax)
www.hhs.state.ne.us

Nevada State Board of Pharmacy
555 Double Eagle Court, Suite 1100
Reno, NV 89521-8991
775-850-1440
775-850-1444 (fax)
http://glsuitewww.glsuite.com/nvbopweb/

New Hampshire Board of Pharmacy, State of
57 Regional Drive
Concord, NH 03301-8518
603-271-2350
603-271-2856 (fax)
www.state.nh.us/pharmacy

New Jersey Board of Pharmacy
124 Halsey Street
P.O. Box 45013
Newark, NJ 07101
973-504-6450
973-648-3355 (fax)
www.state.nj.us/lps/ca/brief/pharm.htm

New Mexico Board of Pharmacy
1650 University Boulevard NE, Suite 400B
Albuquerque, NM 87102
505-841-9102
505-841-9113 (fax)
www.state.nm.us/pharmacy

New York Board of Pharmacy
89 Washington Avenue, Second Floor W
Albany, NY 12234-1000
518-474-3817, x130
518-473-6995 (fax)
www.nysed.gov/prof/pharm.htm

North Carolina Board of Pharmacy
Carrboro Plaza
P.O. Box 459
Carrboro, NC 27510-0459
919-942-4454
919-967-5757 (fax)
www.ncbop.org

North Dakota State Board of Pharmacy
405 East Broadway, Third Floor
P.O. Box 1354
Bismarck, ND 58502-1354
701-328-9535
701-258-9312 (fax)

Ohio State Board of Pharmacy
77 South High Street, Room 1702
Columbus, OH 43215-6126
614-466-4143
614-752-4836 (fax)
www.state.oh.us/pharmacy

Oklahoma State Board of Pharmacy
4545 Lincoln Boulevard, Suite 112
Oklahoma City, OK 73105-3488
405-521-3815
405-521-3758 (fax)
www.pharmacystate.ok.us

Oregon Board of Pharmacy
800 NE Oregon Street #9
State Office Building, Room 425
Portland, OR 97232
503-731-4032
503-731-4067 (fax)
www.pharmacy.state.or.us

Pennsylvania State Board of Pharmacy
124 Pine Street
P.O. Box 2649
Harrisburg, PA 17105-2649
717-783-7156
717-787-7769 (fax)
www.dos.state.pa.us/bpoa/phabd/mainpage.htm

Puerto Rico Board of Pharmacy
Department of Health
Call Box 10200
Santurce, PR 00908
787-725-8161
787-725-7903 (fax)

Rhode Island Board of Pharmacy
3 Capitol Hill, Room 205
Providence, RI 02908
401-222-2837
401-222-2158 (fax)

South Carolina Board of Pharmacy
110 Centerview Drive, Suite 306
Columbia, SC 29211-1927
803-896-4700
803-896-4596 (fax)
www.llr.state.sc.us/pol/pharmacy

South Dakota Board of Pharmacy
4305 South Louise Avenue, Suite 104
Sioux Falls, SD 57106
605-362-2737
605-362-2738 (fax)
www.state.sd.us/dcr/pharmacy

Tennessee Board of Pharmacy
500 James Robertson Parkway, Second Floor
Davy Crockett Tower
Nashville, TN 37243
615-741-2718
615-741-2722 (fax)
www.state.tn.us/commerce/pharmacy

Texas State Board of Pharmacy
333 Guadalupe, Tower 3, Suite 600, Box 21
Austin, TX 78701-3942
512-305-8000
512-305-8082 (fax)
www.tsbp.state.tx.us

Utah Board of Pharmacy
160 East 300 South
P.O. Box 146741
Salt Lake City, UT 84114-6741
801-530-6179
801-530-6511 (fax)
www.commerce.state.ut.us/dopl/dopl1.htm

Vermont Board of Pharmacy
26 Terrace Street, Drawer 09
Montpelier, VT 05609-1106
802-828-2875
802-828-2465 (fax)
www.vtprofessionals.org

Virginia Board of Pharmacy
6606 West Broad Street, Suite 400
Richmond, VA 23230-1717
804-662-9911
804-662-9313 (fax)
www.dhp.state.va.us/pharmacy/default.htm

Washington State Board of Pharmacy
P.O. Box 47863
Olympia, WA 98504-7863
360-236-4825
360-586-4359 (fax)
http://wws2.wa.gov/doh/hpqa-licensing/HPS4/Pharmacy/default.htm

West Virginia Board of Pharmacy
232 Capitol Street
Charleston, WV 25301
304-558-0558
304-558-0572 (fax)

Wisconsin Pharmacy Examining Board
1400 East Washington
P.O. Box 8935
Madison, WI 53708
608-266-2812
608-261-7083 (fax)
www.state.wi.us/agencies/drl

Wyoming State Board of Pharmacy
1720 South Poplar Street, Suite 4
Casper, WY 82601
307-234-0294
307-234-7226 (fax)
http://pharmacyboard.state.wy.us

Canadian Schools and Associations

CANADIAN FACULTIES AND SCHOOLS OF PHARMACY

Alberta

University of Alberta Faculty of Pharmacy and Pharmaceutical Sciences
3118 Dentistry/Pharmacy Centre
Edmonton, Alberta T5G 2N8
780-492-3362
780-492-1217 (fax)
www.pharmacy.ualberta.ca

British Columbia

University of British Columbia
Faculty of Pharmaceutical Sciences
2146 East Mall
Vancouver, British Columbia V6T 1Z3
604-822-2343
604-822-3035 (fax)
www.ubcpharmacy.org

Manitoba

University of Manitoba Faculty of Pharmacy
202 Pharmacy Building
50 Shifton Road
Winnipeg, Manitoba R3T 1Z3
204-474-8794
204-474-7617 (fax)
www.umanitoba.ca/faculties/pharmacy

Newfoundland

Memorial University of Newfoundland
School of Pharmacy
Prince Philip Drive
St. John's, Newfoundland A1B 3V6
709-737-6571
709-737-7044 (fax)
www.pharm.mun.ca

Nova Scotia

Dalhousie University
College of Pharmacy
5968 College Street
Halifax, Nova Scotia B3H 3J5
902-494-2378
902-494-1396 (fax)
www.dal.ca/pharmacy

Ontario

University of Toronto Faculty of Pharmacy
19 Russell Street
Toronto, Ontario M5S 2S2
416-978-2880
416-978-8511 (fax)
www.utoronto.ca/pharmacy

Québec

Université de Montréal Faculté de pharmacie
C.P. 6126, Station Centreville
Montréal, Québec H3C 3J7
514-343-6422
514-343-2102 (fax)
www.pharm.umontreal.ca

Université Laval Faculté de pharmacie
Pavillon Ferdinand-Vandry
Québec, Québec G1K 7P4
418-656-3211
418-656-2305 (fax)
www.pha.ulaval.ca

Saskatchewan

University of Saskatchewan College of Pharmacy and Nutrition
110 Science Place
Saskatoon, Saskatchewan S7N 5C9
306-966-6328
306-966-6377 (fax)
www.usask.ca/pharmacy-nutrition

CANADIAN NATIONAL PHARMACY ASSOCIATIONS

Association of Faculties of Pharmacy of Canada
2609 Eastview
Saskatoon, Saskatchewan S7J 3G7
306-374-6327
306-374-0555 (fax)
www.afpc.info

Canadian Association of Chain Drug Stores
301-45 Sheppard Avenue
Toronto, Ontario M2N 5W9
416-226-9100
416-226-9185 (fax)
www.cacds.com

Canadian Association of Pharmacy Technicians
P.O. Box 1271 Station
Toronto, Ontario M4Y 2V8
www.capt.ca

Canadian Council for Accreditation of Pharmacy Programs
110 Science Place
Thorvaldson Building, Room 123
Saskatoon, Saskatchewan S7J 5C9
306-966-6388
306-966-6377 (fax)
www.napra.ca

Canadian Council on Continuing Education in Pharmacy
3861 Athol Street
Regina, Saskatchewan S4S 3J2
306-584-5703
306-584-5703 (fax)
www.cccep.org

Canadian Pharmacists Association
1785 Alta Vista Drive
Ottawa, Ontario K1G 3Y6
800-917-9489 (inside Canada); 613-523-7877 (outside Canada)
613-523-0445 (fax)
www.cdnpharm.ca

Canadian Society of Hospital Pharmacists
350-1145 Hunt Club Road
Ottawa, Ontario K1V 0Y3
613-736-9733
613-736-5660 (fax)
www.cshp.ca

National Association of Pharmacy Regulatory Authorities
402-222 Somerset Street West
Ottawa, Ontario K2P 2G3
613-569-9658
613-569-9659 (fax)
www.napra.org

Pharmacy Examining Board of Canada
601-415 Yonge Street
Toronto, Ontario M3B 2E7
416-979-2431
416-599-9244 (fax)
www.pebc.ca

CANADIAN PROVINCIAL VOLUNTARY ORGANIZATIONS

Alberta College of Pharmacists
10130-112th Street, Seventh Floor
Edmonton, Alberta T5K 2K4
780-990-0321
780-990-0328 (fax)
www.altapharm.org

Association des pharmaciens des établissements de santé du Québec
1470 rue Peel, Tour B, Bureau 900
Montréal, Québec H3A 1T1
514-286-0776
514-286-1081 (fax)
www.apesquebec.org

Association professionnelle des pharmaciens salariés du Québec
3560 La Vérendrye
Sherbrooke, Québec J1L 1Z6
819-563-6464
819-563-6464 (fax)

Association québécoise des pharmaciens propriétaires
4378 avenue Pierre-de-Coubertin
Montréal, Québec H1V 1A6
514-254-0676; 800-361-7765
514-254-1288 (fax)

British Columbia Pharmacy Association
1503-1200 West Seventy-Third Avenue
Vancouver, British Columbia V6P 6G5
604-261-2092
604-261-2097 (fax)
www.bcpharmacy.ca

College of Pharmacists of British Columbia
200-1765 West Eighth Avenue
Vancouver, British Columbia V6J 1V8
604-733-2440
604-733-2493 (fax)
www.collpharmbc.org

Manitoba Society of Pharmacists
22-90 Garry Street
Winnipeg, Manitoba R3C 4H1
204-956-6680
204-956-6686 (fax)
www.msp.mb.ca

New Brunswick Pharmacists' Association, Inc.
410-212 Queen Street
Fredericton, New Brunswick E3B 1A8
506-459-6008
506-459-0736 (fax)
www.nbnet.nb.ca

Ontario Pharmacist Association
301-23 Lesmill Road
Don Mills, Ontario M3B 3P6
416-441-0788
416-441-0791 (fax)
www.opatoday.com

Pharmacists Association of Alberta
1800-10303 Jasper Avenue NW
Edmonton, Alberta T5J 3N6
780-990-0326
780-990-1236 (fax)
www.altapharm.org

Pharmacy Association of Newfoundland and Labrador
488 Water Street, Apothecary Hall
St. John's, Newfoundland A1E 1B3
709-753-5877
709-753-8615 (fax)

Pharmacy Association of Nova Scotia
1526 Dresden Row
P.O. Box 3214 (S)
Halifax, Nova Scotia B3J 3H5
902-422-9583
902-422-2619 (fax)
www.pans.ns.ca

Pharmacy Society of Yukon
9 Basswood Street
Whitehorse, Yukon Y1A 4P4
867-393-8737

Prince Edward Island Pharmaceutical Association
P.O. Box 1404
Summerside, Prince Edward Island C1N 4K2
902-859-3800
902-422-2619 (fax)

Representative Board of Saskatchewan Pharmacists
700-4010 Pasqua Street
Regina, Saskatchewan S4S 7B9
306-359-7277
306-584-9695 (fax)

CANADIAN PROVINCIAL REGULATORY AUTHORITY

Alberta College of Pharmacists
10130-112th Street, Seventh Floor
Edmonton, Alberta T5K 2K4
780/990-0321
780/990-0328 (fax)
www.altapharm.org

College of Pharmacists of British Columbia
200-1765 West Eighth Avenue
Vancouver, British Columbia V6J 1V8
604/733-2440
604/733-2493 (fax)
www.collpharmbc.org

Manitoba Pharmaceutical Association
187 St. Mary's Road
Winnipeg, Manitoba R2H 1J2
204/233-1411
204/237-3468 (fax)

New Brunswick Pharmaceutical Society
30 Gordon Street, Suite 101
Moncton, New Brunswick E1C 1L8
506/857-8957
506/857-8838 (fax)

Newfoundland Pharmaceutical Association
488 Water Street, Apothecary Hall
St. John's, Newfoundland A1E 1B3
709/753-5877
709/753-8615 (fax)

Northwest Territories Regulatory Authority
P.O. Box 1320
Yellowknife, Northwest Territories X1A 2L9
867/920-8058
867/873-0484 (fax)

Nova Scotia Pharmaceutical Society
1526 Dresden Row
P.O. Box 3363 (S)
Halifax, Nova Scotia B3J 3J1
902/422-8528
902/422-2619 (fax)

Ontario College of Pharmacists
483 Huron Street
Toronto, Ontario M5R 2R4
416/962-4861
416/962-1619 (fax)
www.ocpinfo.com

Ordre des pharmaciens du Québec
266 rue Notre-Dame Ouest, Bureau 301
Montréal, Québec H2Y 1T6
514/284-9588
514/284-3420 (fax)
www.opq.org

Prince Edward Island Pharmacy Board
P.O. Box 89
Crapaud, Prince Edward Island C0A 1J0
902/658-2780
902/658-2198 (fax)

Saskatchewan Pharmaceutical Association
700-4010 Pasqua Street
Regina, Saskatchewan S4S 7B9
306/584-2292
306/584-9695 (fax)

Yukon Regulatory Authority
P.O. Box 2703
Whitehorse, Yukon Y1A 2C6
867/667-5111
867/667-3609 (fax)

Oath of a Pharmacist

At this time, I vow to devote my professional life
to the service of all humankind
through the profession of pharmacy.

I will consider the welfare of humanity
and relief of human suffering
my primary concerns.

I will apply my knowledge, experience, and skills
to the best of my ability
to assure optimal drug therapy outcomes
for the patients I serve.

I will keep abreast of developments
and maintain professional competency
in my profession of pharmacy.

I will maintain the highest principles
of moral, ethical, and legal conduct.

I will embrace and advocate change
in the profession of pharmacy
that improves patient care.

I take these vows voluntarily
with the full realization of the responsibility
with which I am entrusted by the public.

Developed by the American Pharmaceutical Association Academy of Students of Pharmacy/American Association of Colleges of Pharmacy Council of Deans (APhA-ASP/AACP-COD) Task Force on Professionalism, June 26, 1994. Reprinted with permission of the American Association of Colleges of Pharmacy.

Pledge of Professionalism

As a student of pharmacy, I believe there is a need to build and reinforce a professional identity founded on integrity, ethical behavior, and honor. This development, a vital process in my education, will help ensure that I am true to the professional relationship I establish between myself and society as I become a member of the pharmacy community. Integrity must be an essential part of my everyday life and I must practice pharmacy with honesty and commitment to service.

To accomplish this goal of professional development, I, as a student of pharmacy, should:

DEVELOP a sense of loyalty and duty to the profession of pharmacy by being a builder of community, one able and willing to contribute to the well-being of others and one who enthusiastically accepts the responsibility and accountability for membership in the profession.

FOSTER professional competency through lifelong learning. I must strive for high ideals, teamwork, and unity within the profession in order to provide optimal patient care.

SUPPORT my colleagues by actively encouraging personal commitment to the Oath of Maimonides and a Code of Ethics as set forth by the profession.

INCORPORATE into my life and practice dedication to excellence. This will require an ongoing reassessment of personal and professional values.

MAINTAIN the highest ideals and professional attributes to ensure and facilitate the covenantal relationship required of the pharmaceutical caregiver.

Developed by the American Pharmaceutical Association Academy of Students of Pharmacy/American Association of Colleges of Pharmacy Council of Deans (APhA-ASP/AACP-COD) Task Force on Professionalism, June 26, 1994. Reprinted with permission of the American Association of Colleges of Pharmacy.

The profession of pharmacy is one that demands adherence to a set of rigid ethical standards. These high ideals are necessary to ensure the quality of care extended to the patients I serve. As a student of pharmacy, I believe this does not start with graduation; rather, it begins with my membership in this professional college community. Therefore, I must strive to uphold these standards as I advance toward full membership in the profession of pharmacy.

Code of Ethics for Pharmacists

PREAMBLE

Pharmacists are health professionals who assist individuals in making the best use of medications. This Code, prepared and supported by pharmacists, is intended to state publicly the principles that form the fundamental basis of the roles and responsibilities of pharmacists. These principles, based on moral obligations and virtues, are established to guide pharmacists in relationships with patients, health professionals, and society.

I. A pharmacist respects the covenantal relationship between the patient and pharmacist.

Considering the patient-pharmacist relationship as a covenant means that a pharmacist has moral obligations in response to the gift of trust received from society. In return for this gift, a pharmacist promises to help individuals achieve optimum benefit from their medications, to be committed to their welfare, and to maintain their trust.

II. A pharmacist promotes the good of every patient in a caring, compassionate, and confidential manner.

A pharmacist places concern for the well-being of the patient at the center of professional practice. In doing so, a pharmacist considers needs stated by the patient as well as those defined by health science. A pharmacist is dedicated to protecting the dignity of the patient. With a caring attitude and a compassionate spirit, a pharmacist focuses on serving the patient in a private and confidential manner.

Adopted by the membership of the American Pharmaceutical Association, October 27, 1994. Reprinted with permission of the American Pharmacists Association.

III. A pharmacist respects the autonomy and dignity of each patient.

A pharmacist promotes the right of self-determination and recognizes individual self-worth by encouraging patients to participate in decisions about their health. A pharmacist communicates with patients in terms that are understandable. In all cases, a pharmacist respects personal and cultural differences among patients.

IV. A pharmacist acts with honesty and integrity in professional relationships.

A pharmacist has a duty to tell the truth and to act with conviction of conscience. A pharmacist avoids discriminatory practices, behavior, or work conditions that impair professional judgment, and actions that compromise dedication to the best interests of patients.

V. A pharmacist maintains professional competence.

A pharmacist has a duty to maintain knowledge and abilities as new medications, devices, and technologies become available and as health information advances.

VI. A pharmacist respects the values and abilities of colleagues and other health professionals.

When appropriate, a pharmacist asks for the consultation of colleagues or other health professionals or refers the patient. A pharmacist acknowledges that colleagues and other health professionals may differ in the beliefs and values they apply to the care of the patient.

VII. A pharmacist serves individual, community, and societal needs.

The primary obligation of a pharmacist is to individual patients. However, the obligations of a pharmacist may at times extend beyond the individual to the community and society. In these situations, the pharmacist recognizes the responsibilities that accompany these obligations and acts accordingly.

VIII. A pharmacist seeks justice in the distribution of health resources.

When health resources are allocated, a pharmacist is fair and equitable, balancing the needs of patients and society.

Principles of Practice
for Pharmaceutical Care

PREAMBLE

Pharmaceutical Care is a patient-centered, outcomes-oriented pharmacy practice that requires the pharmacist to work in concert with the patient and the patient's other health care providers to promote health, to prevent disease, and to assess, monitor, initiate, and modify medication use to assure that drug therapy regimens are safe and effective. The goal of Pharmaceutical Care is to optimize the patient's health-related quality of life and achieve positive clinical outcomes, within realistic economic expenditures. To achieve this goal, the following must be accomplished:

A. A professional relationship must be established and maintained.

Interaction between the pharmacist and the patient must occur to assure that a relationship based upon caring, trust, open communication, cooperation, and mutual decision making is established and maintained. In this relationship, the pharmacist holds the patient's welfare paramount, maintains an appropriate attitude of caring for the patient's welfare, and uses all his/her professional knowledge and skills on the patient's behalf. In exchange, the patient agrees to supply personal information and preferences and participate in the therapeutic plan. The pharmacist develops mechanisms to assure the patient has access to pharmaceutical care at all times.

B. Patient-specific medical information must be collected, organized, recorded, and maintained.

Pharmacists must collect and/or generate subjective and objective information regarding the patient's general health and activity status, past

Prepared by the APhA Pharmaceutical Care Guidelines Advisory Committee: approved by the APhA Board of Trustees, August 1995. Reprinted with permission of the American Pharmacists Association.

medical history, medication history, social history, diet and exercise history, history of present illness, and economic situation (financial and insured status). Sources of information may include, but are not limited to, the patient, medical charts and reports, pharmacist-conducted health/physical assessment, the patient's family or caregiver, insurer, and other health care providers, including physicians, nurses, midlevel practitioners, and other pharmacists. Since this information will form the basis for decisions regarding the development and subsequent modification of the drug therapy plan, it must be timely, accurate, and complete, and it must be organized and recorded to assure that it is readily retrievable and updated as necessary and appropriate. Patient information must be maintained in a confidential manner.

C. Patient-specific medical information must be evaluated and a drug therapy plan developed mutually with the patient.

Based upon a thorough understanding of the patient and his/her condition or disease and its treatment, the pharmacist must, with the patient and with the patient's other health care providers as necessary, develop an outcomes-oriented drug therapy plan. The plan may have various components which address each of the patient's diseases or conditions. In designing the plan, the pharmacist must carefully consider the psychosocial aspects of the disease as well as the potential relationship between the cost and/or complexity of therapy and patient adherence. As one of the patient's advocates, the pharmacist assures the coordination of drug therapy with the patient's other health care providers and the patient. In addition, the patient must be apprised of (1) various pros and cons (i.e., cost, side effects, different monitoring aspects, etc.) of the options relative to drug therapy and (2) instances where one option may be more beneficial based on the pharmacist's professional judgment. The essential elements of the plan, including the patient's responsibilities, must be carefully and completely explained to the patient. Information should be provided to the patient at a level the patient will understand. The drug therapy plan must be documented in the patient's pharmacy record and communicated to the patient's other health care providers as necessary.

D. The pharmacist assures that the patient has all supplies, information, and knowledge necessary to carry out the drug therapy plan.

The pharmacist providing Pharmaceutical Care must assume ultimate responsibility for assuring that his/her patient has been able to obtain, and is appropriately using, any drugs and related products or equipment called for in the drug therapy plan. The pharmacist must also assure that the patient has a thorough understanding of the disease and the therapy/medications prescribed in the plan.

E. The pharmacist reviews, monitors, and modifies the therapeutic plan as necessary and appropriate, in concert with the patient and health care team.

The pharmacist is responsible for monitoring the patient's progress in achieving the specific outcomes according to strategy developed in the drug therapy plan. The pharmacist coordinates changes in the plan with the patient and the patient's other health care providers as necessary and appropriate in order to maintain or enhance the safety and/or effectiveness of drug therapy and to help minimize overall health care costs. Patient progress is accurately documented in the pharmacy record and communicated to the patient and to the patient's other health care providers as appropriate. The pharmacist shares information with other health care providers as the setting for care changes, thus helping assure continuity of care as the patient moves between the community setting, the institutional setting, and the long-term care setting.

PRACTICE PRINCIPLES

1. Data Collection

1.1 The pharmacist conducts an initial interview with the patient for the purposes of establishing a professional working relationship and initiating the patient's pharmacy record. In some situations (e.g., pediatrics, geriatrics, critical care, language barriers) the opportunity to develop a professional relationship with and collect information directly from the patient may not exist. Under these circumstances, the pharmacist should work directly with the patient's parent, guardian, and/or principal caregiver.

1.2 The interview is organized, professional, and meets the patient's need for confidentiality and privacy. Adequate time is devoted to assure that questions and answers can be fully developed without either party feeling uncomfortable or hurried. The interview is used to systematically collect patient-specific subjective information and to initiate a pharmacy record which includes information and data regarding the patient's general health and activity status, past medical history, medication history, social history (including economic situation), family history, and history of present illness.

The record should also include information regarding the patient's thoughts or feelings and perceptions of his/her condition or disease.

1.3 The pharmacist uses health/physical assessment techniques (blood pressure monitoring, etc.) appropriately and as necessary to acquire necessary patient-specific objective information.

1.4 The pharmacist uses appropriate secondary sources to supplement the information obtained through the initial patient interview and health/physical assessment. Sources may include, but are not limited to, the patient's medical record or medical reports, the patient's family, and the patient's other health care providers.

1.5 The pharmacist creates a pharmacy record for the patient and accurately records the information collected. The pharmacist assures that the patient's record is appropriately organized, kept current, and accurately reflects all pharmacist-patient encounters. The confidentiality of the information in the record is carefully guarded and appropriate systems are in place to assure security. Patient-identifiable information contained in the record is provided to others only upon the authorization of the patient or as required by law.

2. Information Evaluation

2.1 The pharmacist evaluates the subjective and objective information collected from the patient and other sources then forms conclusions regarding (1) opportunities to improve and/or assure the safety, effectiveness, and/or economy of current or planned drug therapy; (2) opportunities to minimize current or potential future drug or health-related problems; and (3) the timing of any necessary future pharmacist consultation.

2.2 The pharmacist records the conclusions of the evaluation in the medical and/or pharmacy record.

2.3 The pharmacist discusses the conclusions with the patient, as necessary and appropriate, and assures an appropriate understanding of the nature of the condition or illness and what might be expected with respect to its management.

3. Formulating the Plan

3.1 The pharmacist, in concert with other health care providers, identifies, evaluates, and then chooses the most appropriate action(s) to (1) improve and/or assure the safety, effectiveness, and/or cost-effectiveness of current or planned drug therapy and/or (2) minimize current or potential future health-related problems.

3.2 The pharmacist formulates plans to effect the desired outcome. The plans may include, but are not limited to, work with the patient as well as with other health providers to develop a patient-specific drug therapy protocol or to modify prescribed drug therapy, develop and/or implement drug therapy monitoring mechanisms, recommend nutritional or dietary modifications, add nonprescription medications or nondrug treatments, refer the patient to an appropriate source of care, or institute an existing drug therapy protocol.

3.3 For each problem identified, the pharmacist actively considers the patient's needs and determines the desirable and mutually agreed upon outcome and incorporates these into the plan. The plan may include specific disease state and drug therapy end points and monitoring end points.

3.4 The pharmacist reviews the plan and desirable outcomes with the patient and with the patient's other health care provider(s) as appropriate.

3.5 The pharmacist documents the plan and desirable outcomes in the patient's medical and/or pharmacy record.

4. Implementing the Plan

4.1 The pharmacist and the patient take the steps necessary to implement the plan. These steps may include, but are not limited to, contacting other health providers to clarify or modify prescriptions; initiating drug therapy; educating the patient and/or caregiver(s); coordinating the acquisition of medications and/or related supplies, which might include helping the patient overcome financial barriers or lifestyle barriers that might otherwise interfere with the therapy plan; or coordinating appointments with other health care providers to whom the patient is being referred.

4.2 The pharmacist works with the patient to maximize patient understanding and involvement in the therapy plan, assures that arrangements for drug therapy monitoring (e.g., laboratory evaluation, blood pressure monitoring, home blood glucose testing, etc.) are made and understood by the patient, and that the patient receives and knows how to properly use all necessary medications and related equipment. Explanations are tailored to the patient's level of comprehension and teaching and adherence aids are employed as indicated.

4.3   The pharmacist assures that appropriate mechanisms are in place to ensure that the proper medications, equipment, and supplies are received by the patient in a timely fashion.

4.4   The pharmacist documents in the medical and/or pharmacy record the steps taken to implement the plan, including the appropriate baseline monitoring parameters, and any barriers which will need to be overcome.

4.5   The pharmacist communicates the elements of the plan to the patient and/or the patient's other health care provider(s). The pharmacist shares information with other health care providers as the setting for care changes, in order to help maintain continuity of care as the patient moves between the ambulatory, inpatient, or long-term care environment.

5. Monitoring and Modifying the Plan/Assuring Positive Outcomes

5.1   The pharmacist regularly reviews subjective and objective monitoring parameters in order to determine if satisfactory progress is being made toward achieving desired outcomes as outlined in the drug therapy plan.

5.2   The pharmacist and patient determine if the original plan should continue to be followed or if modifications are needed. If changes are necessary, the pharmacist works with the patient/caregiver and his/her other health care providers to modify and implement the revised plan as described in "Formulating the Plan" and "Implementing the Plan."

5.3   The pharmacist reviews ongoing progress in achieving desired outcomes with the patient and provides a report to the patient's other health care providers as appropriate. As progress toward outcomes is achieved, the pharmacist should provide positive reinforcement.

5.4   A mechanism is established for follow-up with patients. The pharmacist uses appropriate professional judgment in determining the need to notify the patient's other health care providers of the patient's level of adherence with the plan.

5.5   The pharmacist updates the patient's medical and/or pharmacy record with information concerning patient progress, noting the subjective and objective information which has been considered, his/her assessment of the patient's current progress, the patient's assessment of his/her current progress, and any modifications that are being made to the plan. Communications with other health care providers should also be noted.

APPENDIX

Pharmaceutical care is a process of drug therapy management that requires a change in the orientation of traditional professional attitudes and reengineering of the traditional pharmacy environment. Certain elements of structure must be in place to provide quality pharmaceutical care. Some of these elements are (1) knowledge, skill, and function of personnel; (2) systems for data collection, documentation, and transfer of information; (3) efficient work flow processes; (4) references, resources and equipment; (5) communication skills; and (6) commitment to quality improvement and assessment procedures.

Knowledge, Skill, and Function of Personnel

The implementation of pharmaceutical care is supported by knowledge and skills in the area of patient assessment, clinical information, communication, adult teaching and learning principles, and psychosocial aspects of care. To use these skills, responsibilities must be reassessed and assigned to appropriate personnel, including pharmacists, technicians, automation, and technology. A mechanism of certifying and credentialing will support the implementation of pharmaceutical care.

Systems for Data Collection and Documentation

The implementation of pharmaceutical care is supported by data collection and documentation systems that accommodate patient care communications (e.g., patient contact notes, medical/medication history), interprofessional communications (e.g., physician communication, pharmacist-to-pharmacist communication), quality assurance (e.g., patient outcomes assessment, patient care protocols), and research (e.g., data for pharmacoepidemiology, etc.). Documentation systems are vital for reimbursement considerations.

Efficient Work Flow Processes

The implementation of pharmaceutical care is supported by incorporating patient care into the activities of the pharmacist and other personnel.

Appendix from *Pharmaceutical Care, Principles of Practice,* American Pharmaceutical Association, 2001.

References, Resources, and Equipment

The implementation of pharmaceutical care is supported by tools which facilitate patient care, including equipment to assess medication therapy adherence and effectiveness, clinical resource materials, and patient education materials. Tools may include computer software support, drug utilization evaluation (DUE) programs, disease management protocols, etc.

Communication Skills

The implementation of pharmaceutical care is supported by patient-centered communication. Within this communication, the patient plays a key role in the overall management of the therapy plan.

Quality Assessment/Improvement Programs

The implementation and practice of pharmaceutical care is supported and improved by measuring, assessing, and improving pharmaceutical care activities utilizing the conceptual framework of continuous quality improvement.

This document will not cover each and every situation; that was not the intent of the Advisory Committee. This is a dynamic document and is intended to be revised as the profession adapts to its new role. It is hoped that pharmacists will use these principles, adapting them to their own situation and environments, to establish and implement pharmaceutical care.

Note: Although "drug therapy" typically refers to intended, beneficial effects of pharmacologic drugs, in this document, "drug therapy" refers to the intended, beneficial use of drugs—whether diagnostic or therapeutic—and thus includes diagnostic radiopharmaceuticals, X-ray contrast media, etc., in addition to pharmacologic drugs. Similarly, "drug therapy plan" includes the outcomes-oriented plan for diagnostic drug use in addition to pharmacologic drug use.